D0938607

Comprehensive Virology 2

Comprehensive Virology

Edited by Heinz Fraenkel-Conrat
University of California at Berkeley

and Robert R. Wagner
University of Virginia

Editorial Board

Volume 1: *Descriptive Catalogue of Viruses* — by Heinz Fraenkel-Conrat

Reproduction

Volume 2: *Small and Intermediate RNA Viruses* — Contributors: J.T. August, L. Eoyang, A. Siegel, V. Hariharasubramanian, L. Levintow, E. R. Pfefferkorn, D. Shapiro, and W. K. Joklik

Volume 3: *DNA Animal Viruses* — Contributors: L. Philipson, U. Lindberg, J. A. Rose, N. P. Salzman, G. Khoury, B. Moss, B. Roizman, and D. Furlong

Volume 4: *Large RNA Viruses* — Contributors: P. W. Choppin, R. W. Compans, R. R. Wagner, and J. P. Bader

Volume 5: *Bacterial DNA Viruses* — Contributors: R. Sinsheimer, D. S. Ray, E. P. Geiduschek, M. E. Gottesman, R. Weisberg, and L. M. Kozloff

Structure and Assembly

Contributors include: H. Vasken Aposhian, W. Bauer, D. L. D. Caspar, P. W. Choppin, R. W. Compans, L. V. Crawford, F. A. Eiserling, W. Fiers, John Finch, R. M. Franklin, H. S. Ginsberg, L. Hirth, P. Hung, J. King, Y. Okada, R. R. Rueckert, T. I. Tikchonenko, T. W. Tinsley, J. Vinograd, R. C. Williams, W. B. Wood

Regulation and Genetics

Contributors include: J. Atabekov, D. Baltimore, D. Bishop, G. Bruening, R. Calendar, A. Campbell, P. Cooper, W. Doerfler, W. Eckhart, B. Fields, H. Ginsberg, H. Hanafusa, A. Huang, E. M. J. Jaspars, J. Kates, E. D. Kilbourne, A. Lewis, B. McAuslan, D. Nathans, E. R .Pfefferkorn, C. Pringle, J. R. Roberts, H. L. Sänger, F .W. Stahl, J. H. Subak-Sharpe, W. Szybalski, L. Van Vloten-Doting, and P. Vogt

Interaction of Viruses and Their Hosts

Effects of Physical and Chemical Agents

Comprehensive

Edited by

Heinz Fraenkel-Conrat

Department of Molecular Biology and Virus Laboratory
University of California, Berkeley, California

and

Robert R. Wagner

Department of Microbiology
University of Virginia, Charlottesville, Virginia

Virology

2

Reproduction

Small and Intermediate RNA Viruses

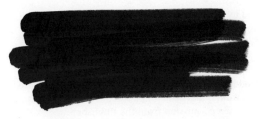

PLENUM PRESS • NEW YORK AND LONDON

Library of Congress Cataloging in Publication Data

Fraenkel-Conrat, Heinz, 1910-
    Reproduction: small and intermediate RNA viruses.

    (Their Comprehensive virology, v. 2)
    Includes bibliographies.
    1. Viruses—Reproduction. I. Wagner, Robert R., 1923-   joint author. II. Title.
III. Series: Fraenkel-Conrat, Heinz, 1910-   Comprehensive virology, v. 2.
QR357.F72 vol. 2 [QR470]   576'.64'08s   [576'.64]
ISBN 0-306-35142-0   74-13471

© 1974 Plenum Press, New York
A Division of Plenum Publishing Corporation
227 West 17th Street, New York, N.Y. 10011

United Kingdom edition published by Plenum Press, London
A Division of Plenum Publishing Company, Ltd.
4a Lower John Street, London W1R 3PD, England

Printed in the United States of America

Foreword

The time seems ripe for a critical compendium of that segment of the biological universe we call viruses. Virology, as a science, having only recently passed through its descriptive phase of naming and numbering, has probably reached that stage at which relatively few new— truly new—viruses will be discovered. Triggered by the intellectual probes and techniques of molecular biology, genetics, biochemical cytology, and high-resolution microscopy and spectroscopy, the field has experienced a genuine information explosion.

Few serious attempts have so far been made to chronicle these events. This comprehensive series, which will comprise some 6000 pages in a total of about 22 volumes, represents a commitment by a large group of active investigators to analyze, digest, and expostulate on the great mass of data relating to viruses, much of which is now amorphous and disjointed and scattered throughout a wide literature. In this way, we hope to place the entire field in perspective as well as to develop an invaluable reference and sourcebook for researchers and students at all levels. This series is designed as a continuum that can be entered anywhere but which also provides a logical progression of developing facts and integrated concepts.

The first volume contains an alphabetical catalogue of almost all viruses of vertebrates, insects, plants, and protists, describing them in general terms. Volumes 2–5 deal primarily, though not exclusively, with the processes of infection and reproduction of the major groups of viruses in their hosts. Volume 2 deals with the simple RNA viruses of bacteria, plants, and animals; the togaviruses (formerly called arboviruses), which share with these only the feature that the virion's RNA is able to act as messenger RNA in the host cell; and the reoviruses of animals and plants, which all share several structurally singular features, the most important being the double-strandedness of their multiple RNA molecules. This grouping, of course, has only slightly more in its favor than others that could have been or indeed were considered.

Volume 3 addresses itself to the reproduction of all DNA-containing viruses of vertebrates, a seemingly simple act of classification, even though the field encompasses the smallest and the largest viruses known.

The reproduction of the larger and more complex RNA viruses represents the subject matter of Volume 4. These share the property of lipid-rich envelopes with the togaviruses included in Volume 2. They share as a group, and with the reoviruses, the presence of enzymes in their virions and the need for their RNA to become transcribed before it can serve messenger functions.

Volume 5 attends to the reproduction of DNA viruses in bacteria, again ranging from small and simple to large and complex.

Aspects of virion structure and assembly of many of these viruses will be dealt with in the following series of volumes, while their genetics, the regulation of their development, viroids, and coviruses will be discussed in subsequently published series. The last volumes will concentrate on host–virus interactions, and on the effects of chemicals and radiation on viruses and their components. At this juncture in the planning of *Comprehensive Virology,* we cannot foresee whether certain topics will become important aspects of the field by the time the final volumes go to press. We envisage the possibility of including volumes on such topics if the need arises.

It is hoped to keep the series at all times up to date by prompt and rapid publication of all contributions, and by encouraging the authors to update their chapters by additions or corrections whenever a volume is reprinted.

Contents

Chapter 2

Reproduction of Small Plant RNA Viruses

Albert Siegel and V. Hariharasubramanian

Chapter 3

Reproduction of Picornaviruses

Leon Levintow

Chapter 4

Reproduction of Togaviruses

Elmer R. Pfefferkorn and Daniel Shapiro

Chapter 5

Reproduction of Reoviridae*

Wolfgang K. Joklik

* See note on page xiv.

NOMENCLATURE OF ANIMAL VIRUS GROUPS

A strong tendency has become evident in recent years to give virus groups names that have more or less self-evident meanings, referring to some structural characteristic of a given group of viruses. Thus the names *picornaviridiae* and *togaviridiae* have become officially recognized for groups of animal viruses, notwithstanding the fact that also very many plant and bacterial viruses are small-RNA viruses and many viruses of other groups contain "mantles" (togas). The term "togaviruses" appeared preferable to the older term "arboviruses" because of the latter's derivation and lack of identifying character. In the same spirit *oncornaviruses* appears justified, even though not all members of the class are truly oncogenic (and "RNA tumor viruses" is no better in this regard), and similar limitations hold for the terms *rhabdoviruses* and *myxoviruses*. The only exception to this terminology based on structure would appear to be the official sanction of the term *reoviridiae*. This word has no meaning to the uninitiated and is erroneous in the eyes of those who know its meaning, since the plant virus members of this group lack a *respiratory-enteric* system and are not *orphans*. *Diplornaviruses* is a good descriptive term for these viruses, since they share the characteristic feature of double-stranded RNA, and the fact that there exist double-stranded-RNA viruses that do not belong to this group is as irrelevant as the fact that the term "picornaviridiae" does not include all small-RNA viruses. However the International Committee of Virus Nomenclature appears to favor the term "reoviridiae," as used by Prof. Joklik.

H. F.-C.

CHAPTER 1

Reproduction of RNA Bacteriophages

L. Eoyang and J. T. August

Department of Molecular Biology
Division of Biological Sciences
Albert Einstein College of Medicine
Bronx, New York 10461

1. INTRODUCTION

Studies on virus replication have been greatly facilitated by the discovery in 1961 of a small RNA-containing bacteriophage (Loeb and Zinder, 1961). The RNA coliphage represents a biological system uniquely reduced to its simplest form. Unlike all other bacterial viruses, the RNA phage does not contain DNA, but rather RNA as its sole genetic material. As a consequence, the RNA must serve a dual function both as a template for nucleic acid synthesis and as a messenger for virus-specific protein synthesis. Due to the size of the genome and the limited number (three) of gene products, it has been possible to elucidate the biological processes of replication and translation as well as the mechanisms by which these events are controlled. Over the past several years, considerable progress has been made in this respect, and though by no means complete, our knowledge of the RNA bacteriophage has become quite extensive. We have attempted to summarize below some of the more recent contributions toward our understanding of the molecular biology of virus replication.

Several reviews on specific aspects of RNA bacteriophages have been published: on replication, Lodish (1968*a*), Erikson (1968), and Stavis and August (1970); on translation, Kozak and Nathans (1972) and Sugiyama *et al.* (1972); on RNA sequence analysis, Gilham (1970); on RNA structure and function, Weissmann *et al.* (1973) and Fiers (1973); on assembly, Hohn and Hohn (1970); and on RNA viruses in general, Zinder (1974).

2. PROPERTIES OF THE RNA PHAGE

2.1. Properties of the Particles

Infection of susceptible bacteria by RNA phages yields 10^3–10^4 viral particles per cell. These particles are composed of a single molecule of RNA, 180 molecules of coat protein, and one molecule of the maturation (A) protein. The RNA genome contains only three genes, those for the coat protein, the maturation protein, and a protein subunit of the phage RNA polymerase. All of the *Escherichia coli* RNA phages that have been isolated are similar in structure and properties. These phages are among the smallest and genetically simplest infectious, self-replicating organisms known.*

An extensive study of over 30 *E. coli* RNA phages has shown that they are all similar and fall into three or possibly four serological groups (Scott, 1965; Watanabe *et al.*, 1967; Sakurai, 1968). Most of the commonly studied phage (f2, MS2, R17, M12, fr, and FH5) are in the same group and the coat protein sequences of these phages differ from each other by only a few amino acids. The Qβ phage is in another group and, although similar in size and many physical properties, has certain distinctive properties, including an RNA genome that appears to be slightly larger than that of other viruses (Boedtker, 1971).

The diameter of these particles is 20–27 nm. They sediment at 75–84 S and have a density of 1.42–1.47 g/ml (Paranchych and Graham, 1962; Enger *et al.*, 1963; Hofschneider, 1963; Marvin and Hoffmann-Berling, 1963; Davern, 1964*a*; Gesteland and Boedtker, 1964; Strauss and Sinsheimer, 1963; Overby *et al.*, 1966). Their particle weight is between 3.6 and 4.2 $\times$ 10^6, a value that agrees with the sum of the molecular weights of the individual components. As determined by X-ray analysis, R17 has a diameter of 27 nm, with an outer shell 3–4 nm thick and a hollow core of about 3 nm in diameter (Fishbach *et al.*, 1965).

---

* Editor's note: The applicability of the term "organism" to a virus may well be questioned [H. F.-C.].

Of the normal products of a bacterial lysate, only a small proportion of the phage particles, 10–20%, produce an infective center. This can be explained either by unsuccessful infection of the bacterium by normal phage or by the possibility that many of the phages are defective in some manner. One type of particle with known low infectivity has been detected as having a buoyant density slightly lower than normal, and is thus termed an L particle (Rohrmann and Krueger, 1970). These L particles appear to have a normal ratio of protein to RNA. They contain A protein and their RNA is infectious in spheroplasts. It is thought that the decreased buoyant density reflects a structural modification in the capsid surface. Another form of defective particle is one that lacks maturation protein. These particles were recognized as products of infection of nonpermissive bacteria by RNA phages which contained an amber mutation in the maturation protein cistron of the genome (Heisenberg and Blessing, 1965; Lodish *et al.,* 1965; Heisenberg, 1966; Argetsinger and Gussin, 1966; Tooze and Weber, 1967). Such particles also appeared after infection of cultures deprived of histidine at a time when polymerase but not maturation protein was synthesized. Under these conditions, defective particles lacking maturation protein were produced (Kaerner, 1969, 1970). These defective particles cannot be distinguished from normal phage by electron microscopy. However, they do not adsorb normally to the bacterial host, and the RNA of the phage is sensitive to attack by RNase (Argetsinger and Gussin, 1966; Heisenberg, 1966). The evidence suggests that in the absence of maturation protein the RNA fails to be packaged correctly and as a consequence protrudes from the particle.

2.2. Physical Properties of the RNA

Each virus particle contains one molecule of single-stranded RNA. The RNA of f2 and similar phages has a molecular weight of $1.1–1.3 \times 10^6$ and a sedimentation coefficient of about 27 S (in 0.1M NaCl) (Strauss and Sinsheimer, 1963; Gesteland and Boedtker, 1964; Overby *et al.,* 1966; Marvin and Hoffmann-Berling, 1963; Mitra *et al.,* 1963; Boedtker, 1971). The $Q\beta$ RNA appears to be slightly larger, with a molecular weight of 1.5×10^6. The four bases are present in nearly equimolar amounts. The RNA is a linear structure since both 5′ and 3′ termini have been detected (*vide infra*). Sedimentation of the RNA under a variety of conditions (Strauss and Sinsheimer, 1968) has failed to show evidence for the potential formation of ring structures.

The radius of gyration, reported as 16 nm (in 0.2M NaCl)

(Strauss and Sinsheimer, 1963) and 19 nm (in 0.1_M NaCl) (Gesteland and Boedtker, 1964), together with the sedimentation coefficient, indicates a compact structure. Thermal denaturation profiles, slow reactivity with formaldehyde (Strauss and Sinsheimer, 1963), and analysis of nucleotide sequences (*vide infra*) indicate extensive hydrogen bonding throughout the molecule. From the change in absorbance upon reaction with formaldehyde, the helical fraction of the RNA was estimated to be about 70% (Mitra *et al.*, 1963; Boedtker, 1967). The RNA probably has a specific secondary structure since limited digestion with ribonuclease at low temperature gives specific cleavage products (Bassel and Spiegelman, 1967; Min Jou *et al.*, 1968; Spahr and Gesteland, 1968; Gould *et al.*, 1969; Thach and Boedtker, 1969).

RNA phages that infect *Pseudomonas* (Feary *et al.*, 1963; Bradley, 1966) and *Caulobacter* (Schmidt and Stanier, 1965; Shapiro and Bendis, 1974) have also been isolated.

2.2.1. Primary Structure

Work on the primary structure of the genome of RNA bacteriophages has been quite extensive in recent years. Much of the sequence analysis has been done on RNA from R17 (Adams *et al.*, 1969a; Steitz, 1969a; Sanger, 1971), MS2 (Fiers *et al.*, 1971), and Qβ (Weissmann *et al.*, 1973), although f2 and M12 RNA have also been studied (Webster *et al.*, 1969; Thirion and Kaesberg, 1970). In addition, small molecules such as Qβ 6 S RNA (Banerjee *et al.*, 1969a) and several classes of variant RNA (Bishop *et al.*, 1968; Kacian *et al.*, 1971) synthesized *in vitro* by the Qβ RNA polymerase (replicase, synthetase) have also been analyzed. As a result of the labors of several groups, over 30% of the genome, or more than 1000 nucleotides of R17 and MS2, and about 15% of Qβ have been sequenced. Of more critical value, however, is that the known sequences include the oligonucleotides at both 5′ and 3′ termini as well as at least part of the cistrons of all three phage-coded proteins. The method of nucleotide sequence analysis essentially involves the specific enzymic cleavage of intact molecules of RNA purified from phage or of RNA fragments synthesized *in vitro* by phage polymerase under limiting conditions (Billeter *et al.*, 1969). Enzymic hydrolysis is usually accomplished by use of the following: T_1 ribonuclease, which specifically cleaves 5′ bonds after Gp residues; U_2 ribonuclease, which splits at purine residues; the carbodiimide method, in which the reagent specifically reacts with guanine and uridine residues and renders the latter resistant to ribonuclease A; ribonuclease A, which splits at cytosine and uridine residues. Separation and sequence analysis of the enzyme digests are generally performed according to the methods developed by Sanger and his colleagues and involve two-dimensional ionophoresis in 8M urea and thin-layer DEAE homochromatography. The detailed techniques of purification, fractionation, and cleavage of the RNA as well as separation and isolation of the polynucleotides have been detailed (Steitz, 1969a; Gilham, 1970; Sanger, 1971) and will not be described here.

2.2.1(a). 5′ Terminus

The 5′ terminus of the RNA from all RNA bacteriophages analyzed thus far is pppGp (DeWachter et al., 1968a,b; Glitz, 1968; Roblin, 1968a,b; Watanabe and August, 1968a). The serologically related phages MS2 and R17 have identical sequences at the 5′ ends for at least the first 125 bases (Adams et al., 1972), whereas f2 has identical sequences for at least the first 74 residues (Ling, 1971) (Table 1). Even RNA from Qβ, which is serologically and chemically distinct, contains 5′-terminal sequences homologous to those of group I phage RNA (Adams et al., 1972). These similarities, however, cannot be related directly to the protein-coding capacity of the RNA. Translation does not occur at or near the 5′ terminus since the initial sequences do not contain either of the formylmethionine codons AUG or GUG necessary for initiation of protein synthesis (DeWachter et al., 1968c; DeWachter and Fiers, 1969; Adams and Cory, 1970; Ling, 1971). In the group I phages, even though AUG and GUG codons appear in preceding residues, translation does not begin until the 130th nucleotide. In Qβ, the first AUG codon is found at the 62nd nucleotide and it is the initiation signal for the translation of the first cistron (Billeter et al., 1969).

As no specificity of base is required, the conservation of primary structure for a long sequence at the 5′ terminus is surprising. It has been suggested by several workers (Adams and Cory, 1970; DeWachter et al., 1971a) that the similarities in sequences may not be fortuitous. Adams and Cory (1970) have hypothesized that the homology of sequence is evidence for the evolution of the RNA phages from a common prototype and that perhaps the 5′-terminal sequence was retained because it may have advantages in natural selection. It was suggested, for instance, that the 5′-terminal sequence protects the molecule from exonucleolytic attack (Kuwano et al., 1970) by its capacity to form tight hydrogen-bonded loops (Fig. 1). In addition, as

TABLE 1

5′-Terminal Sequences in Bacteriophage RNA

RNA	5′ Terminus[a]
f2[b]	pppGGGUUGGGACCCCUUUCGGGGUCCUGCUCAACUUCCUGUCGAGCUAAUGCCAUUUUAAUGUCUUUAGCCGAGACG...
R17[c]	pppGGGUUGGGACCCCUUUCGGGGUCCUGCUCAACUUCCUGUCGAGCUAAUGCCAUUUUAAUGUCUUUAGCCGAGACG...
Qβ[d]	pppGGGGGACCCCCCCUUUAGGGGGUCAC(ACACCUC)AGCAGUACUUCACUGAGUAUAAGAGGACAUAUG...
Qβ minus strand[e]	pppGGGGAGAGAGGGCAAAGCAGAUCCCCUCUCACUCGUAAGAGUAAUUGUG...
Qβ 6 S[f]	pppG...
Qβ "variant" MV-1[g]	pppGGGGAU...

[a] The sequences in parentheses are as yet uncertain.
[b] Ling (1971).
[c] Adams and Cory (1970), Adams et al. (1972).
[d] Billeter et al. (1969).
[e] Goodman et al. (1970).
[f] Banerjee et al. (1969a).
[g] Kacian et al. (1971).

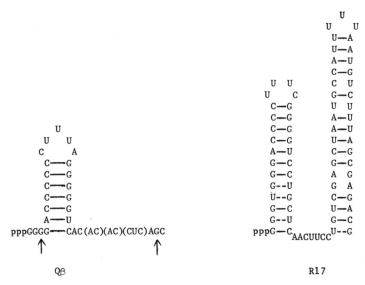

Fig. 1. Possible secondary structure at the 5′ terminus of RNA from Qβ and R17. The Qβ sequence within the arrows indicates a fragment resistant to vigorous digestion by T₁ RNase (Billeter *et al.*, 1969). The sequence for R17 is from Adams and Cory (1970).

suggested by DeWachter *et al.* (1971*a*), the 5′-terminal sequence may serve to specify the 3′ end of the complementary sequence of the minus strand, thereby dictating a similar secondary structure. It may be that a uniquely specific secondary and tertiary structure at the 3′ end of the minus strand is necessary for recognition by the viral RNA polymerase (Fig. 2).

2.2.1(b). 3′ Terminus

The 3′ terminus (Table 2) of all RNA bacteriophages analyzed ends with . . . CCA$_{\overline{OH}}$ (DeWachter and Fiers, 1967; Weith and Gilham, 1967; Dahlberg, 1968), a feature that is also common to plant viral RNA and all tRNA. Terminal cytidine, though to a lesser extent, has also been detected in RNA of f2, MS2, and Qβ (Lee and Gilham, 1965; Rensing and August, 1969). The presence of the 3′-terminal adenosine is curious as the expected base complementary to the guanylate at the 5′ terminus is cytidine. It was demonstrated that if spheroplasts are infected with R17 RNA lacking adenosine at the 3′-OH terminus, the terminal A is restored to progeny RNA (Kamen,

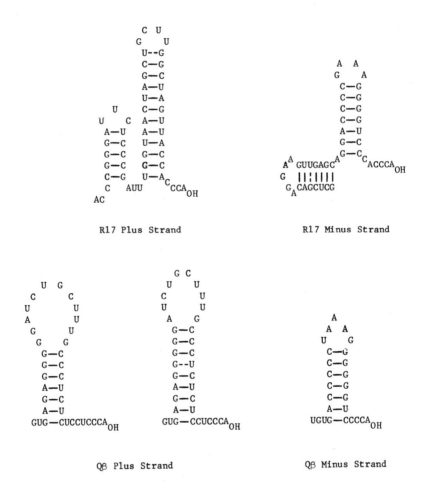

Fig. 2. Possible secondary structure at the 3′ terminus of plus and minus strands of R17 and Qβ RNA. Structures for R17 are from Cory *et al.* (1972). The R17 minus-strand sequence is deduced from the experimentally determined sequence at the 5′ end of R17. The structures for Qβ RNA are from Goodman *et al.* (1970). The second structure for the Qβ plus strand requires a G–U base pair.

1969). In addition, it was found that the terminal A is restored to the RNA product synthesized *in vitro* by the Qβ RNA polymerase even though the template RNA terminates in C_{OH} (Rensing and August, 1969; Weber and Weissmann 1970). Sequential removal of terminal nucleotides both in R17 and Qβ showed that the penultimate cytidylate is required for biological and template activity. Only the terminal adenylate can be removed without destroying the template activity or

TABLE 2

3′-OH-Terminal Sequence of Bacteriophage RNA

RNA	3′ Terminus[a]
f2[b]	. . . UUACCACCCA$_{OH}$
R17[c]	. . . ACCCGGGAUUCUCCCGAUUUGGUAACUAGCUGCUUGGCUAGUUACCACCCA$_{OH}$
Qβ[d]	. . . CCGUGUUCUGGCACCCUACGGGCGUCUUCCAGGGCACGAAGGUUGCGUCUCUCACACGAGGCGUAACCUGGGGGAGGGGCCA
	AUAU(G)GCGCCUAAUUG̲U̲G̲AAUAAAUUAUCACAAUUACUCUUACGAGUGAGGGGGGAUCUGCUUUGCCCUCUCCUCCUCCCCA$_{OH}$
Qβ 6 S[e]	. . . GCC$_{OH}^{A}$G$_{OH}$
Qβ "variant" MV-1[f]	. . . AUCCC$_{OH}$

[a] The underlined triplets indicate possible termination codons.
[b] Weith and Giham (1967), Dahlberg (1968).
[c] Cory et al. (1970, 1972).
[d] Goodman et al. (1970), Weissmann et al. (1973).
[e] Trown and Meyer (1973).
[f] Kacian et al. (1971).

the infectivity of the RNA. It is assumed that the phage enzyme itself adds the terminal adenosine residue.

Just as there is no signal for the initiation of translation at or near the 5′ terminus of phage RNA, neither is there one for termination at or near the 3′ terminus. In R17 RNA, none of the three known termination codons, UAA, UAG, or UGA, are present in the last 10 nucleotides (Dahlberg, 1968). Within the last 51 residues, however, there are three potential termination signals, two UAGs and one UAA (Cory et al., 1972). Of the three, the termination codon (UAG) closest to the 3′ end is precluded from being the normal termination signal by its proximity to the preceding nonsense codon (UAG). It was concluded, that at least the last 25 residues from the 3′ terminus are not translated. In the case of Qβ RNA, no termination codons were found within the last 32 nucleotides at the 3′ terminus (Goodman et al., 1970).

The sequence at the 3′ terminus is of particular interest since RNA synthesis which proceeds in a 5′-triphosphate to a 3′-hydroxyl direction (Banerjee et al., 1969b) initiates near the 3′ end of the template. Viral enzymes like the Qβ RNA polymerase (Haruna and Spiegelman, 1965a; August et al., 1968) recognize only certain templates (Qβ RNA, Qβ complementary strand, Qβ 6 S RNA) for replication. Elucidation of the 3′-terminal sequence, therefore, should provide clues to the specificity of templates. As previously noted the penultimate cytidylate is required for both in vitro and in vivo replication. This cannot be the sole requirement for specificity, however, for the sequence CCCA$_{OH}$ is common to the 3′ termini of almost all viral RNAs analyzed thus far. In R17 RNA (Fig. 2) (Goodman et al., 1970; Cory et al., 1972) the last hexanucleotide (excluding the terminal A) is common to both plus and minus strands, and it is suggested (Cory et al., 1970) that the CCCACC sequence may be part of the recognition site for the R17 polymerase. However, in Qβ RNA there are no such regions of identity between plus and minus strands at the 3′ terminus, so that sequence alone cannot be the critical factor in a specific recognition site. It is known, in fact, that in the purified polymerase system a host factor in required for synthesis of minus strands but not of plus strands (vide infra).

2.2.1(c). Maturation Protein Cistron

Utilizing a unique method previously demonstrated by Takanami et al. (1965), Steitz and others have succeeded in elucidating the se-

quences of the ribosomal binding sites and initiation sites for all three
cistrons of phage RNA. Exploiting the fact that ribosomes bound to
messenger RNA under conditions of polypeptide chain initiation
protect a portion (25–40 nucleotides) of the RNA from nucleolytic attack, they were able to identify initiator regions for the maturation,
coat, and polymerase cistrons (Table 3). The N-terminal amino acid
sequences of the three phage-coded proteins being distinct [the maturation protein beginning with fMet-Arg (Lodish and Robertson,
1969a), the coat protein with fMet-Ala (Weber, 1967; Konigsberg et
al., 1970), and the polymerase with fMet-Ser (Lodish, 1968b; Gesteland and Spahr, 1969; Osborn et al., 1970a)], a comparison of nucleotide sequences immediately following initiator codons with the
known N-terminal amino acid sequences allowed identification of the
cistrons. The efficiency of translation of A protein is quite low compared to the other cistrons, as the ratio of coat, polymerase, and A
protein synthesized is 100:30:5.5, respectively (Lodish, 1968b), and the
yield of fragments containing A protein binding sites is correspondingly
meager.

Taking advantage of the observation by Lodish and Robertson
(1969a) that when ribosomes from *Bacillus stearothermophilus* are
used for *in vitro* translation of f2 RNA only the maturation protein is
initiated and synthesized, Steitz was able to increase the yield of A
protein initiator fragments tenfold over that when *E. coli* ribosomes
were used (Steitz, 1969b). This result and finding an arginine codon
following an AUG initiation sequence allowed her to identify the A
protein sequence. In R17 and in Qβ (Staples et al., 1971) the initiator
codon for all three cistrons is AUG. In MS2, both AUG (Berissi et al.,
1971; DeWachter et al., 1971a) and GUG (Volckaert and Fiers, 1973)
have been reported as the initiator codon for the A protein.

Remaut and Fiers (1972) found that infection by MS2 of an
amber UAG suppressor strain caused the appearance of a fourth viral
protein (A_s) in addition to the three normally found in infected cells. It
was concluded that this protein was an elongation product of the A
protein (addition of 30 amino acids) since no A_s protein was
synthesized after infection of a UAG suppressor strain by a UGA
phage mutant defective in the A protein cistron. Moreover, the efficiency of readthrough was not affected by UGA suppression. It is
likely, therefore, that the termination signal for the maturation protein
cistron of MS2 is a single UAG codon. This conclusion is supported by
the sequence data obtained by Contreras et al. (1973). They reported a
160-nucleotide sequence comprising the residues coding for the last 45
amino acids of the A cistron, the termination codon, and the intercis-

TABLE 3

Sequences of Ribosome Binding Sites of Bacteriophage RNA

Maturation protein

MS2[a]
```
                    fMet Arg Ala Phe Ser
AU·UCC·UAG·GAG·GUU·UGA·CCU·GUG·CGA·GCU·UUU·AGU
```

R17[b]
```
              fMet Arg Ala Phe Ser
CC·UAG·GAG·GUU·UGA·CCU·AUG·CGA·GCU·UUU·AGU·G
```

Qβ[c]
```
           fMet Pro Lys Leu Pro Arg
G·AGU·AUA·AGA·GGA·CAU·AUG·CCU·AAA·UUA·CCG·CGU·G
```

Coat protein

MS2[a]
```
                           fMet Ala Ser Asn Phe Thr
AUA·GAG·CCC·UCA·ACC·GGA·GUU·UGA·AGC·AUG·GCU·UCU·AAC·UUU·ACU
```

R17[b]
```
                    fMet Ala Ser Asn Phe
AC·AGC·CUA·ACC·GGG·GUU·UGA·AGC·AUG·GCU·UCU·AAC·UUU
```

Qβ[e]

fMet Ala Lys Leu glu Thr
AAU·UUG·AUC·AUG·GCA·AAA·UUA·GAG·AC

Polymerase protein

MS2[f]

fMet Ser Lys Thr Thr Lys Lys
UAA·UAG·ACG·CCG·GCC·AUU·CAA·ACA·UGA·GGA·UUA·CCC·AUG·UCG·AAG·ACA·ACA·AAG·AAG

R17[b]

fMet Ser Lys Thr Thr Lys
AA·ACA·UGA·GGA·UUA·CCC·AUG·UCG·AAG·ACA·ACA·AAG

Qβ[g]

fMet Ser Lys Thr Ala
UAA·CUA·AGG·AUG·AAA·UGC·AUG·UCU·AAG·ACA·G(C)

[a] DeWachter et al. (1971b), Volckaert and Fiers (1973).
[b] Steitz (1969b).
[c] Staples et al. (1971).
[d] Min Jou et al. (1972).
[e] Hindley and Staples (1969).
[f] Contreras et al. (1972), Min Jou (1972).
[g] Steitz (1972), Staples and Hindley (1971).

tronic region between the first and second gene. The sequence contains four UAG codons and it was suggested because of the proximities of the preceding three that the fourth codon is the true terminator. The finding by Vandekerckhove *et al.* (1973) that the carboxyl-terminal amino acid of the maturation protein is arginine provides convincing evidence that the last UAG triplet is indeed the termination codon of the maturation protein cistron.

2.2.1(d).   Coat Protein Cistron

The sequence of the initiator region of the coat protein cistron has been determined for f2 (Gupta *et al.,* 1970), R17 (Adams *et al.,* 1969*b*; Robinson *et al.,* 1969; Steitz, 1969*b*), Qβ (Hindley and Staples, 1969; Hindley *et al.,* 1970) and MS2 (Fiers *et al.,* 1971; Min Jou *et al.,* 1971). The entire sequence of the MS2 coat protein gene has been determined by Min Jou *et al.* (1972). They found that 49 different codons specify the sequence of 129 amino acids which constitute the coat protein subunit. Their model of the secondary structure of the coat protein based on the thermodynamic stability (Tinoco *et al.,* 1971) of various base-paired segments suggests that 66% of the nucleotides are involved in helical regions. It was suggested that these regions may serve as structural controls for actual initiator regions. If, for example, the replicase initiation site were sequestered through hydrogen bonding to an early sequence of the coat protein cistron, disruption of this configuration by a translating ribosome would render the replicase cistron accessible to other ribosomes. This mechanism would explain the polarity effect in which a mutation in amino acid position 6 results in decreased synthesis of replicase protein, whereas mutations in positions 50, 54, or 70 do not. If translation of the region around position 6 were critical to the unmasking of the replicase initiator codon, then mutations at later positions would not exert any polarity on the reading of the replicase cistron.

Using an *in vitro* system, Hindley *et al.* (1970) were able to determine the terminal sequence of the coat protein cistron as well as the location of the cistron on the Qβ genome. They prepared full-length Qβ RNA labeled to different extents using purified Qβ RNA polymerase. After binding ribosomes to these RNA preparations, the complexes were digested, isolated, and characterized. Since radioactivity could be recovered only from protected sequences, it was possible to identify the location of the coat protein site. Using this technique, the beginning of the cistron was estimated to be around the 1100–1400th nucleotide.

The nucleotide sequence of the termination region of the coat protein cistron for both R17 (Nichols, 1970) and MS2 (*vide supra*) have been determined. There are three terminator codons: Two adjacent codons, UAA and UAG, immediately follow the codon for the C-terminal amino acid; UGA occurs six triplets later. It is suggested that the normal termination signal is the two adjacent nonsense triplets and that the presence of multiple terminators is to insure the effective termination of translation.

However, in Qβ phage a fourth protein (A_1 or II_b) is detected both *in vitro* and *in vivo* (Garwes *et al.*, 1969; Jockusch *et al.*, 1970; Horiuchi *et al.*, 1971). It has a molecular weight of 36,000–38,000 (Strauss and Kaesberg, 1970; Moore *et al.*, 1971). Evidence indicates that this polypeptide is not the gene product of a fourth cistron but rather a result of faulty translation through the termination signal of the coat protein cistron (Moore *et al.*, 1971; Weiner and Weber, 1971). This possibility is based on the fact that this readthrough protein contains the same N-terminal amino acid sequence as that for coat protein and that this fourth protein is not found in Qβ coat amber mutants which do not induce the synthesis of coat protein (Horiuchi and Matsuhashi, 1970). Additionally, since viruses grown in a UGA suppressor host result in increased amounts of A_1 protein (Weiner and Weber, 1971; Radloff and Kaesberg, 1973), it is likely that the termination signal for coat protein in Qβ is a single UGA codon. If, in Qβ, the coat and replicase genes are separated by at least 600 nucleotides, then the residues of A_1 protein extending beyond the coat cistron need not extend into the replicase gene and may actually be restricted to the intercistronic region preceding it. In fact, as Steitz (1972) has pointed out, faulty translation into the initiator region of the replicase cistron is highly improbable because of the location of four nonsense codons in this region. They are placed such that all three possible phases of translation are obstructed.

2.2.1(e).   Polymerase Protein Cistron

The sequence of the ribosome-binding site for the polymerase cistron has been determined for R17 (Steitz, 1969b), Qβ (Steitz, 1972), and MS2 (Contreras *et al.*, 1972). As observed by Steitz (1969b) for R17 and by Hindley and Staples (1969) for Qβ, ribosomes bind intact RNA predominantly at the coat protein cistron. However, the binding sites of the polymerase protein as well as A-protein cistrons become accessible when the secondary and tertiary structure of the RNA is modified. Staples and Hindley (1971) and Steitz (1972) were able to use RNA fragmented by means of alkali treatment at high ionic strength or autoradiolysis to form initiation complexes with ribosomes. The sequence data (Steitz, 1972) suggest that the $Q\beta$ coat and polymerase genes are separated by a long intercistronic region of at least 600 nucleotides. In group I phages this region extends over only 36 nucleotides. Sequence comparison indicates that the untranslated regions, at least those immediately preceding the initiating codons, are genetically stable within the serologically related phages MS2, R17, and f2 (Robertson and Jeppesen, 1972).

2.2.1(f).   Site of Coat Protein Repression

In an *in vitro* protein-synthesizing system, addition of coat protein to phage RNA inhibits the synthesis of replicase (Sugiyama and Nakada, 1968; Eggen and Nathans, 1969; Spahr *et al.,* 1969; Ward *et al.,* 1969). It has been shown that coat protein acts as a translational repressor of the phage polymerase (Lodish and Zinder, 1966*a*; Lodish, 1968*c*; Sugiyama and Nakada, 1968; Eggen and Nathans, 1969; Nathans *et al.,* 1969; Ward *et al.,* 1969) by specifically inhibiting the initiation of translation of that cistron (Lodish, 1969*a*; Skogerson *et al.,* 1971). The formation of two types of protein–RNA complexes has been observed: Complex I, which consists of 1–6 molecules of coat protein bound to one molecule of phage RNA, sediments at the same rate as free RNA: Complex II, which consists of approximately 180 molecules of coat protein bound to one molar equivalent of RNA, resembles phage but is not infectious (Sugiyama *et al.,* 1967). Digestion of Complex I by RNase T_1 should yield a fragment containing the site of translational repression since this region would be protected against nucleolytic attack by the coat protein. Such a fragment has been isolated and it contains the codon for the last six amino acids of the coat protein, the intercistronic region, and the first codon of the polymerase cistron (Bernardi and Spahr, 1972). Since the R17 RNA–coat protein complex is still capable of directing the *in vitro* synthesis of coat protein, it must be assumed that coat protein does not bind to this region, and the reason this region survives RNase T_1 attack is that it has some degree of secondary structure. Since $Q\beta$ coat protein does not protect R17 RNA just as it does not repress translation of the polymerase cistron in nonhomologous messenger, the binding site for coat protein repression must be presumed to be a specific one. Based on these results, it is suggested that the recognition site for the coat protein consists of the intercistronic region and the first codon of the polymerase cistron.

Evidence by Gralla *et al.* (1974) indicates that in addition to the primary sequence, coat protein recognizes a secondary structure that includes the ribosome-binding site at the beginning of the replicase gene. They found that RNase T_1 digests of R17–coat protein complex yield two major species, the 59-nucleotide fragment characterized by Bernardi and Spahr (1972) and a 29-nucleotide fragment lacking helix *a* (Fig. 3). Measurement of the absorbance change during thermal transition of the large fragment indicates the presence of two hairpin helices which melt independently. This result is consistent with the prediction that the sequence in this region justifies the existence of two hairpin loops. The presence of coat protein is found to retard the rate of melting of the helix containing the replicase initiator codon. Also, T_1 digests of the RNA–coat protein complex sometimes yield the initiator fragment alone, but never only the terminator hairpin. The stoichiometry of binding of coat protein to the protected fragment was found to be an average of one mole of coat protein to one mole of RNA.

Although there is excellent correspondence of sequence in the untranslated termini of related phages, there is less homology in the cistronic regions of the genome. In R17, although the sequence

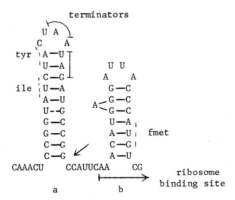

Fig. 3. Sequence of coat protein-protected fragment from R17 RNA. The small arrow indicates the site of T_1 RNase cleavage which produced the 29-nucleotide fragment (Gralla *et al.*, 1974).

GGUUUGA precedes the AUG initiator by 3 nucleotides in both coat and A protein binding sites, no such sequence occurs in the polymerase binding site (Table 3). This similarity of sequence in coat and A protein binding sites does not correlate with the differences in frequency of translation of these two cistrons. The question of recognition sites is as yet an unsolved one, and it is conceivable that its solution will involve the nucleotide sequence around the initiator region, both the secondary and tertiary structure of the RNA, and possible additional nucleotide sequences that the configuration may expose.

2.2.2.   Secondary and Tertiary Structure

As several workers have shown (Cory *et al.*, 1972; Goodman, 1970; Steitz, 1969*b*; Fiers *et al.*, 1971), it is possible to construct stable hairpin loops for several regions of the RNA molecule. The probability that there are regions of extensive base complementarity in phage RNA is supported by the observation that certain regions are resistant to mild attack by degradative enzymes. The secondary and tertiary structure of phage RNA are of significant functional value in transcription as they are in translation (*vide infra*), but as yet the precise configurational requirements for recognition are unknown.

2.3.   Properties of the Phage Proteins

2.3.1.   Properties of the Maturation (A) Protein.

The protein has been isolated as a product of *in vivo* translation from R17 (Osborn *et al.*, 1970*b*; Steitz, 1968*a*) and MS2 (Vandekerckhove *et al.*, 1973) as well as *in vitro* translation (Eggen *et al.*, 1967; Lodish, 1968*b*; Lodish and Robertson, 1969*a*). This histidine-containing protein (Vinuela *et al.*, 1967; Nathans *et al.*, 1966), comprising 1–2% of the total protein produced, has a molecular weight estimated to be 40,000 (Steitz, 1968*b*). The amino acid sequence of 43 C-terminal residues from MS2 maturation protein has been determined (Vandekerckhove *et al.*, 1973).

The maturation protein is probably present in one copy per virion (Steitz, 1968*a*) and is required for adsorption and proper assembly. Infection of nonpermissive bacteria by amber mutants of the maturation protein cistron produces noninfectious defective particles lacking maturation protein. The mutant virus contains intact RNA, but part of the

RNA protrudes from the particle and is consequently sensitive to RNase digestion (Heisenberg, 1966; Steitz, 1968b). It is likely that maturation protein is required for the proper structural conformation of the RNA within the capsid shell.

2.3.2. Properties of the Coat Protein

The capsid of the RNA phage is comprised of 180 coat protein subunits (Vasquez et al., 1966). The complete amino acid sequences of the coat protein of f2 (Konigsberg et al., 1966; Konigsberg, 1966; Weber and Konigsberg, 1967), Qβ (Konigsberg et al., 1970) and R17 (Weber, 1967) have been determined, while nearly complete sequences are known for fr (Wittmann-Liebold, 1966) and ZR (Nishihara et al., 1970). The amino acid compositions of MS2 and M12 are identical (Lin et al., 1967; Vandekerckhove et al., 1969); they differ from that of f2 by substitution of one methionine for leucine, and from that of R17 by substitution of a single glutamic acid or glutamine for lysine (Enger and Kaesberg, 1965). Comparison of terminal residues (Table 4) of the three phage groups indicates that while alanine prevails as the sole amino acid at the amino terminus, tyrosine (group I, III) or alanine (group II) is present at the carboxyl terminus. Coat proteins of group II phages GA and SD lack cysteine and methionine, while Qβ coat protein lacks tryptophan and methionine. All lack histidine. The molecular weight of the coat protein of the known RNA phages is approximately 14,000 (Konigsberg et al., 1970; Weber and Konigsberg,

TABLE 4

Comparison of Coat Protein Sequences from Three Phage Groups*

RNA phage group	Phage	N–terminal sequence[a]	C–terminal sequence
I	f2[b]	Ala–Ser–Asn–Phe–	–Ser–Gly–Ile–Tyr
II	GA[c]	Ala–	–(Tyr, Phe)–Ala
III	Qβ[d]	Ala–Lys–Leu–Glu–	–Asn–Pro–Ala–Tyr

[a] The amino-terminal formylmethionine residue which is incorporated *in vitro* has been shown to be cleaved *in vivo* (Housman et al., 1972; Ball and Kaesberg, 1973).
[b] Weber and Konigsberg (1967).
[c] Nishihara et al. (1969).
[d] Konigsberg et al. (1970).

1967; Enger and Kaesberg, 1965). Depending on how the f2 (129 residues) and Qβ (131 residues) sequences are aligned and whether insertions and deletions are accommodated, 36–48% of residues that differ can be accounted for by a single base change (Konigsberg *et al.*, 1970).

2.3.3. Properties of the Polymerase Protein

The gene product of the third cistron of phage RNA, the polymerase subunit, is the only one not found in the viral particle. The molecular weight of the protein has been estimated to be 70,000 for Qβ (Kondo *et al.*, 1970; Kamen, 1970; August *et al.*, 1973) and 63,000 for f2 (Federoff and Zinder, 1971). The polymerase subunit together with 3 host subunits (*vide infra*) form the active enzyme complex which catalyzes the synthesis of infectious viral RNA. The amino-terminal tripeptide of Qβ polymerase protein synthesized *in vitro* is reported to be fMet-Ser-Lys (Skogerson *et al.*, 1971). Analysis of the phage subunit separated from purified Qβ polymerase isolated from infected *E. coli* extends that sequence to Ser-Lys-Thr-Ala-Ser (Weiner and Weber, 1971).

3. TRANSLATION

The study of gene expression has been greatly facilitated by the discovery of the RNA bacteriophage system. Coupled with the detailed knowledge of protein synthesis in *E. coli,* the genetic and biochemical data on the structure and function of the simple polycistronic messenger RNA have yielded a wealth of information concerning the translational processes of initiation, elongation, and termination, the participation of ribosomes and various cellular factors; and the mechanisms of polarity and suppression as well as those of translational control.

3.1. Regulation of Translation

In the first five minutes after infection the bulk of parental phage RNA is associated with the 30 S ribosome subunits and the polysomes (Godson and Sinsheimer, 1967). An RNA-dependent RNA polymerase activity appears within 10 minutes after infection (August *et al.*, 1963;

Lodish *et al.*, 1964). This phage-induced enzyme catalyzes the synthesis of a complementary minus strand which in turn serves as the template for the synthesis of progeny RNA. The newly synthesized phage RNA is detectable in a seemingly RNase-resistant fraction which appears in the 50 S and polysome fraction (Godson and Sinsheimer, 1967). At 15 minutes post-infection, when large amounts of progeny viral RNA have accumulated but no infectious phage particles have appeared, most of the infectious RNA is associated with the polysomes (Godson, 1968). Newly synthesized RNase-resistant material pulse-labeled 30 minutes after infection is found with the polysomes, particularly the large ones, while little radioactivity is found in free RNA (Godson, 1968; Hotham-Iglewski and Franklin, 1967; Hotham-Iglewski *et al.*, 1968). The localization of this RNA does not seem to correspond to the site of RNA and protein synthesis: most of the RNase-resistant RNA is in the more rapidly sedimenting fractions, whereas the bulk of RNA and protein synthesis is in the lighter fractions (Hotham-Iglewski and Franklin, 1967). The presumption that translation is coupled to transcription is supported by the fact that almost all of the double- and single-stranded phage RNA is associated with ribosomes throughout the latent period. It is likely that the translational events occur on early nascent progeny RNA, as minus strands do not appear to function as messenger (Schwartz *et al.*, 1969). The evidence that in the absence of detergents newly synthesized RNA first appears as a protein–RNA particle in the $30,000 \times g$ sediment indicates that in the cell, RNA and protein synthesis may occur in membrane structures (Haywood and Sinsheimer, 1965; Haywood *et al.*, 1969). These particles, some of which sediment at about 40 S, contain all of the phage-specific proteins (Richelson and Nathans, 1967).

The phage proteins first detected in the infected cell are the polymerase and maturation proteins. Enzyme activity as detected in cell-free extracts appears within 5 to 10 minutes after infection and the activity peaks after 20 to 30 minutes (Weissmann *et al.*, 1963; August *et al.*, 1963; Haruna *et al.*, 1963). The synthesis of maturation protein occurs later than that of polymerase and continues until 30–40 minutes after infection (Sugiyama, 1969; Fromageot and Zinder, 1968). In contrast, the production of coat protein, synthesized in much greater quantity and for a longer time than noncoat histidine-containing proteins, continues at a maximal rate throughout the growth period. This pattern of protein synthesis is also manifest in the requirement for histidine early during infection for the synthesis of noncoat proteins but not later through the latent period when coat protein continues to be synthesized (Cooper and Zinder, 1963).

Many of the studies of phage protein synthesis depended on in-hibition of host protein synthesis by actinomycin D or rifampicin. The results, while not directly applicable to normal phage development be-cause phage yield and RNA synthesis are inhibited (Nathans *et al.*, 1969; Oeschger and Nathans, 1966; Kelly *et al.*, 1965; Haywood and Harris; 1966; Lunt and Sinsheimer, 1966; Marino *et al.*, 1968), have been confirmed in the absence of drugs with the use of the phage R23, which itself markedly inhibits host protein synthesis (Watanabe *et al.*, 1968). Clearly, in the translation of the phage messenger there are mechanisms for control of the amount of protein synthesized and the time of synthesis.

3.2. Polarity

Amber coat protein mutants demonstrate two patterns of protein synthesis, depending upon the site of the mutation. Mutants have been described in which the glutamine codon CAG of the coat protein cis-tron has been substituted by the amber codon UAG at amino acid positions 6 or 70 in f2 (Notani *et al.*, 1965; Lodish and Zinder, 1966*a*) and 6, 50 or 54 in R17 (Tooze and Weber, 1967). The mutation at site 6, but not at the later sites, yields decreased polymerase activity; it is, therefore, considered a polar mutant since it results in decreased syn-thesis of a product of another gene of the same operon (Gussin, 1966; Tooze and Weber, 1967; Lodish and Zinder, 1966*a*). Synthesis of enzymes is not detected by enzyme assay (August *et al.*, 1963; Gussin, 1966), conversion of parental RNA to double-stranded forms (Lodish, 1968*c*; Capecchi, 1967), or by polyacrylamide gel analysis of infected cell extract. The nonpolar mutants distal to position 6 lead to excessive formation of polymerase late in the infectious cycle and to a less marked increase in maturation protein synthesis (Horiuchi and Matsu-hashi, 1970; August *et al.*, 1963; Gussin, 1966, Lodish *et al.*, 1964; Lodish and Zinder, 1966*a*; Nathans *et al.*, 1969; Vinuela *et al.*, 1968).

The observations of a polar effect of certain amber mutants sug-gest that translation of the first part of the coat protein gene is re-quired for translation of the polymerase gene. It has been suggested that translation of the early region of the coat protein cistron modifies the RNA such that the initiation site of the polymerase gene becomes available for ribosome binding (Zinder *et al.*, 1966; Gussin, 1966; En-gelhardt *et al.*, 1967; Lodish, 1968*d*). Such a model is consistent with the observations that fragmentation of phage RNA or changes in its conformation promote *in vitro* synthesis of the polymerase protein (*vide supra*). In line with this evidence is the effect of aurintricarboxylic acid, an inhibitor of the initiation of protein synthesis. If this drug is added early during incubation, i.e., within 2 minutes after the start of coat protein synthesis, there is no synthesis of polymerase (Grubman and Nakada, 1970). By analyzing the time after infection when polymerase synthesis becomes resistant to the drug, it was estimated that the polymerase initiation site becomes available when elongation of the coat polypeptide reaches approximately the 40th amino acid residue (Stewart *et al.*, 1971).

Polarity of translation has not been demonstrated in the translation of other phage cistrons. In cells infected with amber polymerase mutants no phage proteins were detected; with ts polymerase mutants only the enzyme protein was detected (Nathans *et al.*, 1969). These results can be attributed not to a translational mechanism *per se,* but to the fact that synthesis of maturation and coat protein is dependent upon synthesis of progeny RNA. Infection with amber maturation protein mutants did not modify synthesis of polymerase or coat protein.

3.3.   The Repressor Role of Coat Protein

It has been found that infection by nonpolar amber mutants of the coat protein gene results in higher levels of polymerase activity. Moreover, the levels of polymerase produced in permissive strains were inversely related to the amount of functional coat protein produced (Gussin, 1966; Nathans *et al.*, 1969; Garwes *et al.*, 1969; Lodish and Zinder, 1966a). These observations led to the hypothesis that phage coat protein is a "repressor" of the synthesis of the other phage-specific proteins (Gussin, 1966). Such a repressor function of phage coat protein on synthesis of polymerase protein was further elucidated by using RNA complexed with 5–10 molar equivalents of coat protein (Capecchi and Gussin, 1965; Capecchi, 1966; Sugiyama *et al.*, 1967) as a messenger *in vitro*. With homologous mixtures of RNA and coat protein, synthesis of the polymerase protein was specifically repressed, as demonstrated by reduced histidine incorporation and polyacrylamide gel electrophoresis (Sugiyama and Nakada, 1968; Eggen and Nathans, 1969; Robertson *et al.*, 1968; Sugiyama and Nakada, 1967; Ward *et al.*, 1967; Ward *et al.*, 1969). The inhibition occurs at the initiation step of protein synthesis, as shown by lack of formation of the initiation dipeptide (Lodish, 1969a; Roufa and Leder, 1971; Skogerson *et al.*, 1967). A further confirmation of the repressor effect of coat protein has now been obtained by sequence analysis of the coat protein binding site, directly demonstrating coat binding to the initiation site of the polymerase cistron (*vide supra*).

A second possible repressor mechanism has recently been described by which the polymerase–enzyme complex inhibits translation of phage RNA accompanied by the release of ribosomes and cessation of protein synthesis (Kolakofsky and Weissmann, 1971). This has been attributed to the i-factor component of the enzyme acting on the site for ribosome binding to the coat protein initiation site (Groner *et al.*, 1972*a,b*).

3.4. Translation *In Vitro*

The synthesis of phage protein in cell-free extracts was first demonstrated with coat protein, the predominant product of *in vitro* synthesis (Capecchi, 1966; Nathans *et al.,* 1962; Yamazaki and Kaesberg, 1966; Nathans, 1965; Adams and Capecchi, 1966; Webster *et al.,* 1966; Sugiyama and Nakada, 1968). The synthesis of non-coat proteins was indicated as well by the incorporation of histidine, an amino acid absent in the coat protein (Capecchi and Gussin, 1965; Nathans *et al.,* 1962; Nathans, 1965; Ohtaka and Spiegelman, 1963). By use of RNA containing an amber codon in this gene (Capecchi, 1966; Vinuela *et al.,* 1967) it was possible to identify one of these proteins as the product of the polymerase cistron. Identification of the maturation protein was more difficult since little is synthesized *in vitro* (Capecchi, 1966; Adams and Capecchi, 1966; Sugiyama and Nakada, 1968; Vinuela *et al.,* 1967), although material with the same electrophoretic mobility has been found (Eggen *et al.,* 1967; Eggen and Nathans, 1969). However, synthesis of the aminoterminal peptide of the maturation protein was detected by specific labeling with N-formyl-^{35}S-methionine (Lodish, 1968*b*). Also, relatively greater synthesis of this protein was obtained by use of a polar coat mutant RNA complexed with coat protein to reduce the synthesis of coat and polymerase proteins (Lodish and Robertson, 1969*a*) (*vide supra*).

In addition to phage RNA, the strand complementary to R17 RNA and partially double-stranded RNA from f2 infected cells have been tested in the *in vitro* system. The complementary strand does not initiate protein synthesis or bind to ribosomes but stimulates the incorporation of amino acids directed by viral RNA (Schwartz *et al.,* 1969). The partially double-stranded RNA is translated to produce mainly coat protein (Engelhardt *et al.,* 1968).

3.4.1. Initiation of Synthesis

When synthesized *in vitro*, each of the three phage-specific proteins contains N-formylmethionine as the N-terminal amino acid (Lodish, 1968*b,d*; Lodish and Robertson, 1969*a*; Adams and Capecchi, 1966; Webster *et al.*, 1966; Vinuela *et al.*, 1967). In the case of the coat protein of f2, the amino-terminal sequence of the *in vitro* product is fMet-Ala—, in contrast to the natural coat sequence NH_2Ala— (Lodish, 1968*b*; Adams and Capecchi, 1966; Webster *et al.*, 1966; Lodish, 1969*a*). The amino-terminal dipeptide of the f2 maturation protein is fMet-Arg (Lodish, 1969*a*), and that of the polymerase protein is fMet-Ser (Lodish, 1968*b*, 1969*a*).

3.4.2. Effect of Primary and Secondary Structure

The regulation of translation of the phage genome *in vivo* is apparent because coat protein is synthesized in greater quantity and for a longer time than the other phage-specific proteins. Regulation of translation also occurs *in vitro*, as seen both by a temporal order of translation and by greater synthesis of coat protein (Lodish, 1968*b,d*; Ohtaka and Spiegelman, 1963; Engelhardt *et al.*, 1967; Webster and Zinder, 1969). These observations of the relative amounts of viral protein synthesized *in vitro* are dependent upon the integrity and conformation of viral RNA. With intact "native" RNA isolated from phage particles by phenol extraction, ribosomes bind initially only to the coat protein initiation site. This was determined by use of the dipeptide assay for the initiation of synthesis (Lodish, 1968*b*), by nucleotide sequence analysis of the RNA in the initiation complex (Gupta *et al.*, 1970; Hindley and Staples, 1969), by the observations that only one ribosome can attach to phage RNA if polypeptide chain elongation is prevented (Engelhardt *et al.*, 1967; Iwasaki *et al.*, 1968; Lodish and Robertson, 1969*a*; Takanami *et al.*, 1965; Webster *et al.*, 1969; Webster and Zinder, 1969), and by analysis of the protein product of synthesis limited to the single initiation site (Webster *et al.*, 1969; Gupta *et al.*, 1971; Kuechler and Rich, 1970). The specific ribosome binding depends, however, upon the intactness of the RNA, as fragmentation by any one of several procedures or alterations in structural conformation such as formaldehyde treatment allowed the initiation of all three proteins (Lodish, 1968*b,d*, 1969*a*, 1970*a*; Steitz, 1969*b*; Staples and Hindley, 1971; Voorma *et al.*, 1971; Fukami and Imahori, 1971; Gesteland and Spahr, 1969; Lodish and Robertson, 1969*a*).

3.4.3. Ribosome Specificity

Another possible element in the regulation of translation is a specificity of ribosomes for certain RNA sites. This was first made evident by the finding that in contrast to *E. coli* ribosomes, *B. stearothermophilus* ribosomes initiate maturation protein synthesis, but not coat protein or polymerase (Lodish, 1969*b*, 1970*b*; Lodish and Robertson, 1969*b*; Steitz, 1969*b*), while *B. subtilis* is not active with phage RNA (Lodish and Robertson, 1969*b*). Recent work by Steitz (1973) demonstrated that whereas ribosomes from *B. stearothermophilus* bind to the maturation initiation site both in native RNA and in a mixture of the three initiator fragments, *E. coli* ribosomes prefer the maturation protein-initiator fragment over the coat protein region in intact RNA. She suggests that in native RNA the potentially efficient A protein initiator is masked by the remainder of the RNA. It must be presumed then that the species specificity of ribosomes resides in their relative affinities for the coat and polymerase regions.

3.4.4. Specific Initiation Factors

There is also evidence that the initiation factors play a regulatory role. This is suggested by the fact that in the presence of initiation factors from phage T4-infected cells, initiation occurs chiefly at the maturation protein cistron (Steitz *et al.,* 1970), apparently due to a deficiency in IF3 (Lee-Huang and Ochoa, 1971; Pollack *et al.,* 1970). It also has been found that purified fractions of IF3 differ in their ability to direct translation of the different phage proteins (Lee-Huang and Ochoa, 1971; Revel *et al.,* 1970).

3.4.5. Role of Nascent RNA

Another possible component in the regulation of translation is the nascent chain of progeny RNA. A replicative RNA complex consisting of minus-strand RNA as template and one or more nascent progeny RNA chains shows about 5-fold greater initiation of maturation protein relative to total protein than does single-stranded RNA (Robertson and Lodish, 1970). This presumably is because the maturation protein cistron at the 5′ terminus of phage RNA is available for ribosome binding on the nascent chain. Only a few of the maturation protein chains initiated were completed, however, in contrast to coat protein, which was the major product of the reaction. From these observations it was suggested that maturation protein synthesis begins at the 5′ end of the nascent strands of progeny RNA. As RNA synthesis proceeds, however, folding of the RNA chain blocks the maturation protein initiation site, preventing further ribosome binding (Robertson and Lodish, 1970). Thus it was postulated that maturation *in vivo* might occur on nascent RNA chains, consistent with evidence that transcription and translation are coupled.

3.4.6. Summary of the Control of Translation

The first protein synthesized 5–10 minutes after infection is the phage polymerase. This protein must be translated chiefly, if not solely, from parental RNA since normal levels of polymerase do not depend on RNA synthesis. In contrast, normal yields of the other two phage proteins do require synthesis of progeny RNA. Translation of the polymerase gene is dependent, however, on at least partial synthesis of coat protein, as some amber mutants of the coat cistron are polar for polymerase synthesis. After formation of the polymerase protein, the parental RNA is then used as a template for the synthesis of progeny RNA. There is evidence that binding of host subunits of the polymerase complex may also act to prevent further binding of ribosomes to the coat protein initiation site. At 10–20 minutes after infection, maturation and coat protein appear in the infected cell. Shortly thereafter, synthesis of the polymerase protein ceases and the rate of maturation protein synthesis declines. The inhibition of synthesis of polymerase is achieved by a repressor effect of coat protein binding to the parental phage messenger. The synthesis of maturation protein may be regulated by the restricted accessibility of the maturation protein initiation site to ribosome binding in intact RNA. If maturation protein can be translated only from nascent strands (Robertson and Lodish, 1970), then such synthesis would be necessarily limited since the number of intact molecules far exceeds that of nascent chains.

4. REPLICATION

4.1. RNA Replication *In Vivo*

The replication of RNA in RNA bacteriophages is a multistep process which involves the synthesis of complementary RNA in the presence of the parental RNA template and host factors with the subsequent synthesis of progeny RNA from the template complementary strand. Early studies on the mechanism of *in vivo* replication have focused on the isolation of RNA intermediates in the reaction (Erikson, 1968; Lodish, 1968a; Stavis and August, 1970). Three classes of molecules can be distinguished: a completely double-stranded replicative form consisting of a complete plus strand and one minus strand (Ammann *et al.*, 1964; Francke and Hofschneider, 1966a,b; Franklin, 1966, 1967a,b; Granboulan and Franklin, 1966); a replicative intermediate consisting of a complete plus strand and one complete minus strand and one or several partially complete progeny strands (Fenwick *et al.*,1964; Erikson *et al.*, 1964, 1965; Francke and Hofschneider, 1966b; Granboulan and Franklin, 1968; Kelly and Sinsheimer, 1967a); and a small completely RNase-resistant "core" (Billeter *et al.*, 1966a). There are two possible types of replication: semiconservative or conservative. The first is one in which a nascent strand is hydrogen bonded to its complement; as synthesis proceeds it displaces its preexisting counterpart. The second type is one in which a duplex of plus and minus strands remains intact except for a growing point at which the new strand is synthesized; when completed, the progeny strand is displaced (Lodish and Zinder, 1966b; Weissmann *et al.*, 1964a; Fenwick *et al.*, 1964; Kelly and Sinsheimer, 1967a,b; Erikson and Erikson, 1967; Ochoa *et al.*, 1964; Erikson and Franklin, 1966; Billeter *et al.*, 1966b).

It is possible initially to identify parental RNA as part of an RNase-resistant replicative form, and later, during infection, as an RNase-sensitive component of the replicative intermediate (Kelly and Sinsheimer, 1964, 1967a,b; Weissmann *et al.*, 1964a; Kaerner and Hoffmann-Berling, 1964; Erikson and Erikson, 1967; Lodish and Zinder, 1966b). However, contrary to the expectation that all of the labeled RNA in a brief pulse would be in double-stranded form, only approximately 50% of the nascent RNA appears to be RNase-resistant. Since this result is not consistent with a semiconservative mechanism, it has been suggested that replication occurs both conservatively and semiconservatively, with the latter being the prevailing mode (Kelly and Sinsheimer, 1967a). Formaldehyde inactivation of infectious RNA was also used to determine the mechanism of replication. Formaldehyde should inactivate infectious RNA that is a component of a semiconservative structure, while the infectious RNA that is in a conservative-type replicative intermediate should be resistant to formaldehyde treatment. It was found that at least 80% of the infectivity of the replicative intermediate was destroyed by formaldehyde (Francke and Hofschneider, 1969). These results suggest that a majority of replicative-intermediate molecules are of the semiconservative type.

One intriguing observation is that parental RNA is not found in progeny phage (Davis and Sinsheimer, 1963). It is possible that some distinguishing modification (factors perhaps) makes the parental strand the preferential template for the synthesis of minus strands.

Studies on the *in vivo* replication of RNA indicate that the site of RNA synthesis may be membrane associated (Haywood, 1971, 1973; Haywood and Sinsheimer, 1965; Haywood *et al.*, 1969; Hunt *et al.*, 1971). Labeled replicative intermediate was isolated from membrane and membrane eluate, a fraction containing material bound only in the presence of divalent cations. It was found that all replicative RNA was associated with membrane fractions, and that the amount found in the membrane leveled off within 1–2 minutes while that found in the membrane eluate increased with time of labeling. The bulk of the label entering viral RNA came from the replicative intermediate associated with the membrane eluate. It is suggested that the factors required for complementary strand synthesis are bound to membrane. After the replicative RNA is formed it is released into the membrane eluate where polymerase that is no longer bound to factors is capable of making viral RNA (Haywood, 1973).

4.2. RNA Replication *In Vitro*

Infection of *E. coli* by RNA bacteriophage leads to the appearance of an RNA-dependent RNA polymerase, which catalyzes the synthesis of phage RNA. Although phage RNA polymerases have been isolated from several sources (Weissmann *et al.*, 1963, 1964*b*, August *et al.*, 1963, 1965; Haruna *et al.*, 1963; Weissmann, 1965), the system most extensively studied is derived from the bacteriophage Qβ (Watanabe *et al.*, 1967). In the reaction catalyzed by the Qβ RNA polymerase template, Qβ RNA is replicated yielding a product which is infectious in spheroplasts (Spiegelman *et al.*, 1965). In addition to the enzyme and template RNA, the reaction requires host cell factors (August, 1969).

4.2.1. Properties of the Qβ RNA Polymerase

The enzyme, originally isolated from extracts of Qβ-infected cells by Haruna and Spiegelman (1965*a*), has been purified to a high degree of homogeneity (Pace and Spiegelman, 1966; Eoyang and August, 1968, 1971; Kamen, 1972). Purified preparations have specific activities of 200–500 nmoles of GMP incorporated per milligram of enzyme protein per minute at 37°C. The molecular weight of the enzyme has been estimated to be 130,000. The active enzyme complex consists of 4 polypeptides, one of which is the gene product of the replicase cistron of the phage genome (Kondo *et al.*, 1970; Kamen, 1970). Their molecular-weight estimates are: Subunit I, 70,000–74,000; Subunit II, 62,000–65,000; Subunit III, 47,000; Subunit IV, 30,000–35,000 (Kondo *et al.*, 1970; Kamen, 1970; August *et al.*, 1973). Although the molecular weight of the native enzyme as determined by gel filtration, zonal sedimentation, and sedimentation equilibrium centrifugation is 130,000–150,000, the sum of the molecular weights of the four subunits exceeds 200,000. The reason for this discrepancy is as yet unclear, but it is likely that the components actually exist in multiple polymeric forms and that each of these forms exhibit the molecular weight attributed to the active enzyme complex. The finding that simple alterations in ionic environment produce variations in the associative interactions of the four components indicates that the polymerase is not composed of a single active enzyme but a complex of loosely associated protein components.

By virtue of its serological cross-reactivity, its molecular weight, and its equivalency with factor i in the $Q\beta$ RNA reaction, subunit I has been identified as host interference factor i (Kamen *et al.*, 1972; Groner *et al.*, 1972*b*), a bacterial protein which inhibits the translation of the coat protein cistron in native viral mRNA but stimulates the translation of the replicase cistron when it is accessible, e.g., in formaldehyde-treated RNA (Groner *et al.*, 1972*a*). It is presumed that this effect involves the binding of factor i to IF3, a factor which selectively stimulates the binding of ribosomes to the initiation site of the coat protein cistron (Lee-Huang and Ochoa, 1971; Berissi *et al.*, 1971). An intriguing possibility is that an autoregulatory system exists in which, initially, factor i stimulates the synthesis of the replicase subunit. Factor i, together with the replicase subunit and subunits III and IV, is then incorporated into the enzyme complex (Groner *et al.*, 1972*b*).

Subunit II is the virus-specific polypeptide induced upon infection of *E. coli* by RNA phage. It is this polypeptide that confers the specificity of replication to the enzyme complex. Subunits III and IV have been shown to be protein synthesis elongation factors Tu and Ts [for a summary of translational factors, see Lengyel (1969)] on the basis of serological cross-reactivity, the presence of Tu and Ts activities in the $Q\beta$ replicase, identity of aminoterminal residues of subunit IV and Ts, and the recovery of enzymic activity when subunits I and II are reconstituted with authentic Tu and Ts (Blumenthal *et al.*, 1972). As yet the precise role of these two host proteins in Qβ RNA replication is not known. It has been suggested that since Tu and Ts function in the host as intermediaries in the transfer of aminoacyl-tRNA to the ribosome by means of a complex containing Tu, GTP, and aminoacyl-tRNA, subunits III and IV may play an analogous role in Qβ RNA synthesis by binding to the initiation site near the 3′-hydroxyl end of the RNA.

In vivo evidence that at least Ts is required for the poly C-directed poly G polymerase activity associated with Qβ polymerase comes from the isolation of a temperature-sensitive mutant (HAK-88) with a lesion in the Ts cistron (Kuwano *et al.*, 1973). Incubation of enzyme isolated from Qβ-infected HAK-88 cells at the nonpermissive temperature (42°C) shows a marked decrease in enzyme activity compared to that from infected wild-type host.

A unique property of the Qβ polymerase is its template specificity. The only nucleic acids known to serve as template for replication are Qβ RNA (Haruna and Spiegelman, 1965a), Qβ complementary strand (Feix *et al.*, 1968; August *et al.*, 1968; Banerjee *et al.*, 1969b), "variants" of Qβ RNA isolated under various limiting conditions (Mills *et al.*, 1967; Levisohn and Spiegelman, 1968), and a 6 S RNA present in Qβ-infected *E. coli* (Banerjee *et al.*, 1969a).

The specificity of these templates does not reside solely in the primary structure of a limited region since fragments of Qβ RNA do not serve as templates (Haruna and Spiegelman, 1965b). The only known specification for enzyme recognition is the penultimate cytidine at the 3′-OH terminus (Rensing and August, 1969; Kamen, 1969). As described above, the terminal adenosine residue can be removed without affecting the infectivity or template activity of the RNA, but it is the only one that is not crucial to the initiation site. In view of the fact that polycytidylate and synthetic ribocopolymers containing cytidylate also act as template for the enzyme, albeit only for the synthesis of the complementary polymer (Hori *et al.*, 1967), it seems that a string of Cs is one of the recognition requirements for the enzyme. Since other natural messengers such as the RNA of TMV, MS2, and R17 contain C-rich terminal regions as well, it must be presumed that the secondary and tertiary structure of the RNA is also implicated in the specificity of binding sites for the enzyme.

4.2.2. Host Cell Factors

It was found during the course of enzyme purification that other components were required for the recovery of fully active enzyme

(Eikhom *et al.*, 1968; Shapiro *et al.*, 1968). In addition to the polymerase complex, two bacterial proteins not associated with the polymerase and found in both uninfected and infected *E. coli* are required for the synthesis of infectious RNA (Shapiro *et al.*, 1968). Their function is related solely to the template activity of Qβ RNA, as they are not needed for synthesis directed by the Qβ complementary strand or other templates. A factor requirement has also been reported for the f2 poly G polymerase (Federoff and Zinder, 1973). This requirement is observed, however, in the presence of both f2 plus- and minus-strand template. Qβ factors and f2 factor, though functionally analogous, are not interchangeable between the two systems.

4.2.2(a). Factor I

Factor I can be isolated as a homogeneous protein with a molecular weight of 70,000–80,000 (Franze de Fernandez *et al.*, 1968, 1972). SDS-polyacrylamide gel electrophoresis of a boiled, denatured preparation of factor I yields a single band with a molecular weight of approximately 12,000–15,000. This evidence suggests that the active factor is a polymeric protein consisting of 4–6 polypeptides of the same molecular weight. The protein is remarkably resistant to heat (100°C), though it has no unusual constituents. Its amino acid composition has been published (Franze de Fernandez *et al.*, 1972).

The absolute requirement for factor I varies with RNA concentration only, and it is independent of the amount of enzyme in the reaction. Studies on the stoichiometric relationship between factor I and RNA indicate that one molecule of factor I is required per molecule of RNA. Factor I binds to single-stranded RNA (*E. coli* rRNA, R23 RNA, f2 RNA), but not to double-stranded RNA (reovirus RNA) or DNA, either double or single stranded. Analysis of the early steps in the polymerase reaction indicates that neither phosphodiester bond formation nor irreversible binding of 5′-terminal GTP occurs in the absence of factor I. It has been suggested that factor I is required for RNA synthesis at the level of enzyme–RNA binding (Franze de Fernandez *et al.*, 1972).

4.2.2(b). Factor II

The requirement for factor II can be fulfilled by a number of basic polypeptides (Kuo, 1971; Kuo and August, 1972). Aside from many of the basic proteins associated with the structural proteins of ribosomes, factor II activity has been detected in $Q\beta$, R23, and f2 coat protein and lysine-rich and arginine-rich calf thymus histones, as well as salmon sperm protamine sulfate. However, poly-L-lysine, poly-L-arginine, bovine serum albumin, spermine, spermidine, and putrescine are ineffective. Irrespective of the source of factor II, the amount of protein required for maximal activity was the same, 0.1–0.2 μg per μg $Q\beta$ RNA. Factor II proteins bind tightly to RNA, as would be expected considering their basic properties. As measured by the nitrocellulose filter assay, enzyme binding of $Q\beta$ RNA is dependent upon the presence of factor II (Kuo et al., 1974), with the concentration required for binding being the same as that required for RNA synthesis. Analysis of enzyme–RNA binding using equilibrium partition in a two-phase liquid polymer system indicates that while binding of enzyme to different RNA molecules is possible at 0°C, the formation of a specific initiation complex in which one molecule of enzyme binds one molecule of $Q\beta$ RNA occurs only at 37°C and in the presence of GTP and both factors (Silverman, 1973a,b).

The role of the factor proteins is probably to mediate the interaction of polymerase with $Q\beta$ RNA to form an initiation complex. Since enzyme can bind to many sites on the RNA, factor II may function by competing with the enzyme for nonspecific binding regions thereby facilitating enzyme binding to a single specific site. Factor I may possibly act on the RNA initiation site or on the enzyme bound to this site prior to the onset of synthesis.

4.2.3. The Complementary Strand

A strand with a base composition complementary to that of the $Q\beta$ RNA is synthesized early in the reaction, before the appearance of progeny RNA (Feix et al., 1967; Weissmann and Feix, 1966). The minus strand is detected by the appearance of RNase-resistant RNA product after deproteinization (Weissmann et al., 1968). Concomitant with the appearance of RNase-resistant product is the loss in infectivity of the template RNA (Mills et al., 1966). The complementary or minus strand then serves as a template for the synthesis of $Q\beta$ RNA in a reaction that does not require the presence of host factors.

Analysis of the 3′ terminus of the complementary strand shows that A is the predominant terminal residue though C has also been found at the 3′ site (Weber and Weissmann, 1970). Thus, even though both plus and minus strands are terminated by a 3′-adenosine, pppG is the only known residue at the 5′ terminus. Since no adenylate-adding activity has been detected in the purified enzyme (Rensing and August, 1969; August *et al.*, 1973), it must be assumed that the enzyme itself has this capability. The paradox of a terminal adenosine, which is not copied according to the Watson–Crick model of base-pairing, is not a requirement for infectivity or template activity, and yet is added on during replication, remains unresolved.

4.2.4. Synthesis of Viral RNA

The synthesis of infectious viral RNA *in vitro* (Spiegelman *et al.*, 1965) requires, in addition to the phage polymerase, Mg^{2+}, the four ribonucleoside triphosphates, host factors, and $Q\beta$ RNA.

One property of the reaction is the recognition of specific template RNA. In addition to $Q\beta$ RNA, the $Q\beta$ RNA polymerase can utilize only a few natural RNA molecules synthesized *in vivo* and *in vitro*, polyribocytidylic acid, and synthetic ribopolymers which contain cytidylate. There is evidence that the mechanism of this phenomenon resides at least in part in the template-binding properties of the enzyme. Two properties of the enzyme have been distinguished: (1) The recognition of specific templates and (2) binding to a single site on template RNA. At 0°C and in the absence of reaction components required for RNA synthesis, the enzyme reversibly binds to any RNA and to DNA as well (August *et al.*, 1968); as many as 30 enzyme molecules can bind to a single $Q\beta$ RNA molecule (Silverman, 1973*a*). Under these conditions, however, template specificity is manifest by a 10-fold higher affinity of the enzyme for $Q\beta$ RNA than that for other RNAs. It was suggested that such preferential binding to multiple sites could serve *in vivo* to minimize competition for enzyme between phage and cellular RNA. Binding of enzyme to a single site on $Q\beta$ RNA has been observed to require incubation at 37°C in the presence of GTP and host factors (Silverman, 1973*a,b*). The reaction results in the formation of a complex that is not dissociated by high ionic strength or competing RNA, and is specific for $Q\beta$ or other template RNA. The stoichiometry of binding is the same as that for initiation, i.e., a maximum of one molecule of active enzyme is bound per molecule of $Q\beta$ RNA. However, complex formation can be distinguished from initiation of synthesis as the latter is dependent on the presence of Mg^{2+} ions. It was hypothesized that the role of the basic protein factor II in this reaction is to compete with enzyme for the nonspecific binding sites thus facilitating enzyme binding to the specific site. Presumably the binding site is that which specifies the initiation of synthesis at the 3′-OH terminus of the template.

The first RNA to be synthesized is the complementary strand. The subsequent synthesis of viral RNA can be described by two possible models: (1) a double-stranded intermediate consisting of a plus strand and a newly completed minus strand serves as the template, and (2) free complementary minus strand serves as template. Although there has been much work on the isolation of these double-stranded structures from both *in vivo* and *in vitro* sources (Weissmann *et al.*, 1964*a*; Weissmann and Borst, 1963; Weissmann, 1965; Mills *et al.*, 1966; Bishop *et al.*, 1967*a,b*; Pace *et al.*, 1967, 1968), it is not clear whether they are direct precursors of the viral product or artifacts of the isolation procedure. Since detection of double-stranded structures is based on their resistance to RNase and extraction procedures such as phenol may artifactually confer double-stranded characteristics to the RNA, evidence that they are intermediates in replication is not conclusive. More persuasive evidence that free complementary strands may indeed be the true template for viral RNA synthesis is the fact that neither replicative-form RNA (one plus and one minus strand) nor replicative-intermediate RNA (one plus, one minus, and one or more nascent plus chains) has been found to serve as template, while free complementary minus strand serves quite well (Weissmann *et al.*, 1967, 1968). There are, however, no data to explain how the potentially hydrogen-bonded complementary strands are maintained free or are denatured in the course of the reaction.

Based on the available data, it is possible to construct the following scheme for the replication of phage RNA. Specific recognition of Qβ RNA results from the high-affinity reversible binding of enzyme to template. In the presence of GTP and host factors, the enzyme selectively and irreversibly binds to a single site, possibly initiated by factors binding to competing RNA sites. Synthesis is initiated in the presence of Mg^{2+} and the four nucleoside triphosphates, beginning at the penultimate C residue and ending with the addition of the 3′-terminal adenosine to yield the complementary strand. The newly synthesized complementary strand acts as the template for the synthesis of viral RNA, with the enzyme again initiating at the penultimate C and completing the molecule by the addition of an A residue.

4.2.5. Replication of Other Templates

In addition to Qβ RNA and its complementary strand, two other classes of RNA are replicated by the polymerase *in vitro*. These are not infectious nor do they require the presence of factors for their synthesis. One class of small RNA molecules replicated *in vitro* is the $Q\beta$ 6 S RNA isolated from infected cells (Banerjee *et al.*, 1969*b*; Prives and Silverman, 1972). This double-stranded molecule has a chain length of 130 nucleotides. As they do not have the same terminal sequences, they are considered (Trown and Meyer, 1973) to be distinct from the "variant" RNA. Variant RNA molecules (Mills *et al.*, 1967, 1968; Levisohn and Spiegelman, 1968, 1969) originally derived from $Q\beta$ RNA have been isolated by selecting for molecules which are differentiated either by virtue of the selective advantage of being able to replicate rapidly or by survival under limiting conditions, i.e., low concentrations of substrate or in the presence of inhibitors (Saffhill *et al.*, 1971). Several such variants have been isolated, the smallest of which contains only 6% of the genetic material found in phage $Q\beta$ (Kacian *et al.*, 1972).

5. ADSORPTION AND PENETRATION

Infection by RNA phage particles can occur only in male bacteria (Loeb and Zinder, 1961), but phage RNA is infectious in both male and female spheroplasts. Male cells are distinguished by the presence of F pili, phenotypic expressions of the fertility (F) factor (Crawford and Gesteland, 1964; Caro and Schnös, 1966; Brinton *et al.*, 1964; Valentine and Strand, 1965). These filamentous appendages, one or two of which are present on the surface of male cells (Brinton *et al.*, 1964), are flexible rods, 85 nm in diameter, and from less than 1 μm to 80 μm long (Brinton and Beer, 1967). As shown in electron micrographs, the virus particles adsorb to the pilus in large numbers along its entire length (Crawford and Gesteland, 1964; Caro and Schnös, 1966; Brinton *et al.*, 1964; Valentine and Strand, 1965), but infection is carried out by only one or a few particles; this evidence suggests the existence of either a few unique binding sites or an exclusion process which prevents multiple infections. Phage attachment to F pili is presumed to be mediated by the maturation protein (Roberts and Steitz, 1967) since phage mutants defective in maturation protein do not adsorb to bacteria (Lodish *et al.*, 1965). These mutants are characterized by their sensitivity to RNase, and it is thought that the loss of infectivity is a consequence of RNA degradation. There is, however, another class (class III) of defective particles found in R17 phage preparations which lack the maturation protein, are unable to adsorb to pili, and yet are resistant to RNase (Krahn and Paranchych, 1971). It would seem, therefore, that the maturation protein has a dual function affecting both the stability of the phage and its ability to adsorb to the host.

The adsorption of phage to the cell triggers a series of events during the initial five minutes of the infectious cycle. This eclipse period parallels the release of maturation protein from the viral capsid, a marked decrease in the cellular levels of nucleoside triphosphates, and the release of free pili into the medium (Paranchych *et al.*, 1971). The RNA separates from the coat protein leaving the empty shell outside (Edgell and Ginoza, 1965). At the separation stage the RNA becomes sensitive to RNase. The separation reaction is energy dependent, requires host metabolic activity (Danziger and Paranchych, 1970*a*), but does not require divalent metal ions (Paranchych, 1966; Danziger and Paranchych, 1970*b*).

After separating from the coat, the RNA then penetrates the host cell. This reaction is dependent on the presence of divalent cations (Paranchych, 1966) and is blocked by the addition of EDTA (Silverman and Valentine, 1969). It has been suggested that penetration is facilitated by a structural modification of the F pilus in which the pilus becomes fragmented (Paranchych *et al.*, 1971).

6. ASSEMBLY

Phage RNA together with homologous or heterologous coat protein is capable of forming several types of complexes that resemble phage particles (Sugiyama *et al.*, 1967; Eggen and Nathans, 1969; Hung *et al.*, 1969). Although there is RNA–protein interaction between phage RNA and heterologous protein, there seems to be a specificity of interaction between homologous protein and RNA. A complex of a few heterologous or homologous protein subunits and phage RNA can be converted into phagelike particles only upon addition of the same protein (Hung *et al.*, 1969). It has been shown that during *in vitro* self-assembly Qβ and MS2 protein do not interact to form mixed particles (Ling *et al.*, 1969). Further evidence for the specificity of assembly was the finding that double infection of *E. coli* with MS2 and Qβ does not produce hybrid or mixed-coat particles (Ling *et al.*, 1970).

Studies of defective particles produced by amber mutants of the maturation protein cistron (Argetsinger and Gussin, 1966; Hohn, 1967) and reconstitution experiments (Hung and Overby, 1969; Roberts and Steitz, 1967) demonstrate that self-assembly of complete phage particles requires biologically competent RNA, coat protein, and maturation protein. It has been suggested that maturation protein is required at an early step in the packaging of the phage particle and it may involve the correct assembly of viral RNA into the viral particle (Kaerner, 1970; Cramer and Sinsheimer, 1971). In view of the observations that newly synthesized maturation protein is found to be associated with viral RNA (Richelson and Nathans, 1967) in infected cells, that the protein penetrates the host cell during infection, and that it enters the cell complexed with the infecting RNA (Kozak and Nathans, 1971; Krahn *et al.*, 1972), it is likely that it functions both in adsorption to F pili and in assembly of the mature phage particle.

Three models of the mechanism of phage assembly have been proposed: (1) RNA is packaged into an empty shell formed by the aggregation of protein subunits. (2) An assemblage of protein subunits is constructed around an RNA core. (3) RNA and protein condense cooperatively, perhaps in a two-step reaction in which first, an initiation complex is formed by a few protein molecules and RNA, and second, the particle is completed by the subsequent aggregation of additional coat subunits. The observations that empty shells do not react with RNA (Hohn, 1969), that capsid formation is not specific to the size or composition of RNA, and that initiation complexes of the types described have been isolated would seem to preclude the first two models of phage assembly.

The final events in phage infection, that of phage release and cell lysis, have not as yet been well defined. It is known, however, that cell lysis is not an absolute and necessary prerequisite for phage release since at reduced temperatures phage particles can be released from intact bacterial cells (Engelberg and Soudry, 1971; Hoffmann-Berling and Maze, 1964). Zinder and Lyons (1968) have suggested that coat protein causes the lysis of the host cell when infected with phage f2. The f2 mutants that are blocked in coat protein synthesis or produce defective coat protein do not lyse host bacteria. However, since in phage $Q\beta$ maturation protein mutants do not cause host cell lysis (Horiuchi and Matsuhashi, 1970) and no lytic activity of coat protein has been detected (Zinder and Lyons, 1968), it would seem that the function of coat protein in cell lysis is less direct.

7. THE RELATION OF PHAGE INFECTION AND HOST METABOLISM

7.1. Host Metabolism Required for Phage Synthesis

Although DNA synthesis is not required for RNA phage replication, as shown by the inability of inhibitors of DNA synthesis to block phage multiplication (Cooper and Zinder, 1962; Watanabe and August, 1967, 1968b), phage growth does require the maintenance of some host metabolic functions. Thus, alteration of the host DNA by ultraviolet irradiation or thymine starvation abolishes the cell's susceptibility to infection (Neubauer and Zavada, 1965; Rappaport, 1965; Zavada et al., 1966). Evidence for the requirement for host-DNA-dependent RNA synthesis is the finding that actinomycin D, a known inhibitor of cellular metabolism markedly inhibits phage growth when added either before or up to 10–16 minutes after infection (Vinuela et al., 1967; Haywood and Sinsheimer, 1965; Oeschger and Nathans, 1966; Haywood and Harris, 1966; Lunt and Sinsheimer, 1966). The inhibition of phage yield is accompanied by a decreased synthesis of 27 S progeny RNA. Total RNA synthesis is increased, however, and there is an accumulation of a 6–10 S phage-specific RNase-resistant RNA. The significance of the synthesis of the "aberrant" RNA is unknown, but it can also be observed under abnormal conditions such as UV irradiation (Kelly et al., 1965; Nonoyama and Ikeda, 1964) or infection by a coat protein or maturation protein mutant of f2 (Lodish and Zinder, 1966a). It is known that an RNase-resistant 6 S RNA can be replicated in vitro by the Qβ polymerase (vide supra).

The use of actinomycin D to inhibit host protein synthesis has been complicated by the fact that the cell must be pretreated to enhance its permeability to this drug, thus making interpretation of the data less satisfactory. The discovery that rifampicin inhibits cellular RNA and protein synthesis (Hartmann et al., 1967) presumably by binding to the β subunit of the DNA-dependent RNA polymerase (Zillig et al., 1970; Heil and Zillig, 1970) has led to further studies on the effect of this drug on host–phage interactions. RNA phage replication is blocked by rifampicin if it is added prior to infection (Fromageot and Zinder, 1968; Marino et al., 1968). It is suggested that the block occurs after the penetration of the phage RNA. Subsequent studies on Qβ and MS2 prompted suggestions that the effect of rifampicin is on a host factor essential for phage assembly (Passent and Kaesberg, 1971) or the release of phage particles (Engelberg and Soudry, 1971).

Although it is generally accepted that host protein synthesis is required for phage replication, the precise mechanism involved is as yet unknown. Studies with the Qβ polymerase reaction indicate that in vitro synthesis of phage RNA is not inhibited by rifampicin (Bandle and Weissmann, 1970). However, in MS2-infected cells, while rifampicin only reduces the rate of minus-strand synthesis, it completely abolishes progeny RNA synthesis (Engelberg, 1972). It has been suggested that the synthesis of host factors necessary for $Q\beta$ RNA synthesis *in vitro* may be involved. The possibility that protein synthesis elongation factors Tu and Ts are the affected proteins has also been suggested (Meier and Hofschneider, 1972), though in view of the fact that Tu and Ts comprise at least 2% of the soluble protein in *E. coli* (Miller and Weissbach, 1970), this possibility seems less likely. Alternatively, consideration must be given to the possibility that factor i, identified also as host subunit I of the $Q\beta$ polymerase–enzyme complex (*vide supra*), is the protein being depleted.

The presence of an analogue of uracil, 5-fluorouracil (Cooper and Zinder, 1962; Davern 1964b; Shimura and Nathans, 1964; Shimura *et al.*, 1965), has been found to also inhibit phage growth. Addition of the drug up to 13 minutes after infection results in a yield of MS2 about three orders of magnitude less than that found in untreated cells. When added later in infection, the effect is less dramatic and the particle yield is about 50% despite an approximately 80% replacement of uracil by 5-fluorouracil. It appears that some necessary early function of phage or host is highly susceptible to the presence of 5-fluorouracil. The effect of 5-fluorouracil cannot be explained by perturbation of specific base complementarity since highly substituted phage lose little infectivity compared to those grown in the presence of the analogue (Shimura *et al.*, 1965).

RNA phage replication is also inhibited by colicine E_2 or superinfection with $\phi X174$ or T-even DNA phages (Neubauer and Zavada, 1965; Hattman and Hofschneider, 1967; Yarosh and Levinthal, 1967; Huppert *et al.*, 1967; Fujimura, 1966). The effect appears to require the expression of the DNA phage genome in the synthesis of DNA phage protein. It is suggested that inhibition of f2 multiplication by superinfection with T4 phage is due to the induction of a specific endoribonuclease which degrades f2 RNA and thus prevents phage protein synthesis (Goldman and Lodish, 1971). Superinfection by T4 DNA-free ghosts can also block RNA phage replication but, unlike the effect by T4 viable phage, inhibition by ghosts cannot be blocked by rifampicin (Goldman and Lodish, 1973). It seems, therefore, that whereas inhibition of RNA phage replication by intact T4 is due to induction of expression of T4 gene function, inhibition caused by T4 ghosts may be due to suppression of host function by affecting the pools of DNA, RNA, or protein precursors (Duckworth, 1970). Since phage RNA synthesis is known to be dependent on host metabolism, attempts have been made to pinpoint the specific host gene expression required. By measuring infectious RNA uptake rather than uracil uptake to monitor phage RNA synthesis, phage RNA replication was compared in rel^+ (relaxed) and rel (stringent) strains of *E. coli* deprived of a required amino acid. No effect of amino acid starvation was observed (Siegel and Kjeldgaard, 1971). This suggests that the rel gene may not be a control for the synthesis of phage RNA as had been previously thought (Friesen, 1965, 1969).

7.2. Phage-Induced Changes in Host Metabolism

Changes in cellular metabolism upon RNA phage infection vary according to the infecting phage. With f2 and Qβ, for instance, synthesis of bacterial RNA is only slightly affected upon infection, with less than half of the protein and RNA synthesized after infection being recoverable in phage particles (Watanabe *et al.*, 1968). In contrast, despite their physical and chemical similarities, infection with R17, R23, and ZIK/1 results in a marked inhibition of bacterial protein and ribosomal RNA synthesis (Ellis and Paranchych, 1963; Hudson and Paranchych, 1967; Bishop, 1965; Yamazaki, 1969). During R23 infection, 60% of the RNA synthesized is encapsulated into phage particles and almost all protein synthesized late in infection is coat protein (Watanabe *et al.*, 1968).

Induction of β-galactosidase is inhibited when cells are infected with β and R23 and to a lesser extent when f2 or Qβ is used (Nonoyama *et al.*, 1963; Watanabe *et al.*, 1968). No inhibition is seen, however, when addition of inducer precedes infection. Coat protein synthesis is not required for this inhibition, as protein synthesis is also reduced in cells infected with a nonpolar amber mutant of the coat protein gene, while a lesion in the phage polymerase gene blocks the expression of this inhibitory effect. The inhibition of ribosomal RNA synthesis can not be correlated with the ability of infecting R17 to produce either coat or maturation protein. Phage-induced inhibition of host rRNA synthesis has been observed only when the infecting phage is able to produce viral polymerase (Spangler and Iglewski, 1972). Since inhibition of host protein and RNA synthesis can also occur at high multiplicities of infection with ultraviolet-inactivated phage or when penetration is blocked by EDTA (Yamazaki, 1969; Watanabe and Watanabe, 1968), it would appear that there are several mechanisms by which host metabolism is inhibited and some of them may not require the expression of a phage cistron.

8.   CONCLUSION

The RNA bacteriophage has been the model system for the study of replication because of the simplicity of its genetic material. The same molecule serves both as a messenger for transcription and translation. The size of the genome is limited to three cistrons and consequently only three gene products need be monitored. The simplicity, however, has proven to be deceptive, for although our knowledge of the transcriptional and translational processes as well as the mechanisms by which these processes are controlled has advanced remarkably, the elucidation of these mechanisms is far from complete: While the physical structure of the phage particle is known, there is uncertainty as to how the component parts are assembled; while considerable progress has been made in sequencing the three cistrons and their surrounding regions, the unique recognition sequences and configurations that specify translation or transcription are unknown; while the three enzyme-associated host proteins required for *in vitro* replication have been identified, their function in the synthesis reaction has not been defined. Thus, although many of the major uncertainties in RNA phage replication have been resolved, the task is as yet unfinished.

ACKNOWLEDGMENTS

This work was supported in part by the National Institute of General Medical Sciences, National Institutes of Health Grants GM 1191 and GM 11301. This is Communication No. 315 from the Joan and Lester Avnet Institute of Molecular Biology. The kindness of colleagues who made available their papers both published and in press is gratefully acknowledged.

9.   REFERENCES

Adams, J. M., and Capecchi, M. R., 1966, N-Formylmethionyl-sRNA as the initiator of protein synthesis, *Proc. Natl. Acad. Sci. USA* **55,** 147.

Adams, J. M., and Cory, S., 1970, Untranslated nucleotide sequence at the 5′-end of R17 bacteriophage RNA, *Nature (Lond.)* **227,** 570.

Adams, J. M., Jeppesen, P. G. N., Sanger, F., and Barrell, B. G., 1969a, Nucleotide sequences from fragments of R17 bacteriophage RNA, *Cold Spring Harbor Symp. Quant. Biol.* **34,** 611.

Adams, J. M., Jeppesen, P. G. N., Sanger, F., and Barrell, B. G., 1969b, Nucleotide sequence from the coat protein cistron of R17 bacteriophage RNA, *Nature (Lond.)* **223,** 1009.

Adams, J. M., Spahr, P. -F., and Cory, S., 1972, Nucleotide sequence from the 5′-end to the first cistron of R17 bacteriophage RNA, *Biochemistry* **11**, 976.

Ammann, J., Delius, H., and Hofschneider, P. H., 1964, Isolation and properties of an intact phage-specific replicative form of RNA phage M12, *J. Mol. Biol.* **10**, 557.

Argetsinger, J. E., and Gussin, G., 1966, Intact ribonucleic acid from defective particles of bacteriophage R17, *J. Mol. Biol.* **21**, 421.

August, J. T., 1969, Mechanism of synthesis of bacteriophage RNA, *Nature (Lond.)* **222**, 121.

August J. T., Cooper, S., Shapiro, L., and Zinder, N. D., 1963, RNA phage-induced RNA polymerase, *Cold Spring Harbor Symp. Quant. Biol.* **23**, 95.

August, J. T., Shapiro, L., and Eoyang, L., 1965, Replication of RNA viruses. I. Characterization of a viral RNA-dependent RNA polymerase, *J. Mol. Biol.* **11**, 257.

August, J. T., Banerjee, A. K. Eoyang, L., Franze de Fernandez, M. T., Hori, K., Kuo, C. H., Rensing, U., and Shapiro, L., 1968, Synthesis of bacteriophage Qβ RNA, *Cold Spring Harbor Symp. Quant. Biol.* **33**, 73.

August, J. T., Eoyang, L., Franze de Fernandez, M. T., Hayward, W. S., Kuo, C. H., and Silverman, P., 1973, Host proteins in the replication of bacteriophage RNA, *in* "Gene Expression and Its Regulation" Vol. I (F. T. Kenney, B. A. Hamkalo, G. Favelukes, and J. T. August, eds.), pp. 29–41, Plenum Press, New York.

Ball, L. A., and Kaesberg, P., 1973, Cleavage of the N-terminal formylmethionine residue from a bacteriophage coat protein *in vitro, J. Mol. Biol.* **79**, 531.

Bandle, E., and Weissmann, C., 1970, Rifampicin and the replication of the RNA-containing bacteriophage Qβ, *Biochim. Biophys. Acta* **199**, 551.

Banerjee, A. K., Rensing, U., and August, J. T., 1969a, Replication of RNA viruses. X. Replication of a natural 6 S RNA by the Qβ RNA polymerase, *J. Mol. Biol.* **45**, 181.

Banerjee, A. K., Kuo, C. H., and August, J. T., 1969b, Replication of RNA viruses. VIII. Direction of chain growth in the Qβ RNA polymerase reaction, *J. Mol. Biol.* **40**, 445.

Bassel, B. A., and Spiegelman, S., 1967, Specific cleavage of Qβ RNA and identification of the fragment carrying the 3′-OH terminus, *Proc. Natl. Acad. Sci. USA* **58**, 1155.

Berissi, H., Groner, Y., and Revel, M., 1971, Effect of a purified initiation factor F3(B) on the selection of ribosomal binding sites on phage MS2 RNA, *Nat. New Biol.* **234**, 44.

Bernardi, A., and Spahr, P. F., 1972, Nucleotide sequence at binding site for coat protein of R17, *Proc. Natl. Acad. Sci. USA* **69**, 3033.

Billeter, M. A., Wiessmann, C., and Warner, R. C., 1966a, Replication of viral ribonucleic acid. IX. Properties of double-stranded RNA from *Escherichia coli* infected with bacteriophage MS2, *J. Mol. Biol.* **17**, 145.

Billeter, M. A., Libonati, M., Vinuela, E., and Weissmann, C., 1966b, Replication of viral ribonucleic acid. X. Turnover of virus-specific double-stranded ribonucleic acid during replication of phage MS2 in *Escherichia coli, J. Biol. Chem.* **241**, 4750.

Billeter, M. A., Dahlberg, J. E., Goodman, H. M., Hindley, J., and Weissmann, C., 1969, Sequence of the first 175 nucleotides from the 5′-terminus of Qβ RNA synthesized *in vitro, Nature (Lond.)* **224**, 1083.

Bishop, D. H. L., 1965, Ribonucleic acid synthesis by *Escherichia coli* C3000/L after infection by the ribonucleic acid coliphage Z1K/1, and properties of coliphage Z1K/1 ribonucleic acid, *Biochem. J.* **97**, 17.

Bishop, D. H. L., Claybrook, J. R., Pace, N. R., and Spiegelman, S., 1967a, An analysis by gel electrophoresis of Qβ RNA complexes formed during the latent period of an *in vitro* synthesis, *Proc. Natl. Acad. Sci. USA* **57**, 147.

Bishop, D. H. L., Claybrook, J. R., and Spiegelman, S., 1967b, Electrophoretic separation of viral nucleic acids on polyacrylamide gels, *J. Mol. Biol.* **26**, 373.

Bishop, D. H. L., Mills, D. R., and Spiegelman, S., 1968, The sequence at the 5′-terminus of a self-replicating variant of viral Qβ ribonucleic acid, *Biochemistry* **7**, 3744.

Blumenthal, T., Landers, T. A., and Weber, K., 1972, Qβ replicase contains protein biosynthesis EF Tu and EF Ts, *Proc. Natl. Acad. Sci. USA* **69**, 1313.

Boedtker, H., 1967, The reaction of ribonucleic acid with formaldehyde. I. Optical absorbance studies, *Biochemistry.* **6**, 2718.

Boedtker, H., 1971, Conformation independent MW determinations of RNA by gel electrophoresis, *Biochim. Biophys. Acta* **240**, 448.

Bradley, D. E., 1966, The structure and infective process of a *Pseudomonas aeruginosa* bacteriophage containing ribonucleic acid, *J. Gen. Microbiol.* **45**, 83.

Brinton, C. C., and Beer, H., 1967, The interaction of male-specific bacteriophages with F. pili, *in* "The Molecular Biology of Viruses" (J. S. Colter and W. Paranchych, eds.), pp. 251–289, Academic Press, New York.

Brinton, C. C., Gemski, P., and Carnahan, J., 1964, A new type of bacterial pilus genetically controlled by the fertility factor of *E. coli* K12 and its role in chromosome transfer, *Proc. Natl. Acad. Sci. USA* **52**, 776.

Capecchi, M. R., 1966, Cell-free protein synthesis programmed with R17 RNA: Identification of two phage proteins, *J. Mol. Biol.* **21**, 173.

Capecchi, M. R., 1967, Polarity *in vitro*, *J. Mol. Biol.* **30**, 213.

Capecchi, M. R., and Gussin, G. N., 1965, Suppression *in vitro*: Identification of a serine-sRNA as a "nonsense" suppressor, *Science (Wash., D.C.)* **149**, 417.

Caro, L. G., and Schnös, M., 1966, The attachment of the male-specific bacteriophage F1 to sensitive strains of *Escherichia coli, Proc. Natl. Acad. Sci. USA* **56**, 126.

Contreras, R., Vandenberghe, A., Volckaert, G., Min Jou, W., and Fiers, W., 1972, Studies on the bacteriophage MS2—Some nucleotide sequences from the RNA-polymerase gene, *FEBS (Fed. Eur. Biochem. Soc.) Lett.* **24**, 339.

Contreras, R., Ysebaert, M., Min Jou, W., and Fiers, W., 1973, Bacteriophage MS2 RNA: Nucleotide sequence of the end of the A protein and the intercistronic region, *Nat. New Biol.* **241**, 99.

Cooper, S., and Zinder, N. D., 1962, The growth of an RNA bacteriophage: The role of DNA synthesis, *Virology* **18**, 405.

Cooper, S., and Zinder, N. D., 1963, The growth of an RNA bacteriophage: The role of protein synthesis, *Virology* **20**, 605.

Cory, S., Spahr, P., and Adams, J., 1970, Untranslated nucleotide sequences in R17 bacteriophage RNA, *Cold Spring Harbor Symp. Quant. Biol.* **35**, 1.

Cory, S., Adams, J., Spahr, P., and Rensing, U., 1972, Sequence of 51 nucleotides at 3′ end of R17, *J. Mol. Biol.* **63**, 41.

Cramer, J. H., and Sinsheimer, R. L., 1971, Replication of bacteriophage MS2. X. Phage specific ribonucleoprotein particles found in MS2-infected *E. coli, J. Mol. Biol.* **62**, 189.

Crawford, E. M., and Gesteland, R. F., 1964, The adsorption of bacteriophage R17, *Virology* **22**, 165.

Dahlberg, J. E., 1968, Terminal sequences of bacteriophage RNAs, *Nature (Lond.)* **220**, 548.

Danziger, R. E., and Paranchych, W., 1970a, Stages in phage R17 infection. III. Energy requirements for the F-pili mediated eclipse of viral infectivity, *Virology* **40**, 554.

Danziger, R. E., and Paranchych, W., 1970b, Stages in phage R17 infection. II. Ionic requirements for phage R17 attachment to F-pili, *Virology* **40**, 547.

Davern, C. I., 1964a, The isolation and characterization of an RNA bacteriophage, *Aust. J. Biol. Sci.* **17**, 719.

Davern, C. I., 1964b, The inhibition and mutagenesis of an RNA bacteriophage by 5′-fluorouracil, *Aust. J. Biol. Sci.* **17**, 726.

Davis, J. E., and Sinsheimer, R. L., 1963, The replication of bacteriophage MS2. I. Transfer of parental nucleic acid to progeny phage, *J. Mol. Biol.* **6**, 203.

DeWachter, R., and Fiers, W., 1967, Studies on the bacteriophage MS2. IV. The 3′-OH terminal undecanucleotide sequence of the viral RNA chain, *J. Mol. Biol.* **30**, 507.

DeWachter, R., and Fiers, W., 1969, Sequences at the 5′-terminus of bacteriophage Qβ RNA, *Nature (Lond.)* **221**, 233.

DeWachter, R., Verhassel, J. P., and Fiers, W., 1968a, The 5′-terminal end group of the RNA of the bacteriophage MS2, *Biochim. Biophys. Acta* **157**, 195.

DeWachter, R., Verhassel, J. -P., and Fiers, W., 1968b, Studies on the bacteriophage MS2. V. The 5′-terminal tetranucleotide sequence of the viral RNA chain, *FEBS (Fed. Eur. Biochem. Soc.) Lett.* **1**, 93.

DeWachter, R., Verhassel, J. -P., and Fiers, W., 1968c, The 5′-terminal tetranucleotide sequence of bacteriophage MS2 ribonucleic acid, *Arch. Int. Physiol.* **76**, 580.

DeWachter, R., Merregaert, J., Vandenberghe, A., Contreras, R., and Fiers, W., 1971b, Studies on MS2—Untranslated 5′-terminal sequence preceding first cistron, *Eur. J. Biochem.* **22**, 400.

DeWachter, R., Vandenberghe, A., Merregaert, J., Contreras, R., and Fiers, W., 1971a, Leader sequence from 5′-terminus to A protein initiation codon in MS2, *Proc. Natl. Acad. Sci. USA* **68**, 585.

Duckworth, D. H., 1970, The metabolism of T4 phage ghost-infected cells. I. Macromolecular synthesis and transport of nucleic acid and protein precursors, *Virology* **40**, 673.

Edgell, M. H., and Ginoza, W., 1965, The fate during infection of the coat protein of the spherical bacteriophage R17, *Virology* **27**, 23.

Eggen, K., and Nathans, D., 1969, Regulation of protein synthesis directed by coliphage MS2 RNA. II. *In vitro* repression by phage coat protein, *J. Mol. Biol.* **39**, 293.

Eggen, K., Oeschger, M. P., and Nathans, D., 1967, Cell-free protein synthesis directed by coliphage MS2 RNA: Sequential synthesis of specific phage proteins, *Biochem. Biophys. Res. Commun.* **28**, 587.

Eikhom, T. S., Stockley, D. J., and Spiegelman, S., 1968, Direct participation of a host protein in the replication of viral RNA *in vitro*, *Proc. Natl. Acad. Sci. USA* **59**, 506.

Ellis, D. B., and Paranchych, W., 1963, Synthesis of ribonucleic acid and protein in bacteria infected with an RNA bacteriophage, *J. Cell. Comp. Physiol.* **62**, 207.

Engelberg, H., 1972, Inhibition of RNA bacteriophage replication by rifampicin, *J. Mol. Biol.* **68**, 541.

Engelberg, H., and Soudry, E., 1971, RNA bacteriophage release: Requirement for host-controlled protein synthesis, *J. Virol.* **8**, 257.

Engelhardt, D. L., Webster, R. E., and Zinder, N. D., 1967, Amber mutants and polarity *in vitro, J. Mol. Biol.* **29**, 45.

Engelhardt, D. L., Robertson, H. D., and Zinder, N. D., 1968, *In vitro* translation of multistranded RNA from *Escherichia coli* infected by bacteriophage f2, *Proc. Natl. Acad. Sci. USA* **59**, 972.

Enger, M. D., and Kaesberg, P., 1965, Comparative studies of the coat proteins of R17 and M12 bacteriophages, *J. Mol. Biol.* **13**, 260.

Enger, M. D., Stubbs, E. A., Mitra, S., and Kaesberg, P., 1963, Biophysical characteristics of the RNA-containing bacterial virus R17, *Proc. Natl. Acad. Sci. USA* **49**, 857.

Eoyang, L., and August, J. T., 1968, Phage Qβ RNA polymerase, *in* "Methods in Enzymology," Vol. 12B (L. Grossman and K. Moldave, eds.), pp. 530–540, Academic Press, New York.

Eoyang, L., and August, J. T., 1971, Qβ RNA polymerase from phage Qβ-infected *E. coli, in* "Procedures in Nucleic Acid Research," (G. L. Cantoni and D. R. Davies, eds.), pp. 829–839, Harper and Row, New York.

Erikson, R. L., 1968, Replication of RNA viruses, *Annu. Rev. Microbiol.* **22**, 305.

Erikson, R. L., and Erikson, E., 1967, Structure and function of bacteriophage R17 replicative intermediate ribonucleic acid. II. Properties of the parental labeled molecule, *J. Virol.* **1**, 523.

Erikson, R. L., and Franklin, R. M., 1966, Symposium on replication of viral nucleic acids. I. Formation and properties of a replicative intermediate in the biosynthesis of viral ribonucleic acid, *Bacteriol. Rev.* **30**, 267.

Erikson, R. L., Fenwick, M. L., and Franklin, R. M., 1964, Replication of bacteriophage RNA: Studies on the fate of parental RNA, *J. Mol. Biol.* **10**, 519.

Erikson, R. L., Fenwick, M. L., and Franklin, R. M., 1965, Replication of bacteriophage RNA: Some properties of the parental labeled replicative intermediate, *J. Mol. Biol.* **13**, 399.

Feary, T. W., Fisher, Jr., E., and Fisher, T. N., 1963, A small RNA-containing *Pseudomonas aeruginosa* bacteriophage, *Biochem. Biophys. Res. Commun.* **10**, 359.

Federoff, N. V., and Zinder, N. D., 1971, Structure of the poly G polymerase component of the bacteriophage f2 replicase, *Proc. Natl. Acad. Sci. USA* **68**, 1838.

Federoff, N. N., and Zinder, N. D., 1973, Factor requirement of the bacteriophage f2 replicase, *Nat. New Biol.* **241**, 105.

Feix, G., Slor, H., and Weissmann, C., 1967, Replication of viral RNA. XIII. The early product of phage RNA synthesis *in vitro, Proc. Natl. Acad. Sci. USA* **57**, 1401.

Feix, G., Pollet, R., and Weissmann, C., 1968, Replication of viral RNA. XVI. Enzymatic synthesis of infectious viral RNA with noninfectious Qβ minus strands as template, *Proc. Natl. Acad. Sci. USA* **59**, 145.

Fenwick, M. L., Erikson, R. L., and Franklin, R. M., 1964 Replication of the RNA of bacteriophage R17, *Science (Wash., D.C.)* **146**, 527.

Fiers, W., 1973, The structure of viral RNA, *in* "Physico-Chemical Properties of Nucleic Acids" (J. Duchesne, ed.), pp. 213–234, Academic Press, New York.

Fiers, W., Contreras, R., DeWachter, R., Haegeman, G., Merregaert, J., Min Jou,

W., and Vandenberghe, A., 1971, Recent progress in sequence of MS2 RNA, *Biochimie* **53,** 495.

Fischbach, F. A., Harrison, P. M., and Anderegg, J. W., 1965, An X-ray scattering study of the bacterial virus R17, *J. Mol. Biol.* **13,** 638.

Francke, B., and Hofschneider, P. H., 1966*a*, Über infektiiöse Substrukturen aus *Escherichia coli* Bakteriophagen. VII. Formation of a biologically intact replicative form in ribonucleic acid bacteriophage (M12)-infected cells, *J. Mol. Biol.* **16,** 544.

Francke, B., and Hofschneider, P. H., 1966*b*, Infectious nucleic acids of *E. coli* bacteriophages. IX. Sedimentation constants and strand integrity of infectious M12 phage replicative-form RNA, *Proc. Natl. Acad. Sci. USA* **56,** 1883.

Francke, B., and Hofschneider, P. H., 1969, Infectious nucleic acids of *E. coli* bacteriophages. XI. Differentiation between conservatively and semiconservatively replicating RNA intermediates of the bacteriophage M12 by formaldehyde inactivation, *J. Mol. Biol.* **40,** 45.

Franklin, R. M., 1966, Purification and properties of the replicative intermediate of the RNA bacteriophage R17, *Proc. Natl. Acad. Sci. USA* **55,** 1504.

Franklin, R. M., 1967*a*, Replication of bacteriophage ribonucleic acid: Some physical properties of single-stranded, double-stranded, and branched viral ribonucleic acid, *J. Virol.* **1,** 64.

Franklin, R. M., 1967*b*, Replication of bacteriophage ribonucleic acid: Some properties of native and denatured replicative intermediate, *J. Virol.* **1,** 514.

Franze de Fernandez, M. T., Eoyang, L., and August, J. T., 1968, Factor fraction required for the synthesis of bacteriophage Qβ RNA, *Nature (Lond.)* **219,** 588.

Franze de Fernandez, M. T., Hayward, W. S., and August, J. T., 1972, Bacterial proteins required for replication of Qβ RNA: Purification and properties of factor I, *J. Biol. Chem.* **247,** 824.

Friesen, J. D., 1965, Control of bacteriophage RNA synthesis in *Escherichia coli, J. Mol. Biol.* **13,** 220.

Friesen, J. D., 1969, Dependence of f2 bacteriophage RNA replication on amino acids, *J. Mol. Biol.* **46,** 349.

Fromageot, H. P. M., and Zinder, N. D., 1968, Growth of bacteriophage f2 in *E. coli* treated with rifampicin, *Proc. Natl. Acad. Sci. USA* **61,** 184.

Fujimura, R. K., 1966, Effect of colicine E2 on the biosynthesis of bacteriophage R17, *J. Mol. Biol.* **17,** 75.

Fukami, H., and Imahori, K., 1971, Control of translation by conformation of messenger RNA, *Proc. Natl. Acad. Sci. USA* **68,** 570.

Garwes, D., Sillero, A., and Ochoa, S., 1969, Virus-specific proteins in *Escherichia coli* infected with phage Qβ, *Biochim. Biophys. Acta* **186,** 166.

Gesteland, R. F., and Boedtker, H., 1964, Some physical properties of bacteriophage R17 and its ribonucleic acid, *J. Mol. Biol.* **8,** 496.

Gesteland, R. F., and Spahr, P. F., 1969, Translation of R17 RNA fragments, *Cold Spring Harbor Symp. Quant. Biol.* **34,** 707.

Gilham, P., 1970, RNA sequence analysis, *Annu. Rev. Biochem.* **39,** 227.

Glitz, D. G., 1968 The nucleotide sequence at the 3′-linked end of bacteriophage MS2 ribonucleic acid, *Biochemistry* **7,** 927.

Godson, G. N., 1968, Site of synthesis of viral ribonucleic acid and phage assembly in MS2-infected *Escherichia coli, J. Mol. Biol.* **34,** 149.

Godson, G. N., and Sinsheimer, R. L., 1967, The replication of bacteriophage MS2. VI. Interaction between bacteriophage RNA and cellular components in MS2-infected *Escherichia coli, J. Mol. Biol.* **23,** 495.

Goldman, E., and Lodish, H., 1971, Inhibition of replication of ribonucleic acid bacteriophage f2 by superinfection with bacteriophage T4, *J. Virol.* **8,** 417.

Goldman, E., and Lodish, H., 1973, T4 phage and T4 ghosts inhibit f2 phage replication by different mechanisms, *J. Mol. Biol.* **74,** 151.

Goodman, H. M., Billeter, M., Hindley, J., and Weissmann, C., 1970, The nucleotide sequence at the 5′-terminus of the Qβ RNA minus strand, *Proc. Natl. Acad. Sci. USA* **67,** 921.

Gould, H. J., Pinder, J. C., and Matthews, H. R., 1969, Fractionation of low-molecular-weight fragments of ribosomal and viral RNA by polyacrylamide gel electrophoresis, *Anal. Biochem.* **29,** 1.

Gralla, J., Steitz, J., and Crothers, D., 1974, Direct physical evidence for secondary structure in an isolated fragment of R17 bacteriophage messenger RNA, *Nature,* in press.

Granboulan, N., and Franklin, R. M., 1966, Electron microscopy of viral RNA replicative form, and replicative intermediate of the bacteriophage R17, *J. Mol. Biol.* **22,** 173.

Granboulan, N., and Franklin, R. M., 1968, Replication of bacteriophage ribonucleic acid: Analysis of the ultrastucture of the replicative form and the replicative intermediate of bacteriophage R17, *J. Virol.* **2,** 129.

Groner, Y., Pollack, Y., Berissi, H., and Revel, M., 1972a, Cistron specific translation control protein in *E. coli, Nat. New Biol.* **239,** 16.

Groner, Y., Schelps, R., Kamen, R., Kolakofsky, D., and Revel, M., 1972b, Host subunit of Qβ replicase is translation factor i, *Nat. New Biol.* **239,** 19.

Grubman, M. J., and Nakada, D., 1970, Translation of MS2 phage RNA cistrons *in vitro, Bacteriol. Proc.,* P172.

Gupta, S. L., Chen, J., Schaefer, L., Lengyel, P., and Weissman, S. M., 1970, Nucleotide sequence of a ribosome attachment site of bacteriophage f2 RNA, *Biochem. Biophys. Res. Commun.* **39,** 883.

Gupta, S. L., Waterson, J., Sopori, M. L., Weissman, S. M., and Lengyel, P., 1971, Movement of the ribosome along the messenger ribonucleic acid during protein synthesis, *Biochemistry* **10,** 4410.

Gussin, G. N., 1966, Three complementation groups in bacteriophage R17, *J. Mol. Biol.* **21,** 435.

Hartmann, G., Honikel, K. O., Knusel, F., and Neusch, J., 1967, The specific inhibition of the DNA-directed RNA synthesis rifamycin, *Biochim. Biophys. Acta* **145,** 843.

Haruna, I., and Spiegelman, S., 1965a, Specific template requirements of RNA replicases, *Proc. Natl. Acad. Sci. USA* **54,** 579.

Haruna, I., and Spiegelman, S., 1965b, Recognition of size and sequence by an RNA replicase, *Proc. Natl. Acad. Sci. USA* **54,** 1189.

Haruna, I., Nozu, K., Ohtaka, Y., and Spiegelman, S., 1963, An RNA "replicase" induced by and selective for a viral RNA: Isolation and properties, *Proc. Natl. Acad. Sci. USA* **50,** 905.

Hattman, S., and Hofschneider, P. H., 1967, Interference of bacteriophage T4 in the reproduction of RNA-phage M12, *J. Mol. Biol.* **29,** 173.

Haywood, A. M., 1971, Cellular site of *Escherichia coli* ribosomal RNA synthesis, *Proc. Natl. Acad. Sci. USA* **68,** 435.

Haywood, A. M., 1973, Two classes of membrane binding of replicative RNA bacteriophage MS2, *Proc. Natl. Acad. Sci. USA* **70,** 2381.

Haywood, A. M., and Harris, J. M., 1966, Actinomycin inhibition of MS2 replication, *J. Mol. Biol.* **18,** 448.

Haywood, A. M., and Sinsheimer, R. L., 1965, The replication of bacteriophage MS2. V. Proteins specifically associated with infection, *J. Mol. Biol.* **14,** 305.

Haywood, A. M., Cramer, J. H., and Shoemaker, N. L., 1969, Host–virus interaction in RNA bacteriophage infected *E. coli.* I. Location of "late" MS2-specific RNA synthesis, *J. Virol.* **4,** 364.

Heil, A., and Zillig, W., 1970, Reconstitution of bacterial DNA-dependent RNA-polymerase from isolated subunits as a tool for the elucidation of the role of the subunits in transcription, *FEBS (Fed. Eur. Biochem. Soc.) Lett.,* **11,** 165.

Heisenberg, M., 1966, Formation of defective bacteriophage particles by fr amber mutants, *J. Mol. Biol.* **17,** 136.

Heisenberg, M., and Blessing, J., 1965, Unvollstandige viruspartikel als folge von mu-tationen in genom des bacteriophagen fr, *Z. Naturforsch.* **20B,** 859.

Hindley, J., and Staples, D. H., 1969, Sequence of a ribosome binding site in bacterio-phage Qβ RNA, *Nature (Lond.)* **224,** 964.

Hindley, J., Staples, D. H., and Billeter, M. A., 1970, Location of the coat cistron on the RNA of phage Qβ, *Proc. Natl. Acad. Sci. USA* **67,** 1180.

Hoffmann-Berling, H. and Maze, H., 1964, Release of male-specific bacteriophage from surviving host bacteria. *Virology* **22,** 305.

Hofschneider, Von, P. H., 1963, Untersuchungen über kleine *E. coli* K12 Bakterio-phagen, *Z. Naturforsch.* **18B,** 203.

Hohn, T., 1967, Self-assembly of defective particles of the bacteriophage fr, *Eur. J. Biochem.* **2,** 152.

Hohn, T., 1969, The assembly of protein particles of the RNA bacteriophage fr in absence of RNA, *Biochem. Biophys. Res. Commun.* **36,** 7.

Hohn, T., and Hohn, B., 1970, Structure and assembly of simple RNA bacterio-phages, *Adv. Virus Res.* **16,** 43.

Hori, K., Banerjee, A. K., Eoyang, L., and August, J. T., 1967, Replication of RNA viruses. V. Template activity of synthetic ribocopolymers in the Qβ RNA polymerase reaction, *Proc. Natl. Acad. Sci. USA* **57,** 1790.

Horiuchi, K., and Matsuhashi, S., 1970, Three cistrons in bacteriophage Qβ, *Virology* **42,** 49.

Horiuchi, K., Webster, R. E., and Matsuhashi, S., 1971, Gene products of Qβ, *Virology* **45,** 429.

Hotham-Iglewski, B., and Franklin, R. M., 1967, Replication of bacteriophage ribonu-cleic acid: Alterations in polyribosome patterns patterns and association of double-stranded RNA with polyribosomes in *Escherichia coli* infected with bacteriophage R17, *Proc. Natl. Acad. Sci. USA* **58,** 743.

Hotham-Iglewski, B., Phillips, L. A., and Franklin, R. M., 1968, Viral RNA transcription–translation complex in *Escherichia coli* infected with bacteriophage R17, *Nature (Lond.)* **219,** 700.

Housman, D., Gillespie, D., and Lodish, H., 1972, Removal of formyl-methionine residue from nascent bacteriophage f2 protein, *J. Mol. Biol.* **65,** 163.

Hudson, J. B., and Paranchych, W., 1967, Effect of bacteriophage R17 infection on host-directed synthesis of ribosomal ribonucleates, *J. Virol.* **1,** 529.

Hung, P. P., and Overby, L. R., 1969, The reconstitution of infective bacteriophage Qβ, *Biochemistry* **8,** 820.

Hung, P. P., Ling, C. M., and Overby, L. R., 1969, Self-assembly of Qβ and MS2 phage particles: Possible function of initiation complexes, *Science* (*Wash., D.C.*) **166**, 1638.

Hunt, D., Saito, Y., and Watanabe, M., 1971, Membrane bound RNA in *E. coli* infected with RNA bacteriophage R23, *J. Biol. Chem.* **246**, 4151.

Huppert, J., Blum-Emerique, L., and Breugnon, M., 1967, Mixed infection of *Escherichia coli* by RNA and DNA bacteriophages. I. Inhibition of RNA phage multiplication by superinfection with DNA phages, *Virology* **33**, 307.

Iwasaki, K., Sabol, S., Wahba, A. J., and Ochoa, S., 1968, Translation of the genetic message. VII. Role of initiation factors in formation of the chain initiation complex with *Escherichia coli* ribosomes, *Arch. Biochem. Biophys.* **125**, 542.

Jockusch, H., Ball, L. A., and Kaesberg, P., 1970, Synthesis of polypeptides directed by the RNA of phage Qβ, *Virology* **42**, 401.

Kacian, D., L. Mills, D. R., and Spiegelman, S., 1971, The mechanism of Qβ replication: sequence at the 5′-terminus of 6 S RNA template, *Biochim. Biophys. Acta* **238**, 212.

Kacian, D. L., Mills, D. R., Kramer, F. R., and Spiegelman, S., 1972, Replicating RNA molecule suitable for detailed analysis of extracellular evolution and replication, *Proc. Natl. Acad. Sci. USA* **69**, 3038.

Kaerner, H. C., 1969, Translation control of viral RNA in *Escherichia coli, J. Mol. Biol.* **42**, 259.

Kaerner, H. C., 1970, Sequential steps in the *in vivo* assembly of the RNA bacteriophage, *J. Mol. Biol.* **53**, 515.

Kaerner, H. C., and Hoffmann-Berling, H., 1964, Synthesis of double-stranded RNA in RNA-phage infected *E. coli* cells, *Nature* (*Lond.*) **202**, 1012.

Kamen, R., 1969, Infectivity of bacteriophage R17 RNA after sequential removal of 3′-terminal nucleotides, *Nature* (*Lond.*) **221**, 321.

Kamen, R., 1970, Characterization of the subunits of Qβ replicase, *Nature* (*Lond.*) **228**, 527.

Kamen, R., 1972, A new method of purification of Qβ polymerase, *Biochim. Biophys. Acta* **262**, 88.

Kamen, R., Kondo, M., Romer, W., and Weissmann, C., 1972, Reconstitution of Qβ replicase lacking subunit α with protein synthesis interference factor i, *Eur. J. Biochem.* **31**, 44.

Kelley, R. B., and Sinsheimer, R. L., 1964, A new RNA component in MS2-infected cells, *J. Mol. Biol.* **8**, 602.

Kelley, R. B., and Sinsheimer, R. L., 1967*a*, The replication of bacteriophage MS2. IX. Structure and replication of the replicative intermediate, *J. Mol. Biol.* **29**, 237.

Kelley, R. B., and Sinsheimer, R. L., 1967*b*, The replication of bacteriophage MS2. VII. Non-conservative replication of double-stranded RNA, *J. Mol. Biol.* **26**, 169.

Kelley, R. B., Gould, J. L., and Sinsheimer, R. L., 1965, The replication bacteriophage MS2. IV. RNA components specifically associated with infection, *J. Mol. Biol.* **11**, 562.

Kolakofsky, D., and Weissmann, C., 1971, Qβ replicase as repressor of Qβ RNA directed protein synthesis, *Biochim. Biophys. Acta* **246**, 596.

Kondo, M., Gallerani, R., and Weissmann, C., 1970, Subunit structure of Qβ replicase, *Nature* (*Lond.*) **228**, 525.

Konigsberg, W., 1966, The arrangement of the tryptic peptides in the coat protein of the f2 bacteriophage, *J. Biol. Chem.* **241**, 4534.

Konigsberg, W., Weber, K., Notani, G., and Zinder, N. D., 1966, The isolation and characterization of the tryptic peptides from the f2 bacteriophage coat protein. *J. Biol. Chem.* **241**, 2579.

Konigsberg, W., Maita, T., Katze, J., and Weber, K., 1970, Amino acid sequence of the Qβ coat protein, *Nature (Lond.)* **227**, 271.

Kozak, M., and Nathans, D., 1971, Fate of maturation protein during infection of *E. coli, Nat. New Biol.* **234**, 209.

Kozak, M., and Nathans, D., 1972, Translation of genome of RNA bacteriophage, *Bacteriol. Rev.* **36**, 109.

Krahn, P. M., and Paranchych, W., 1971, Heterogeneous distribution of A protein in R17 phage preparations, *Virology* **43**, 533.

Krahn, P. M., O'Callaghan, R., and Paranchych, W., 1972, Stages in phage R17 infection. VI. Infection of A protein and RNA into host cell, *Virology* **47**, 628.

Kuechler, E., and Rich, A., 1970, Position of the initiator and peptidyl sites in the *E. coli* ribosome, *Nature (Lond.)* **225**, 920.

Kuo, C. H., 1971, Host cell factor II for synthesis of Qβ RNA, *in* "Procedures in Nucleic Acid Research" (G. L. Cantoni and D. R. Davies, eds.), pp. 846–850, Harper and Row, New York.

Kuo, C. H., and August, J. T., 1972, Histone or bacterial basic protein required for replication of bacteriophage RNA, *Nat. New Biol.* **237**, 105.

Kuo, C. H., Eoyang, L., and August, J. T., 1974, Protein factors required for the replication of phage Qβ RNA *in vitro, in* "RNA Phages" (N. D. Zinder, ed.), Plenum Press, New York.

Kuwano, M., Apirion, D., and Schlessinger, D., 1970, Ribonuclease V of *Escherichia coli*: Susceptibility of heated ribosomal RNA and stability of R17 phage RNA, *Science (Wash., D.C.)* **168**, 1225.

Kuwano, M., Ono, M., Yamamoto, M., Endo, H., Kamiya, T., and Hori, K., 1973, Elongation factor T altered in a temperature-sensitive *E. coli* mutant, *Nat. New Biol.* **244**, 107.

Lee, J. C., and Gilham, P. T., 1965, Determination of terminal sequences in viral and ribosomal ribonucleic acids, *J. Am. Chem. Soc.* **87**, 4000.

Lee-Huang, S., and Ochoa, S., 1971, Messenger discriminating species of initiation factor F₃, *Nat. New Biol.* **234**, 236.

Lengyel, P., 1969, The process of translation in 1969, *Cold Spring Harbor Symp. Quant. Biol.* **34**, 828.

Levisohn, R., and Spiegelman, S., 1968, The cloning of a self-replicating RNA molecule, *Proc. Natl. Acad. Sci. USA* **60**, 866.

Levisohn, R., and Spiegelman, S., 1969, Further extracellular Darwinian experiments with replicating RNA molecules: Diverse variants isolated under different selective conditions, *Proc. Natl. Acad. Sci. USA* **63**, 805.

Lin, J.-Y., Tsung, C. M., and Fraenkel-Conrat, H., 1967, The coat protein of the RNA bacteriophage MS2, *J. Mol. Biol.* **24**, 1.

Ling, C. M., Hung, P. P., and Overby, L. R., 1969, Specificity in self-assembly of bacteriophages Qβ and MS2, *Biochemistry* **8**, 4464.

Ling, C. M., Hung, P. P., and Overby, L. R., 1970, Independent assembly of Qβ and MS2 phages in doubly infected *E. coli, Virology* **40**, 920.

Ling, V., 1971, Sequence at the 5′-end of bacteriophage f2 RNA, *Biochem. Biophys. Res. Commun.* **42**, 82.

Lodish, H. F., 1968a, The replication of RNA-containing bacteriophages, *Progr. Biophys.* **18**, 285.

Lodish, H. F., 1968b, f2 RNA: Control of translation and gene order, *Nature (Lond.)* **220**, 345.

Lodish, H. F., 1968c, Polar effects of an amber mutation in f2 bacteriophage, *J. Mol. Biol.* **32**, 47.

Lodish, H. F., 1968d, Independent translation of the genes of bacteriophage f2 RNA, *J. Mol. Biol.* **32**, 681.

Lodish, H. F., 1969a, Independent initiation of translation of two bacteriophage f2 proteins, *Biochem. Biophys. Res. Commun.* **37**, 127.

Lodish, H. F., 1969b, Species specificity of polypeptide chain initiation, *Nature (Lond.)* **224**, 867.

Lodish, H. F., 1970a, Secondary structure of bacteriophage f2: Ribonucleic acid and the initiation of *in vitro* protein biosynthesis, *J. Mol. Biol.* **50**, 689.

Lodish, H. F., 1970b, Specificity in bacterial protein synthesis: Role of initiation factors and ribosomal subunits, *Nature (Lond.)* **226**, 705.

Lodish, H. F., and Robertson, H. D., 1969a, Cell-free synthesis of bacteriophage f2 maturation protein, *J. Mol. Biol.* **45**, 9.

Lodish, H. F., and Robertson, H. D., 1969b, Regulation of *in vitro* translation of bacteriophage f2 RNA, *Cold Spring Harbor Symp. Quant. Biol.* **34**, 655.

Lodish, H. F., and Zinder, N. D., 1966a, Mutants of the bacteriophage f2. VIII. Control mechanisms for phage-specific synthesis, *J. Mol. Biol.* **19**, 333.

Lodish, H. F., and Zinder, N. D., 1966b, Semi-conservative replication of bacteriophage f2 RNA, *J. Mol. Biol.* **21**, 207.

Lodish, H. F., Cooper, S., and Zinder, N. D., 1964, Host-dependent mutants of the bacteriophage f2. IV. On the biosynthesis of a viral RNA polymerase, *Virology* **24**, 60.

Lodish, H. F., Horiuchi, K., and Zinder, N. D., 1965, Mutants of the bacteriophage f2. V. On the production of noninfectious phage particles, *Virology* **27**, 139.

Loeb, T., and Zinder, N. D., 1961, A bacteriophage containing RNA, *Proc. Natl. Acad. Sci. USA* **47**, 282.

Lunt, M. R., and Sinsheimer, R. L., 1966, Inhibition of ribonucleic acid bacteriophage growth by actinomycin D, *J. Mol. Biol.* **18**, 541.

Marino, P., Baldi, M. I., and Tocchini-Valentini, G. P., 1968, Effect of rifampicin on DNA-dependent RNA polymerase and on RNA phage growth, *Cold Spring Harbor Symp. Quant. Biol.* **33**, 125.

Marvin, D. A., and Hoffmann-Berling, H., 1963, Physical and chemical properties of two new small bacteriophages, *Nature (Lond.)* **197**, 517.

Meier, D., and Hofschneider, P., 1972, Effect of rifampicin on the growth of RNA bacteriophage M12, *FEBS (Fed. Eur. Biochem. Soc.) Lett.* **25**, 179.

Miller, D. L., and Weissbach, H., 1970, Studies on the purification and properties of factor Tu from *E. coli, Arch. Biochem. Biophys.* **141**, 26.

Mills, D. R., Pace, N. R., and Spiegelman, S., 1966, The *in vitro* synthesis of a noninfectious complex containing biologically active viral RNA, *Proc. Natl. Acad. Sci. USA* **56**, 1778.

Mills, D. R., Peterson, R. L., and Spiegelman, S., 1967, An extracellular Darwinian experiment with a self-duplicating nucleic acid molecule, *Proc. Natl. Acad. Sci. USA* **58**, 217.

Mills, D. R., Bishop, D. H. L., and Spiegelman, S., 1968, The mechanism and direction of RNA synthesis templated by free minus strands of a "little" variant of $Q\beta$ RNA, *Proc. Natl. Acad. Sci. USA* **60**, 713.

Min Jou, W., Hindley, J., and Fiers, W., 1968, Limited enzymatic degradation of bacteriophage MS2 RNA, *Arch. Intern. Physiol. Biochim.* **76**, 194.

Min Jou, W., Haegeman, G., and Fiers, W., 1971, Studies on the bacteriophage MS2 nucleotide fragments from the coat protein cistron, *FEBS (Fed. Eur. Biochem. Soc.) Lett.* **13**, 105.

Min Jou, W., Haegeman, G., Ysebaert, M., and Fiers, W., 1972, Nucleotide sequence of gene coding for the bacteriophage MS2 coat protein, *Nature (Lond.)* **237**, 82.

Mitra, S., Enger, M. D., and Kaesberg, P., 1963, Physical and chemical properties of RNA from the bacterial virus R17, *Proc. Natl. Acad. Sci. USA* **50**, 68.

Moore, C. H., Farron, F., Bohnert, and Weissmann, C., 1971, Possible origin of a minor virus-specific protein (A₁), *Nat. New Biol.* **234**, 50.

Nathans, D., 1965, Cell-free protein synthesis directed by coliphage MS2 RNA: Synthesis of intact viral coat protein and other products, *J. Mol. Biol.* **13**, 521.

Nathans, D., Notani, G., Schwartz, J. H., and Zinder, N. D., 1962, Biosynthesis of the coat protein of coliphage f2 by *E. coli* extracts, *Proc. Natl. Acad. Sci. USA* **48**, 1424.

Nathans, D., Oeschger, M. P., Eggen, K., and Shimura, Y., 1966, Bacteriophage-specific proteins in *E. coli* infected with an RNA bacteriophage, *Proc. Natl. Acad. Sci. USA* **56**, 1844.

Nathans, D., Oeschger, M. P., Polmar, S. K., and Eggen, K., 1969, Regulation of protein synthesis directed by coliphage MS2 RNA. I. Phage protein and RNA synthesis in cells with suppressible mutants, *J. Mol. Biol.* **39**, 279.

Neubauer, Z., and Zavada, V., 1965, The capacity of the bacterial host for the reproduction of the RNA phage f2, *Biochem. Biophys. Res. Commun* **20**, 1.

Nichols, J. L., 1970, Nucleotide sequence from the polypeptide chain termination region of the coat protein cistron in bacteriophage R17 RNA, *Nature (Lond.)* **225**, 147.

Nishihara, T., Haruna, I., Watanabe, I., Nozu, Y., and Okada, Y., 1969, Comparison of coat proteins from three groups of RNA phages, *Virology* **37**, 153.

Nishihara, T., Nozu, Y., and Okada, Y., 1970, Amino acid sequence of the coat protein of the RNA phage ZR, *J. Biochem.* **67**, 403.

Nonoyama, M., and Ikeda, Y., 1964, Ribonuclease-resistant RNA found in cells of *Escherichia coli* infected with RNA phage, *J. Mol. Biol.* **9**, 763.

Nonoyama, M., Yuki, A., and Ikeda, Y., 1963, On some properties of phage β, a new RNA-containing phage, *J. Gen. Appl. Microbiol.* **9**, 299.

Notani, G. W., Engelhardt, D. L., Konigsberg, W., and Zinder, N. D., 1965, Suppression of a coat protein mutant of the bacteriophage f2, *J. Mol. Biol.* **12**, 439.

Ochoa, S., Weissman, C., Borst, P., Burdon, R. H., and Billeter, M. A., 1964, Replication of viral RNA, *Fed. Proc.* **23**, 1285.

Oeschger, M. P., and Nathans, D., 1966, Differential synthesis of bacteriophage-specific proteins in MS2-infected *Escherichia coli* treated with actinomycin, *J. Mol. Biol.* **22**, 235.

Ohtaka, Y., and Spiegelman, S., 1963, Translational control of protein synthesis in a cell-free system directed by a polycistronic viral RNA, *Science (Wash., D.C.)* **142**, 493.

Osborn, M., Weber, K. and Lodish, H. F., 1970a, Amino-terminal peptides of RNA phage proteins synthesized in the cell-free system, *Biochem. Biophys. Res. Commun.* **41**, 748.

Osborn, M., Weiner, A., and Weber, K., 1970b, Large-scale purification of A protein from bacteriophage R17, *Eur. J. Biochem.* **17**, 63.

Overby, L. R., Barlow, G. H., Doi, R. H., Jacob, M., and Spiegelman, S., 1966, Comparison of two serologically distinct ribonucleic acid bacteriophages. I. Properties of the viral particles, *J. Bacteriol.* **91**, 442.

Pace, N. R., and Spiegelman, S., 1966, The synthesis of infectious RNA with a replicase purified according to its size and density, *Proc. Natl. Acad. Sci. USA* **55**, 1608.

Pace, N. R., Bishop, D. H. L., and Spiegelman, S., 1967, The kinetics of product appearance and template involvement in the *in vitro* replication of viral RNA, *Proc. Natl. Acad. Sci. USA* **58**, 711.

Pace, N. R., Bishop, D. H. L., and Spiegelman, S., 1968, The immediate precursor of viral RNA in the Qβ-specific reaction, *Proc. Natl. Acad. Sci. USA* **59**, 139.

Paranchych, W., 1966, Stages in phage R17 infection: The role of divalent cations, *Virology* **28**, 90.

Paranchych, W., and Graham, F., 1962, Isolation and properties of an RNA-containing bacteriophage, *J. Cell. Comp. Physiol.* **60**, 199.

Paranchych, W., Ainsworth, S. K., Dick, A. J., and Krahn, P. M., 1971, Stages in phage R17 infection, phage eclipse and role of F pili, *Virology* **45**, 615.

Passent, J., and Kaesberg, P., 1971, Effect of rifampin on development of RNA phage Qβ, *J. Virol.* **8**, 286.

Pollack, Y., Groner, Y., Aviv (Greenshpan), H., and Revel, M., 1970, Role of initiation factor B (F3) in the preferential translation of T4 late messenger RNA in T4 infected *E. coli, FEBS (Fed. Eur. Biochem. Soc.) Lett.* **9**, 218.

Prives, C., and Silverman, P., 1972, Replication of RNA viruses: Structure of a 6 S RNA synthesized by Qβ RNA polymerase, *J. Mol. Biol.* **71**, 657.

Radloff, R., and Kaesberg, P., 1973, Electrophoretic and other properties of Qβ: Effect of variable number of read through patterns, *J. Virol.* **11**, 116.

Rappaport, I., 1965, Some studies of the infectious process with MS2 bacteriophage, *Biochim. Biophys. Acta* **103**, 486.

Remaut, E., and Fiers, W., 1972, Studies on bacteriophage MS2—termination on signal of A protein cistron, *J. Mol. Biol.* **71**, 243.

Rensing, U., and August, J. T., 1969, The 3′-terminus and the replication of phage RNA, *Nature (Lond.)* **224**, 853.

Revel, M., and Aviv, H., Groner, Y., and Pollack, Y., 1970, Fractionation of translation initiation factor B (F3) into cistron specific species, *FEBS (Fed. Eur. Biochem. Soc.) Lett.* **9**, 213.

Richelson, E., and Nathans, D., 1967, Association of bacteriophage proteins and RNA in *E. coli* infected with MS2, *Biochem. Biophys. Res. Commun.* **29**, 842.

Roberts, J. W., and Steitz, J. E., 1967, The reconstitution of infective bacteriophage R17, *Proc. Natl. Acad. Sci. USA* **58**, 1416.

Robertson, H. D., and Jeppesen, P. G., 1972, Extent and variation in three related bacteriophage RNA molecules, *J. Mol. Biol.* **68**, 417.

Robertson, H. D., and Lodish, H. F., 1970, Messenger characteristics of nascent bacteriophage RNA, *Proc. Natl. Acad. Sci. USA* **67**, 710.

Robertson, H. D., Webster, R. E., and Zinder, N. D., 1968, Bacteriophage coat protein as repressor, *Nature (Lond.)* **218**, 533.

Robinson, W. E., Frist, R. H., and Kaesberg, P., 1969, Genetic coding: Oligonucleotide coding for first six amino acid residues of the coat protein of R17 bacteriophage, *Science (Wash., D.C.)* **166**, 1291.

Roblin, R., 1968a, The 5′-terminus of bacteriophage R17 RNA; pppGp, *J. Mol. Biol.* **31**, 51.

Roblin, R., 1968b, Nucleotides adjacent to the 5′-terminus of bacteriophage R17 RNA, *J. Mol. Biol.* **36**, 125.

Rohrmann, G. F., and Krueger, R. G., 1970, The self-assembly of RNA-free protein subunits from bacteriophage MS2, *Biochem. Biophys. Res. Commun.* **38**, 406.

Roufa, D. J., and Leder, P., 1969, Biosynthesis of phage-specific initiation dipeptides, *J. Biol. Chem.* **246**, 3160.

Saffhill, R., Schneider-Bernloehr, H., Orgel, L. E., and Spiegelman, S., 1971, *In vitro* selection of Qβ RNA variants resistant to ethnidium bromide, *J. Mol. Biol.* **51**, 531.

Sakurai, T., Miyake, T., Shiba, T., and Watanabe, I., 1968, Isolation of a possible fourth group of RNA phage, *Jap. J. Microbiol.* **12**, 544.

Sanger, F., 1971, Nucleotide sequences in bacteriophage RNA, *Biochem. J.* **124**, 833.

Schmidt, J. M., and Stanier, R. J., 1965, Isolation and characterization of bacteriophages active against stalked bacteria, *J. Gen. Microbiol.* **39**, 95.

Schwartz, J. H., Iglewski, W. J., and Franklin, R. M., 1969, The lack of messenger activity of ribonucleic acid complementary to the viral ribonucleic acid of bacteriophage R17, *J. Biol. Chem.* **244**, 736.

Scott, D. W., 1965, Serological cross-reactions among the RNA-containing coliphages, *Virology* **26**, 85.

Shapiro, L., and Bendis, I., 1974, RNA phage of bacteria other than *E. coli, in* "RNA Phages" (N. D. Zinder, ed.), Plenum Press, New York.

Shapiro, L., Franze de Fernandez, M. T., and August, J. T., 1968, Resolution of two factors required in the Qβ RNA polymerase reaction, *Nature (Lond.)* **220**, 478.

Shimura, Y., and Nathans, D., 1964, The preparation of coliphage MS2 containing 5-fluorouracil, *Biochem. Biophys. Res. Commun.* **16**, 116.

Shimura, Y., Moses, R. E., and Nathans, D., 1965, Coliphage MS2 containing 5-fluorouracil. I. Preparation and physical properties, *J. Mol. Biol.* **12**, 266.

Siegel, J., Kjeldgaard, N., 1971, Effect of *rel* locus on Qβ RNA synthesis, *J. Mol. Biol.* **57**, 147.

Silverman, P. M., 1973a, Replication of RNA viruses: Analysis by liquid polymer phase partition of binding Qβ RNA, *Arch. Biochem. Biophys.* **157**, 234.

Silverman, P. M., 1973b, Replication of RNA viruses: Specific binding of Qβ RNA polymerase to Qβ RNA, *Arch. Biochem. Biophys.* **157**, 222.

Silverman, P. M., and Valentine, R. C., 1969, The RNA injection step of bacteriophage f2 infection, *J. Gen. Virol.* **4**, 111.

Skogerson, K., Roufa, D., and Leder, P., 1971, Characterization of the initial peptide of Qβ RNA polymerase and control of its synthesis, *Proc. Natl. Acad. Sci. USA* **68**, 276.

Spahr, P. F., and Gesteland, R. F., 1968, Specific cleavage of bacteriophage R17 RNA by an endonuclease isolated from *E. coli* MRE 600, *Proc. Natl. Acad. Sci. USA* **59**, 876.

Spahr, P. F., Farber, M., and Gesteland, R. F., 1969, Binding site on R17 RNA for coat protein, *Nature (Lond.)* **222**, 455.

Spangler, V. L., and Iglewski, W. J., 1972, Effect of R17 bacteriophage-specific proteins on ribosomal ribonucleic acid synthesis of *Escherichia coli, J. Virol.* **9**, 792.

Spiegelman, S., Haruna, I., Holland, I. B., Beaudreau, G., and Mills, D., 1965, The synthesis of a self-propagating and infectious nucleic acid with a purified enzyme, *Proc. Natl. Acad. Sci. USA* **54**, 919.

Staples, D. H., and Hindley, J., 1971, Ribosome binding site of Qβ RNA polymerase cistron, *Nat. New Biol.* **234**, 211.

Staples, D. H., Hindley, J., Billeter, M. A., and Weissman, C., 1971, Localization of
    Qβ maturation cistron ribosome binding site, *Nat. New Biol.* **234**, 202.
Stavis, R. L., and August, J. T., 1970, The biochemistry of RNA bacteriophage rep-
    lication, *Annu. Rev. Biochem.* **39**, 527.
Steitz, J. A., 1968a, Isolation of the A protein from bacteriophage R17, *J. Mol. Biol.*
    33, 937.
Steitz, J. A., 1968b, Identification of the A protein as a structural component of bac-
    teriophage R17, *J. Mol. Biol.* **33**, 923.
Steitz, J. A., 1969a, The nucleotide sequences of the ribosomal binding sites of bac-
    teriophage R17 RNA, *Cold Spring Harbor Symp. Quant. Biol.* **34**, 621.
Steitz, J. A., 1969b, Polypeptide chain initiation: Nucleotide sequences of the three
    ribosomal binding sites in bacteriophage R17 RNA, *Nature (Lond.)* **224**, 957.
Steitz, J., 1972, Oligonucleotide sequence of replicase initiation site in Qβ RNA, *Nat.
    New Biol.* **236**, 71.
Steitz, J., 1973, Discriminatory ribosome rebinding of isolated regions of protein syn-
    thesis initiation from the ribonucleic acid of bacteriophage R17, *Proc. Natl. Acad. Sci.
    USA* **70**, 2605.
Steitz, J. A., Dube, S. K., and Rudland, P. S., 1970, Control of translation by T4
    phage: Altered ribosome binding at R17 initiation sites, *Nature (Lond.)* **226**, 824.
Stewart, M. L., Grollman, A. P., and Huang, M.-T., 1971, Aurintricarboxylic acid:
    Inhibitor of initiation of protein synthesis, *Proc. Natl. Acad. Sci. USA* **68**, 97.
Strauss, E., and Kaesberg, P., 1970, Acrylamide gel electrophoresis of bacteriophage
    Qβ: Electrophoresis of the intact virions and of the viral proteins, *Virology* **42**, 437.
Strauss, J. H., Jr., and Sinsheimer, R. L., 1963, Purification and properties of bac-
    teriophage MS2 and of its ribonucleic acid, *J. Mol. Biol.* **7**, 43.
Strauss, J. H., Jr., and Sinsheimer, R. L., 1968, Initial kinetics of degradation of MS2
    ribonucleic acid by ribonuclease heat and alkali and the presence of configurational
    restraints in this ribonucleic acid, *J. Mol. Biol.* **34**, 453.
Sugiyama, T., 1969, Translational control of MS2 RNA cistrons, *Cold Spring Harbor
    Symp. Quant. Biol.* **34**, 687.
Sugiyama, T., and Nakada, D., 1967, Control of translation of MS2 RNA cistrons by
    MS2 coat protein, *Proc. Natl. Acad. Sci. USA* **57**, 1744.
Sugiyama, T., and Nakada, D., 1968, Translational control of bacteriophage MS2
    RNA cistrons by MS2 coat protein: Polyacrylamide gel electrophoresis analysis and
    proteins synthesized *in vitro, J. Mol. Biol.* **31**, 431.
Sugiyama, T., Herbert, R. R., and Hartman, K. A., 1967, Ribonucleoprotein com-
    plexes formed between bacteriophage MS2 RNA and MS2 protein *in vitro, J. Mol.
    Biol.* **25**, 455.
Sugiyama, T., Korant, B. D., and Lonberg-Holm, K. K., 1972, RNA virus gene
    expression and its control, *Annu. Rev. Microbiol.* **26**, 467.
Takanami, M., Yan, Y., and Jukes, T. H., 1965, Studies on the site of ribosomal
    binding of f2 bacteriophage RNA, *J. Mol. Biol.* **12**, 761.
Thach, S., Boedtker, H., 1969, High molecular weight fragments of R17 bacterio-
    phage RNA produced by pancreatic ribonuclease, *J. Mol. Biol.* **45**, 451.
Thirion, J.-P., and Kaesberg, P., 1970, Base sequences of polypurine region of the
    RNAs of bacteriophages R17 and M12, *J. Mol. Biol.* **47**, 193.
Tinoco, I., Uhlenbeck, O., and Levine, M., 1971, Estimation of secondary structure in
    ribonucleic acids, *Nature (Lond.)* **230**, 362.

Tooze, J., and Weber, K., 1967, Isolation and characterization of amber mutants of bacteriophage R17, *J. Mol. Biol.* **28**, 311.

Trown, P. W., and Meyer, P. L., 1973, Recognition of template RNA by Qβ polymerase: Sequence at the 3′-terminus of Qβ 6 S RNA, *Arch. Biochem. Biophys.* **154**, 250.

Valentine, R. C., and Strand, M., 1965, Complexes of F-pili and RNA bacteriophage, *Science (Wash., D.C.)* **148**, 511.

Vandekerckhove, J., Francq, H., and Van Montagu, M., 1969, The amino acid sequence of the coat protein of the bacteriophage MS-2 and localization of the amber mutation in the coat mutants growing on a su_3^+ suppressor, *Arch. Intern. Physiol. Biochem.* **77**, 175.

Vandekerckhove, J., Nolf, F., and Van Montagu, M., 1973, Amino acid sequence at carboxyl terminus of maturation protein of MS2, *Nat. New Biol.* **241**, 102.

Vasquez, C., Granboulan, N., and Franklin, R. M., 1966, Structure of the ribonucleic acid bacteriophage R17, *J. Bacteriol.* **92**, 1779.

Vinuela, E., Algranati, I. D., and Ochoa, S., 1967, Synthesis of virus-specific proteins in *Escherichia coli* infected with the RNA bacteriophage MS2, *Eur. J. Biochem.* **1**, 3.

Vineuela, E., Algranati, I. D., Feix, G., Garwes, D., Weissmann, C., and Ochoa, S., 1968, Virus-specific proteins in *Escherichia coli* infected with some amber mutants of phage MS2, *Biochim. Biophys. Acta* **155**, 558.

Volckaert, G., and Fiers, W., 1973, Studies on the bacteriophage MS2: GUG as initiation codon of the A-protein cistron, *FEBS (Fed. Eur. Biochem. Soc.) Lett.* **35**, 91.

Voorma, H. O., Benne, R., and den Hertog, T. J. A., 1971, Binding of aminoacyl-tRNA to ribosomes programmed with bacteriophage MS2-RNA, *Eur. J. Biochem.* **18**, 451.

Ward, R., Shive, K., and Valentine, R. C., 1967, Capsid protein of f2 as translational repressor, *Biochem. Biophys. Res. Commun.* **29**, 8.

Ward, R., Strand, M., and Valentine, R. C., 1969, Translational repression of f2 protein synthesis, *Biochem. Biophys. Res. Commun.* **30**, 310.

Watanabe, H., and Watanabe, M., 1968, Effect of infection with ribonucleic acid bacteriophage R23 on the inducible synthesis of β-galactosidase in *Escherichia coli, J. Virol.* **2**, 1400.

Watanabe, I., Miyake, T., Sakurai, T., Shiba, T., and Ohno, T., 1967, Isolation and grouping of RNA phages, *Proc. Jap. Acad.* **43**, 204.

Watanabe, M., and August, J. T., 1967, Methods for selecting RNA bacteriophage, *in* "Methods in Virology," Vol. III (K. Maramorosch and H. Kaprowski, eds.), pp. 337–350, Academic Press, New York.

Watanabe, M., and August, J. T., 1968a, Identification of guanosine triphosphate as the 5′-terminus of RNA from bacteriophage Qβ and R23, *Proc. Natl. Acad. Sci. USA* **59**, 513.

Watanabe, M., and August, J. T., 1968b, Replication of RNA bacteriophage R23. II. Inhibition of phage-specific RNA synthesis by phleomycin, *J. Mol. Biol.* **33**, 21.

Watanabe, M., Watanabe, H., and August, J. T., 1968, Replication of RNA bacteriophage R23. I. Quantitative aspects of phage RNA and protein synthesis, *J. Mol. Biol.* **33**, 1.

Weber, H., and Weissmann, C., 1970, The 3′-termini of Qβ plus and minus strands, *J. Mol. Biol.* **51**, 215.

Weber, K., 1967, Amino acid sequence studies on the tryptic peptides of the coat protein of the bacteriophage R17, *Biochemistry* **6**, 3144.

Weber, K., and Konigsberg, W., 1967, Amino acid sequence of the f2 coat protein, *J. Biol. Chem.* **242**, 3563.

Webster, R. E., and Zinder, N. D., 1969, Fate of the message—Ribosome complex upon translation of termination signals, *J. Mol. Biol.* **42**, 425.

Webster, R. E., Engelhardt, D. L., and Zinder, N. D., 1966, *In vitro* protein synthesis: Chain initiation, *Proc. Natl. Acad. Sci. USA* **55**, 155.

Webster, R. E., Robertson, H. D., and Zinder, N. D., 1969, The 5′-terminus of f2 RNA and the coat protein gene, *Cold Spring Harbor Symp. Quant. Biol.* **34**, 675.

Weiner, A. M., and Weber, K., 1971, Natural read-through at the UGA termination signal of Qβ coat protein cistron, *Nat. New Biol.* **234**, 50.

Weissmann, C., 1965, Replication of viral RNA. VII. Further studies on the enzymatic replication of MS2 RNA, *Proc. Natl. Acad. Sci. USA* **54**, 202.

Weissmann, C., and Borst, P., 1963, Double-stranded ribonucleic acid formation *in vitro* by MS2 phage-induced RNA synthetase, *Science (Wash., D.C.)* **142**, 1188.

Weissmann, C., and Feix, G., 1966, Replication of viral RNA. XI. Synthesis of viral "minus" strands *in vitro, Proc. Natl. Acad. Sci. USA* **55**, 1264.

Weissmann, C., Simon, L., and Ochoa, S., 1963, Induction by an RNA phage of an enzyme catalyzing incorporation of ribonucleotides into ribonucleic acid, *Proc. Natl. Acad. Sci. USA* **49**, 407.

Weissmann, C., Borst, P., Burdon, R. H., Billeter, M. A., and Ochoa, S., 1964*a*, Replication of viral RNA. III. Double-stranded replicative form of MS2 phage RNA, *Proc. Natl. Acad. Sci. USA* **51**, 682.

Weissmann, C., Borst, P., Burdon, R. H., Billeter, M. A., and Ochoa, S., 1964*b*, Replication of viral RNA. IV. Properties of RNA synthetase and enzymatic synthesis of MS2 phage RNA, *Proc. Natl. Acad. Sci. USA* **51**, 890.

Weissmann, C., Feix, G., Slor, H., and Pollet, R., 1967, Replication of viral RNA. XIV. Single-stranded minus strands as template for the synthesis of viral plus strands *in vitro, Proc. Natl. Acad. Sci. USA* **57**, 1870.

Weissmann, C., Feix, G., and Slor, H., 1968, *In vitro* synthesis of phage RNA: The nature of the intermediates, *Cold Spring Harbor Symp. Quant. Biol.* **33**, 83.

Weissmann, C., Billeter, M., Goodman, H., Hindley, J., and Weber, H., 1973, Structure and function of phage RNA, *Annu. Rev. Biochem.* **42**, 303.

Weith, H. L., and Gilham, P. T., 1967, Structural analysis of polynucleotides by sequential base elimination. The sequence of the terminal decanucleotide fragment of the ribonucleic acid from bacteriophage f2, *J. Am. Chem. Soc.* **89**, 5473.

Wittmann-Liebold, B., 1966, Aminosäuresequenzen im Hüllenprotein des RNS-Bakteriophagen fr, *Z. Naturforsch.* **21b**, 1249.

Yamazaki, H., 1969, The mechanism of early inhibition by an RNA phage of protein and RNA synthesis in infected cells, *Virology* **37**, 429.

Yamazaki, H., and Kaesberg, P., 1966, Analysis of products of protein synthesis directed by R17 viral RNA, *Proc. Natl. Acad. Sci. USA* **56**, 624.

Yarosh, E., and Levinthal, C., 1967, Exclusion of RNA bacteriophages and interference with their RNA replication by bacteriophage T4, *J. Mol. Biol.* **30**, 329.

Zavada, V., Fikotova, J., Koutecka, E., Heubauer, Z., and Raskova, M., 1966, The capacity of the bacterial host for the reproduction of the RNA phage f2. II. Its UV sensitivity in 5-BU-labeled host and the effect of the thymineless death, *Biochem. Biophys. Res. Commun.* **22**, 480.

Zillig, W., Zechel, K., Rabussay, D., Schachner, M., Sethi, V. S., Palm, P., Heil, A., and Seifert, W., 1970, On the role of different subunits of DNA-dependent RNA polymerase from *E. coli* in the transcription process, *Cold Spring Harbor Symp. Quant. Biol.* **35,** 47.

Zinder, N., ed., 1974, "RNA Phages," Plenum Press, New York (in press).

Zinder, N. D. and Lyons, L. B., 1968, Cell lysis: another function of coat protein of the bacteriophage f2. *Science (Wash., D.C.)* **159,** 84.

Zinder, N. D., Engelhardt, D. L., and Webster, R. E. 1966, Punctuation in the genetic code, *Cold Spring Harbor Symp. Quant. Biol.* **31,** 251.

Reproduction of Small Plant RNA Viruses*

Albert Siegel and V. Hariharasubramanian

Biology Department
Wayne State University
Detroit, Michigan 48202

1. INTRODUCTION

Plant cells appear to be no different from bacterial and animal cells in their capacity to support virus replication and, indeed, tobacco mosaic virus was the first infectious entity to be identified as what we now consider to be virus (Iwanowski, 1892; Beijerinck, 1898). In this chapter we shall describe current knowledge concerning replication of the class of small single-stranded RNA-containing viruses which use cells of higher plants as host. Reference is made to the recent treatises by Matthews (1970) and Kado and Agrawal (1972) for more complete coverage of principles of and techniques used in plant virology.

Evidence derived mostly from study of bacterial and animal viruses leads to the following broad outline of the strategy of replication for most of the small RNA-containing viruses. Upon infection, viral RNA is released from its capsid into cellular protoplasm whereupon it is both translated and replicated. It is generally assumed that the cell lacks the complete enzymatic apparatus necessary to repli-

* Some of the work reported herein and preparation of this chapter was supported in part by AEC contract AT(11-1)-2384 and a grant from the National Science Foundation.

cate viral RNA and, thus, that the viral RNA contains a coding sequence for an RNA replicase (or at least a part of such an enzyme) which must be translated before replication can proceed. Replication then proceeds via double-stranded RNA intermediates in a manner reminiscent of DNA replication but modified to produce an excess of new single-stranded viral RNA molecules. These combine with other translation products, primarily capsid protein, to yield newly assembled infectious virus particles (as reviewed by Sugiyama *et al.,* 1972).

In the past few years plant virus workers have begun to examine the infection process with the view towards ascertaining whether the above general scheme is valid for plant viruses and, in addition, to determine the particulars of the replication process as it occurs in plant cells infected with different types of viruses.

Understanding of the replication of plant viruses is not as well advanced as that for some of the bacterial and animal RNA viruses, probably because the nature of the host–virus system presents a peculiar set of experimental difficulties. Chief among these difficulties has been the inability to study the events of infection in a population of cells in which all could be infected simultaneously and in which the subsequent events of infection could be maintained in synchrony. Other problems are presented by the fact that most plant cells are composed of only a thin layer of protoplasm bounded on the outside by a plasma membrane and rigid cell wall and on the inside by a tonoplast which encloses a large vacuole which frequently contains noxious substances. The preparation of cell-free systems and fractions is made difficult because forces necessary to break the tough cell wall can cause damage to organelles, and also because disruption of the cell dilutes the protoplasm and causes it to come into contact with vacuolar substances.

Advances in plant cell culture have been made recently which may overcome some of the difficulties previously encountered by plant virus investigators. It has been found that leaf cells may be separated from each other by pectinases and that cell walls may be removed by a mixture of enzymes containing cellulase. The resultant protoplasts can be maintained in viable condition in hypertonic solutions so that they resemble animal cells in their lack of a large central vacuole. The protoplasts can be treated with either virus or viral RNA under conditions in which the majority become infected and thus, the promise is great that they will prove an extremely useful tool for study of the infection process (Takebe and Otsuki, 1969; Cocking, 1966; Zaitlin and Beachy, 1974; Coutts *et al.,* 1972; Aoki and Takebe, 1969).

2. NATURE OF THE HOST–VIRUS SYSTEM

2.1. Types and Properties of Plant Viruses

The types of plant viruses which have been identified so far and some of their features are listed in Table 1. Most plant viruses can be considered picornaviruses because they consist of a single-stranded RNA genome encapsidated with protein subunits to form either a nucleoprotein particle with icosahedral symmetry or a rodlike structure (sometimes flexuous) with helical symmetry. There are, however, a number of other types of plant viruses in addition to the small ones which contain single-stranded RNA. A group typified by lettuce necrotic yellow virus (Wolanski *et al.*, 1967) and potato yellow dwarf virus (Macleod *et al.*, 1966) can be classified as rhabdoviruses (Howatson, 1970), having a single-stranded RNA genome in a complex bacilliform, or bullet-shaped, lipid-membrane-containing particle. Wound tumor virus (Black and Markham, 1963) is an example of a virus with a segmented, double-stranded RNA genome (Reddy and Black, 1973) similar to that of the reoviruses (Shatkin *et al.*, 1968). There are several, such as cauliflower mosaic virus (Shepherd *et al.*, 1968), which are small viruses that contain double-stranded DNA. Finally, there is the large, complex, membrane-containing tomato spotted wilt virus which has not been fully characterized (Joubert *et al.*, 1974; Mohamed *et al.*, 1973).

The primary concern in this chapter, as already stated, will be the small, RNA-containing, plant viruses. Although many of these resemble some of the animal and bacterial picornaviruses in structural organization, others have particular features of interest. A disease agent, termed "viroid," so far unique to higher plants and responsible for diseases such as potato spindle tuber and citrus exocortis (Diener and Raymer, 1969; Semancik and Weathers, 1972), has been characterized as an 80,000-dalton RNA molecule which lacks a protein capsid. It has been postulated that a viroid may be responsible for a number of "slow" animal virus diseases such as scrapie (Diener, 1972).

A fairly large number of plant viruses have a split genome, characterized by two or more single-stranded RNA molecules separately encapsidated. An example is brome mosaic virus, which consists of three nucleoprotein particles, all of which are necessary for initiation of infection and which have identical protein capsids. Two of the particles each contain a single RNA molecule of molecular weights 1.1 and 1.0 × 10⁶, the third two RNA molecules of 0.7 and 0.3 × 10⁶

TABLE 1

Classification of Plant Viruses[a]

Virus type	Virus group	Number of particles	S value	Particle size, nm	% RNA	Number of RNA species	RNA mol. wt. × 10⁶	Protein mol. wt. × 10³	RNA components required for replication
Rod-shaped virus, undivided genome, single-stranded RNA	Tobamovirus, TMV	1	190	280	5	1	2	17.5	1
	Potexvirus, potato virus X	1	118	480–580	6	1	2.1	23 or 27	1
	Carlavirus, e.g., carnation latent virus	1		620–690	6	1			1
	Potyvirus, potato virus Y	1		720–800		1		28 or 34	1
Rod-shaped virus, divided genome, single-stranded RNA	Tobravirus, tobacco rattle virus	2; long + short	Long = 300; short = variable	180–210; short variable	5	2	2.3; short = variable	24	The RNA from long particle is infectious but cannot produce capsid protein which is encoded by the short RNA
	Barley stripe mosaic virus	3				2–4	1.4; 1.17, 1.04; 0.93		More than one
Single-stranded RNA virus, bullet-shaped, virions showing RNA polymerase activity	Rhabdovirus								
	Lettuce necrotic yellow virus	1	940	227 × 66		1	4		
	Potato yellow dwarf	1	810–950	380 × 75		1	4.3	78, 56, 33, 22	

									Insect transmitted
Double-stranded RNA, divided genome with virions showing RNA polymerase activity	Reovirus, wound tumor virus	1	514 ± 10	60–80	20–23	12	2.65, 2.20, 2.0, 1.68, 1.65, 1.05, 0.95, 0.88, 0.57, 0.56, 0.54, 0.33		
Single-stranded RNA virus requiring helper virus	Satellite tobacco necrosis virus	1	50	17	20	1	0.4	20	1 + helper
	Satellite tobacco ringspot virus	1	91–126	30		14–26	0.086[b]	Coded by helper TRSV	1 + helper
Isometric virus, undivided genome, single-stranded RNA	Tombusvirus, tomato bushy stunt virus	1	132	30	17	1	1.6	40 and 28	1
	Tobacco necrosis virus	1	118	28	20	1	1.5	30	1
	Tymovirus, e.g., turnip yellow virus	2	118, 50	30	35, 0	1	2	20	1
Isometric virus, divided genome, single-stranded RNA	Comovirus, e.g., cowpea mosaic virus	3	115, 95, 58	30	33, 22, 0	2	2.5; 1.5	49 and 25	2, bottom and middle component alone required
	Neopovirus, tobacco ringspot virus	3	126, 91, 53	30	35, 25, 0	2	2.3; 1.4	57	2, bottom and middle component alone required

TABLE 1—Continued

Virus type	Virus group	Number of particles	S value	Particle size, nm	% RNA	Number of RNA species	RNA mol. wt. $\times 10^6$	Protein mol. wt. $\times 10^3$	RNA components required for replication
Isometric virus, divided genome, single-stranded RNA (*continued*)	Pea enation mosaic virus	2	112, 99	29	28, 28	2	1.6; 1.3	22	2
	Bromovirus	3	87 (all three)	26	20, 20 20	4	1.09; 0.99, 0.75, 0.28	20	3, the smallest RNA species not required
	Alfalfa mosaic virus[c]	4	99, 89, 75, 68	60, 50, 40, 30; bascilliform particles of different sizes $\times$ 18 diameter	18, 18, 18, 18	4	1.27; 1.0; 0.76; 0.33	30, 27, or 24	4, bottom, middle, top *b*, and coat protein
Pleomorphic myxovirus[a]	Tomato spotted wilt virus[d]							220, 84, 50, 29	
DNA virus	Cauliflower mosaic virus	1	220	50	16	1 (DNA)	4.5	33,000	1

[a] The classification used here is essentially based on Harrison *et al.* (1971). In addition to those listed here, there is also the "viroid" group which consists of potato spindle tuber virus, exocortis virus, and chrysanthemum stunt virus where the infectious entity is a small piece of nucleic acid of 85,000–110,000 daltons. The nucleic acid has a lot of secondary structure.

[b] The molecular weight when estimated by S value was 86,000 daltons; however, by polyacrylamide electrophoresis the molecular weight was estimated to be about 80,000 daltons. Recent estimates by electron microscopy give a value of 116,000 daltons (Sego *et al.*, 1974).

[c] The numbers and molecular weights of AMV proteins are disputed.

[d] There is a good deal of controversy regarding TSWV; in view of this, although data regarding S value and particle size are available, these are not given here.

daltons (Lane and Kaesberg, 1971). The three largest RNA species are necessary to initiate infection, while the fourth, which proves to be an excellent *in vitro* messenger for the capsid protein subunit, has a nucleotide sequence which is identical to part of that in the third largest RNA (Shih *et al.*, 1972). Several other split-genome viruses resemble brome mosaic virus in the nature of their components, whereas others are somewhat different.

A more complete description and classification of the known plant viruses can be found in the following references: Gibbs *et al.*, 1970–1971; Harrison and Murant, 1972–1973); Harrison *et al.*, 1971; and Brown and Hull, 1973.

2.2. Some General Features of Infection

Virus replication generally begins in a primary infected cell, and infection may then spread to uninfected cells by either of two methods: to adjacent cells probably via plasmodesmata (thin protoplasmic connections between most adjacent plant cells), or to distantly located cells via the conducting elements of the plant. Symptoms, which appear as a consequence of virus infection and which are frequently reflected in the names of viruses, are specific to virus–host combinations and cultural conditions. There can be either no apparent symptom, lack of full chlorophyll development in some portions of the host, malformed growth, tumor formation, death of either the host or parts of the host, or other manifestations of infection. Taking TMV as an example, no apparent symptoms develop when mature leaves of most cultivars of tobacco (*Nicotiana tabacum* L.) are inoculated with the common strain although the virus replicates to extremely high titers in these leaves. Symptoms do develop, however, on leaves that were immature at the time of inoculation; depending primarily on position of the leaf, age of the plant, and cultural conditions, these symptoms may take the form of a disappearance or lack of development of chlorophyll (mottling) particularly along the veins of the leaf (vein clearing), malformation (blistering), or a mosaic of light green and dark green areas (the symptom from which the virus is named). When *N. glutinosa,* the tobacco cultivar *Xanthi* n.c., or several other hypersensitive species are inoculated with the same virus, however, an entirely different symptom appears: necrotic spots which develop only on the inoculated leaf (local lesions). The number of these spots is a function of the concentration of virus in the inoculum; thus, a basis for an infectivity bioassay is provided which is similar in many respects to the plaque assay for bacterial and animal viruses although, in the case of plant virus infection, the "efficiency of plating" is very low.

Replication of virus in plant cells is frequently accompanied by the appearance of characteristic intracellular inclusion bodies, the nature and content of which vary depending upon the host–virus system (Rubio-Huertos, 1972). The inclusions may consist of crystalline or pseudocrystalline arrays of virus particles (Steere and Williams, 1953; Sheffield, 1939); tubes composed of an array of capsid protein (Hitchborn and Hills, 1968); a complex of sheets of non-capsid protein (Edwardson *et al.,* 1968; Hiebert and McDonald, 1973); or a complex mixture of virus, endoplasmic reticulum, ribosomes, and filaments (Esau and Cronshaw, 1967).

The question of host range for individual viruses presents an enigma; although it is observed that a virus will infect some plant species easily and others with difficulty or not at all, it is known that successful inoculation depends on a number of factors, not all of which have been well studied (Kado, 1972). It is difficult to conclude that a plant species might have an absolute immunity to a particular virus either because virus replication might be inapparent or because proper inoculation conditions for initiation of infection might not have been discovered. Two examples of the difficulties in establishing host range follow. (1) The U2 strain of tobacco mosaic virus produces no visible signs of infection on pinto bean when this host is maintained under certain cultural conditions. If, however, the leaves are heat-shocked a few hours after inoculation, large local necrotic lesions appear to signify virus replication (Rappaport and Wu, 1963). (2) Cowpea chlorotic mottle virus multiplies only to a limited extent in the inoculated leaves of a tobacco plant and does not become systemic in this host. It is surprising to find, therefore, that tobacco protoplasts provide an excellent substrate for replication of this virus (Motoyoshi *et al.,* 1973*b*).

A large number of plant viruses are not transmitted vertically, either through female or male gametes. This is not a general rule, however, because other plant viruses are transmitted through seed to a greater or lesser extent, dependent on the host and other factors. There exists also a group of viruses which are pollen transmitted. This topic has recently been reviewed (Shepherd, 1972; Bennett, 1969).

2.3. Virus Transmission

Virus infection is transmitted from host to host in nature by a number of living vectors, the insects being of primary importance. Of the insects, aphids probably transmit the largest number of different viruses (Watson, 1972), but other insect groups, among which are leaf hoppers (Whitcomb, 1972), white flies, mealybugs, flea beetles, thrips, bugs, and psyllas (Gibbs, 1969), also contain members which serve as plant virus vectors. In addition to insects, other organisms such as mites (Slykhuis, 1972), fungi (Teakle, 1972), nematodes (Taylor, 1972), and dodder, a parasitic higher plant (Bennett, 1967), have been found to transmit particular plant viruses.

No vector has yet been found for a considerable number of plant viruses. These, as well as most of the viruses with known vectors, can be transmitted by mechanical inoculation or grafting. Infection by mechanical inoculation is generally accomplished by mild injury to a host in the presence of a virus-containing suspension. Techniques and principles of mechanical inoculation have recently been reviewed by Kado (1972). Until quite recently, studies of plant-virus replication have generally been performed with tissue that had been inoculated mechanically. During the past several years, however, studies have appeared in which plant protoplasts have been infected under strictly defined conditions, generally with the aid of poly-L-ornithine (i.e., Sakai and Takebe, 1972).

2.4. Early Events of Infection

Most of the available information on the initiation of infection has been derived from experiments in which leaves of a hypersensitive host have been inoculated mechanically. Several days following inoculation, such leaves develop necrotic lesions as a consequence of localized virus replication. The following principles concerning initiation of infection have been found to apply in several host–virus systems.

1. Tissue must be abraded if it is to become infected. High-titer virus suspensions can be applied to leaf tissue without effect unless the surface of the leaf is rubbed or otherwise traumatized. It is not known how abrasion causes a leaf to become susceptible, but it has been found empirically that mild abrasives such as carborundum or diatomaceous earth will increase the number of infections obtained with a given inoculum. One can speculate that abrasion causes localized damage to cuticle and cellulose cell wall, thus permitting virus particles to come into contact with the cell membrane or with ectodesmata (Brants, 1965; Merkens *et al.,* 1972), but, actually, little is known about how virus particles or their nucleic acids get into cells.

2. Infectible sites appear on the surface of a leaf as a conse-

quence of abrasion. These sites are defined operationally, and little is known of their physical nature. Generally, they can be most easily infected (converted to an infective center) if virus particles are present at the time of abrasion. The infectible sites disappear as the time is extended between abrasion and exposure to virus, although in some systems there is an initial increase in their number (Siegel, 1966; Furumoto and Wildman, 1963; Jedlinski, 1956). Analysis of the relationship between the number of infections and the inoculum concentrations leads to the conclusion that infectible sites probably vary in their susceptibility to infection (Kleczkowski, 1950; Furumoto and Mickey, 1967).

3.   The efficiency of infection is low. Under the best of circumstances, between 10^4 and 10^5 virus particles need to be applied to a leaf for each infection (Steere, 1955). However, since most of such virus can be recovered in infective form by washing of the inoculated leaf, the actual efficiency is several orders of magnitude higher (Fraenkel-Conrat et al., 1964). The reason for low efficiency is unknown, and it is true even when plant protoplasts are exposed to virus in liquid suspension (Takebe and Otsuki, 1969; Motoyoshi et al., 1973b).

4.   A single infectious virus particle is sufficient to establish infection despite the low efficiency of infection. This is deduced from the relationship between inoculum concentration and local-lesion number and applies to those viruses which have an unsplit genome. The relative efficiency of infection with a split-genome virus, upon dilution, is lower (Van Kammen, 1968; Van Vloten-Doting et al., 1968); this is as would be expected since a split-genome virus depends on the simultaneous presence of the component parts of the genome at an infectible site (Fulton, 1962).

5.   Probably only a single infectious unit can initiate and participate in an infection, even when an infectible site is exposed to many such units. This conclusion is open to some question and is based partially on the quantitative interference between strains of a virus in establishing infection (Lauffer and Price, 1945; Siegel, 1959) and partially on the observation that infective centers are inactivated exponentially by ultraviolet light soon after their formation (Rappaport and Wu, 1962).

6.   An early and necessary process which follows upon establishment of an infected site is the release of viral nucleic acid from its capsid. The manner in which this occurs is unknown, but a number of methods have been used to estimate how long it takes. One such method is based on the fact that infection can be induced with viral nu-

cleic acid as well as with virus particles (Fraenkel-Conrat et al., 1957). Several investigators have observed that necrotic local lesions appear sooner when the inoculum contains nucleic acid rather than virus, the difference, about two hours under certain conditions, being attributed to the time for uncoating (i.e., Kassanis, 1960). Another method which yields the same conclusion observes the time it takes for infective centers induced by either nucleic acid or virus particles to change in sensitivity to inactivation by ultraviolet light (Siegel et al., 1957; Kassanis, 1960).

7. A peculiar feature found in some virus-host combinations is that under certain conditions the interaction of a virus particle and an infectible site will not lead to productive infection. The infection process will proceed to a certain point and then stop. Sometimes, such "blocked" sites can be activated by a treatment such as heat shock (Yarwood, 1961; Wu, 1963).*

3. REPLICATION OF VIRAL NUCLEIC ACID

3.1. Some Properties of Plant Virus RNA

RNA virus genomes possess several properties which distinguish them from nonviral RNA species found in uninfected hosts. It is generally thought that the virus genome should contain minimally: (1) a recognition sequence for an RNA replicase enzyme, (2) a coding sequence for a replicase enzyme, or at least part of a replicase enzyme, and (3) a coding sequence for at least one type of capsid protein.

Many plant viruses contain RNA molecules which can be considered complete genomes because it can be inferred that they contain the three features listed above. It has become apparent in recent years, however, that a number of plant viruses contain RNA molecules which lack one or two of the above properties. Listed in Table 2 are a number of pertinent viral RNAs together with indications as to which of the three properties they probably contain.

Viroid RNA. The smallest RNA listed represents a type of infectious agent responsible for several plant diseases, among them potato spindle tuber (Diener and Raymer, 1969), citrus exocortis (Semancik and Weathers, 1972), and chrysanthemum stunt (Diener

---

* Editor's note: The interactions of plant viruses with host cell components is an active field of research that will be dealt with in greater detail in a future chapter of *Comprehensive Virology* [H. F.-C.].

TABLE 2

Selected Properties of Some RNAs Found in Plant Viruses

RNA	Size, daltons $\times 10^{-5}$	Recognition sequence for replicase	Cistron for replicase	Cistron for capsid protein
Viroid	0.8	+	−	−
Tobacco ringspot virus satellite RNA	0.8–1.16[a]	+	−	−
Brome mosaic virus RNA #4, alfalfa mosaic virus top a RNA	3	−[b]	−	+
Tobacco necrosis virus satellite RNA	4	+	−	+
Tobacco rattle virus short RNA	6	+	−	+
Tobacco rattle virus long RNA	23	+	+	−
Tobacco necrosis virus RNA	12	+	+	+
Tobacco mosaic virus RNA, turnip yellow mosaic virus RNA	20	+	+	+

[a] See Table 1.
[b] It has not been established whether or not brome mosaic virus #4 RNA is replicated or whether it appears only as an enzymatic digestion product of brome mosaic virus #3 RNA.

and Lawson, 1973). This RNA has a molecular weight of about 80,000 daltons (Diener and Smith, 1973; Semancik *et al.,* 1973), which means that it is constituted of only about 250 nucleotide residues. This RNA probably does not contain a coding sequence for capsid protein because of its small size and because no capsid has been found (Zaitlin and Hariharasubramanian, 1972). It apparently exists as a free nucleic acid with considerable secondary structure. It is unlikely, moreover, because of its small size that it contains a coding sequence for any protein, although the possibility has not been eliminated that it may code for a small peptide which imparts specificity to a replicase. If this RNA does indeed lack genes for a capsid protein and a replicase component, then it is left with only one of the three features of viral RNA: the ability to recognize a replicase enzyme.

Because of its unique features, this disease agent has been given the appelation viroid (Diener, 1971) to distinguish it from typical viruses. It is interesting to note that the viroid is only slightly larger than midvariant-1, the well-characterized RNA which is one of the smallest molecules known to be replicated by Qβ replicase (Mills *et al.,*

1973). The question arises as to the source of replicase enzyme for viroid RNA. One possible source is the partially characterized RNA replicase that has been found in extracts of leaves from apparently healthy plants, the *in vivo* function and activity of which remain to be elucidated (Duda *et al.*, 1973; Astier-Manifacier and Cornuet, 1971). A peculiar feature of this enzyme is that more of it is found in extracts of tissue infected with a virus than in healthy tissue, although it is questionable whether this enzyme plays any role in the replication of the viral RNAs.

Tobacco Ringspot Satellite RNA. This RNA has about the same molecular weight as viroid RNA but differs from it by being dependent on the presence of another virus, tobacco ringspot, for its replication. It is encapsidated by the tobacco ringspot virus protein; 12–25 satellite RNA molecules are found in the same type of protein shell that normally contains tobacco ringspot virus RNA (Schneider *et al.*, 1972). As with viroid RNA, ringspot satellite RNA appears to be too small to contain structural genetic information, but it is reasonable to assume that it contains a recognition site for and is replicated by an enzyme coded for by the ringspot virus genome.

Brome Mosaic Virus (BMV) RNA #4 and Alfalfa Mosaic Virus (AMV) top a RNA. A number of plant viruses have split genomes. One of the examples described in the introduction and listed in Tables 1 and 2 is brome mosaic virus, which consists of 4 RNA species encapsidated in three identical protein shells with icosahedral symmetry (Lane and Kaesberg, 1971). Several other viruses are similarly constituted (Hull, 1972; Peden and Symons, 1973), e.g., the well-studied cowpea chlorotic mottle virus (Bancroft, 1971; Bancroft and Flack, 1972). Either the three nucleoprotein particles or the three largest RNA molecules are required for infection; the fourth or smallest RNA molecule is the next viral RNA to be listed in Table 2. This 300,000-dalton-molecular-weight species, although encapsidated, is not required for infection. Its genetic information is redundant, as it is also contained in the next largest encapsidated RNA (component 3–700,00 daltons) (Shih *et al.*, 1972). Evidence to date indicates that component 4 is probably not replicated, but that it may be formed as a specific nuclease product of component 3; it has been found to be an excellent *in vitro* messenger for the capsid protein (Shih and Kaesberg, 1973). The larger RNA component, 3, which also contains the gene for coat protein, is not as efficient a messenger for the coat protein, at least in the system tested. We conclude, therefore, that BMV #4 contains the gene for coat protein but probably lacks either the gene for a replicase or a replicase recognition site.

A similar situation exists for alfalfa mosaic virus although the details differ. This virus has 4 RNA species, but in this case each of the four is encapsidated separately in capsids of different sizes and configurations (Van Vloten-Doting *et al.,* 1970). The nucleoprotein particles have been named, in decreasing size order: bottom, middle, top *b,* and top *a.* The three largest particles, but not top *a,* are required for initiating infection. A peculiar situation exists, however, when the RNA molecules are used as inoculum. Either all four RNA species are required to initiate infection or capsid protein can substitute for the smallest RNA, that contained in top *a* (Bol *et al.,* 1971). It is suspected that the RNA contained in top *a* is an efficient messenger for capsid protein in a manner similar to brome mosaic virus RNA #4 (Bol and Van Vloten-Doting, 1973). The evidence indicates that top *a* RNA is translated but not replicated and that its nucleotide sequence is also present in the third largest RNA component, top *b* (Dingjan-Versteegh *et al.,* 1972). It is not clear why RNA components such as BMV #4 and AMV top *a* are encapsidated. It may be that they contain a recognition site for capsid protein or that they facilitate infection under natural conditions.

Satellite Tobacco Necrosis Virus RNA. The next larger RNA listed in Table 2 is the 400,000-dalton RNA molecule found in the tobacco necrosis satellite virus (Reichmann, 1964). This virus is dependent for its multiplication on a concurrent infection with tobacco necrosis virus, but the converse is not true (Kassanis, 1962). This RNA is similar to that of the tobacco ringspot satellite virus in that it lacks a replicase-specifying gene but it differs in that it is somewhat larger and that is contains a gene for its own unique capsid protein which is different from that of the necrosis virus (Kassanis and Nixon, 1961; Klein *et al.,* 1972). It differs from the BMV #4 and AMV top *a* RNAs in being replicated and, thus, it contains a replicase recognition sequence. It is probably replicated by the tobacco necrosis RNA-specified replicase.

Tobacco Rattle Virus Short RNA. Tobacco rattle virus is another split-genome virus that is somewhat different from the others so far considered. It consists of two rod-shaped nucleoprotein particles of different lengths (Paul and Bode, 1955; Harrison and Woods, 1966). Different strains of this virus all have long rods of about the same length, 188–197 nm, which contain RNA of about 2.3×10^6 daltons (Tollin and Wilson, 1971). The shorter rods have different lengths, from 43 to 114 nm, depending on the strain. Listed in Table 2 is the RNA from the shortest short rod. It has a molecular weight of 600,000 daltons and resembles the tobacco necrosis satellite virus RNA in lacking a replicase-specifying gene and in possessing both a gene for coat protein and a replicase recognition sequence. It differs from satellite RNA in being somewhat larger and in the fact that the capsid protein specified is that for the long RNA as well as for the short RNA. It is dependent for multiplication on a replicase specified by the long RNA. The long RNA, in contrast to the short RNA, lacks a cistron for capsid protein and can initiate infection by itself; in this case, however, no nucleoprotein virus particles are produced, only infectious nucleic acid (Lister, 1966; Frost *et al.*, 1967; Sänger, 1968).

Other than the long tobacco rattle virus, no component of a split-genome virus has been shown to be capable of initiating infection. It is not known why this is so but it may be that in some systems RNA replication may require the concurrent synthesis of capsid or other viral-related protein or because the genetic information for a presumed multicomponent replicase is distributed among the different RNA species. An observation which supplies support for the former argument is the odd requirement for either virus protein or the presumed viral protein messenger for initiation of infection by the three largest RNA components of alfalfa mosaic virus. On the other hand, in addition to the long tobacco rattle RNA, at least two viral RNAs have been shown to replicate in the absence of functional virus protein. These are the unsplit, single-stranded genomes of certain mutant strains of tobacco mosaic (PM 1–6), and tobacco necrosis viruses which code for aberrant, nonfunctional coat proteins (Siegel *et al.*, 1962; Babos and Kassanis, 1962; Kassanis and Welkie, 1963).

Plant viral RNA species have so far been described which lack one or another of the three basic properties which are necessary to constitute the genome of a nucleoprotein virus capable of independent replication. These by no means constitute a complete catalogue of such RNA species because all of the RNA components of the split-genome viruses fall into this class. The reader is referred to the recent comprehensive review by Van Kammen (1972) for further details of the split-genome viruses and their nucleic acids (see also Coviruses in Vol. 1 of *Comprehensive Virology*).

The Single-Stranded RNA Complete Genomes. Several examples are listed in Table 2 of RNA molecules which constitute a complete viral genome and which presumably contain genes for capsid protein and replicase in addition to a replicase recognition site. The size range of such single-stranded complete genomes is narrowly restricted; the smallest, that found in tobacco necrosis virus, being 1.2×10^6 daltons (Kaper and Waterworth, 1973) and the largest, as in the well-studied tobacco mosaic and turnip yellow mosaic viruses, being about 2×10^6

daltons. Apparently, a nucleic acid molecule composed of fewer than about 4000 nucleotides is not sufficiently large to contain all of the information and structure necessary for successful infection of a plant cell (or, at least, none such has as yet been found), and there exists an unknown restriction which makes a complete, single-stranded RNA genome longer than about 6400 nucleotides unlikely.

Different kinds of viral RNA have been discussed so far in relation to three properties; replicase recognition site, genes for capsid protein, and genes for replicase. There are several other properties of viral RNA which may or may not be of significance in the replication process. A genomic recognition site(s) for capsid protein or for aggregates of capsid protein may be necessary for regulation of replication and/or translation (Hohn and Hohn, 1970; Sugiyama et al., 1972) as well as to ensure efficient and specific encapsidation of viral RNA. Such recognition sites have been identified for the RNAs of tobacco mosaic (Butler and Klug, 1971; Thouvenel et al , 1971; Ohno et al., 1971), tobacco rattle virus (Abou Haidar et al., 1973), and alfalfa mosaic virus (Van Vloten-Doting and Jaspars, 1972), and it may be that other viral RNAs also contain regions of high specific affinity for capsid protein.

Several viral RNAs have been found to resemble transfer RNAs in their capability to become amino-acylated in the presence of appropriate tRNA synthetase enzymes. This property is specific in that the RNAs with this property each will accept only a particular amino acid. To date, it has been found that the RNA of some strains of tobacco mosaic virus will accept histidine (Litvak et al., 1973), the RNA from turnip yellow mosaic and related viruses will accept valine (Pinck et al., 1970, 1972), and brome mosaic virus RNA will accept tyrosine (Hall et al., 1972). A further indication that viral RNA may have considerable secondary structure is the unconfirmed report that fragments of TMV RNA can be charged with either serine or methionine, dependent on Mg^{2+} ion concentration (Sela, 1972).

Whereas some plant virus RNAs have, or tend to form, a tRNA-like 3′-terminal structure and have been shown not to contain a polyadenylic acid sequence (Siegel et al., 1973; Fraser, 1973), this is not true in all cases. Cowpea mosaic virus, a two-component split-genome virus, contains two RNA species, each of which has a 200-member polyadenylic acid 3′-terminal sequence (El Manna and Bruening, 1973) similar to that of a number of animal virus RNAs (Armstrong et al., 1972; Green and Cartas, 1972; Johnston and Bose, 1972). Only a few of the plant virus RNAs have as yet been examined for the nature of their 3′-terminal structure and, thus, not enough information is available for generalization or speculation concerning the significance of a 3′ terminal which may be tRNA-like, polyadenylated or, perhaps, neither.

3.2. Virus-Related RNA Found in Infected Tissue

Infected cells contain unique virus-induced RNA species in addition to those encapsidated in virus particles. Two of these are similar to the double-stranded replicative form (RF) and the partially double-stranded replicative intermediate (RI) found in infected bacterial and animal cells. The third is a low-molecular-weight species (LMC) identified primarily in tissue infected with tobacco mosaic virus and perhaps also in extracts of broad bean mottle virus-infected tissue (Romero, 1972).

3.2.1. RF

Soon after the discovery of a double-stranded form of RNA in encephalomyocarditis-infected mouse ascites tumor cells by Montagnier and Sanders (1963), such forms were identified in extracts of a number of tissues or cells infected with other RNA viruses (Ralph, 1969; Bishop and Levintow, 1971). Among these were extracts of plant tissue infected with tobacco mosaic virus, turnip yellow mosaic virus, and a number of other plant viruses (Shipp and Haselkorn, 1964; Burdon et al., 1964; Mandel et al., 1964; Ralph et al., 1965). Perhaps the best-characterized plant virus RF to date is that extracted from tobacco mosaic virus-infected tissue. It resembles that of poliovirus RF (Bishop and Koch, 1967) in being composed of an unbroken strand of viral RNA (plus strand) annealed to complementary RNA (minus strand) (Nilsson-Tillgren, 1970; Jackson et al., 1971). Like the RFs of several bacterial virus RNAs (Francke and Hofschneider, 1966) and in contrast to poliovirus RF (Pons, 1964), the tobacco mosaic virus RF is not infectious but becomes so when the strands are separated (Jackson et al., 1971). The only detectable double-stranded RNA in extracts of tobacco mosaic virus-infected tissue is RF of molecular weight ca. 4×10^6 daltons (Siegel et al., 1973) and RI of a somewhat higher molecular weight (see below). Minus strand has not been detected to exist free in extracts but only as a component of the double-stranded forms (Siegel et al., 1973).

Tissues infected with unsplit-genome viruses have been found to contain a single, homogeneous RF component. In contrast, it has been

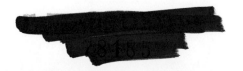

observed that split-genome viruses induce the appearance of multiple RF species, generally one RF species for each genome component. Extracts of tissue infected with the following viruses have been found to contain multiple RF species: cowpea mosaic virus (Van Griensven and Van Kammen, 1969), alfalfa mosaic virus (Pinck and Hirth, 1972), brome mosaic virus (Lane and Kaesberg, 1971), and barley stripe mosaic virus (Pring, 1972; Jackson and Brakke, 1973). Although it is clear that cells infected with split-genome viruses contain multiple RF species, individual RF species have not as yet been definitively matched to particular genome components.

In almost all cases examined to date, RF species identified in extracts of infected leaves appear to be of a size to contain an unbroken strand of viral RNA and its complement. A notable exception to this generality is the RF found in extracts of leaves infected with tobacco ringspot virus; it is considerably smaller than expected and rather heterogeneous (Rezaian and Francki, 1973). The significance of the low-molecular-weight double-stranded tobacco ringspot virus RNA for viral RNA replication remains to be elucidated.

3.2.2. RI

A form of RNA that is partially double-stranded and partially single-stranded is present in cells infected with bacterial and animal RNA viruses (Franklin, 1966; Baltimore, 1968). This form, called replicative intermediate (RI), is believed to be composed of a double-stranded core, the same length as RF, and to have single-stranded tails which presumably are mostly plus strands in the process of being synthesized. RI has also been isolated from extracts of tobacco mosaic virus-infected tobacco leaves and has been partially characterized. It is somewhat larger than RF as evidenced by its sedimentation behavior in sucrose gradient and its electrophoretic mobility in polyacrylamide gel. It is intermediate between viral RNA and RF in bouyant density (in cesium sulfate), and it is converted to a form closely resembling RF upon mild ribonuclease treatment (Nilsson-Tillgren, 1970; Jackson *et al.*, 1971).

3.2.3. LMC

A low-molecular-weight (*ca.* 350,000 daltons), single-stranded RNA species has been detected in total extracts of tobacco mosaic

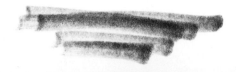

virus-infected tobacco leaf cells (Jackson *et al.*, 1972; Fraser, 1969; Hirai and Wildman, 1969) and has been identified as a fragment of viral RNA. It does not contain the 5´-terminal end of viral RNA and it is present in low concentration, being detectable only after labeling of cellular RNA with radioactive isotopes (Siegel *et al.*, 1973). A low-molecular-weight fragment of viral RNA has also been detected in association with ribosomes of tobacco mosaic virus-infected tissue (Babos, 1969, 1971), but it has not yet been determined whether the RNA fragment detected in the total RNA extract of infected cells is the same as that found in association with ribosomes.

3.3. Mechanism of RNA Replication

3.3.1. Evidence from *In Vivo* Studies

In Sect. 3.2 we reviewed evidence for the presence of the double-stranded RNA forms RF and RI in plant virus tissue. In this section we will describe the work done so far to determine whether and in what manner these forms serve as intermediates in the synthesis of viral RNA. Although there is uncertainty concerning the functional conformation of these forms inside the cell (Weissmann *et al.*, 1968; Bové *et al.*, 1968), the experiments with plant-virus systems have not yet proceeded to the point where this can be a matter of concern. It is assumed, by analogy with evidence from bacterial and animal systems, that the double-stranded forms are indeed involved in replication of plant virus RNA; the few experiments performed to date support this assumption.

Ralph *et al.* (1965) observed that when double-stranded RNA is extracted from turnip yellow mosaic virus-infected leaves labeled with ^{32}P for a short time (0.5–4 hours), the plus strand (viral RNA) is probably labeled to a greater extent than its complement, indicating asymmetric rapid synthesis of plus strands. In contrast, when the double-stranded RNA was labeled for 4 days before extraction, it appeared that both strands had become equally labeled. In agreement with these results, Nilsson-Tillgren (1970) observed that most of the label in tobacco mosaic virus RI was in plus strand after a one-hour labeling period. However, experiments performed under somewhat different conditions and employing a different method of analysis revealed that both strands of tobacco mosaic virus RF were almost equally labeled following only a two-hour exposure of infected tissue to ^{3}H-uridine (Siegel *et al.*, 1973). A more-refined temporal analysis is needed on uniform experimental material to define the relative rates of synthesis of plus and minus strands of plant virus RF and RI.

A study designed to determine the rate of appearance of plus and minus strands in tobacco leaf cells which approach synchronous infection with tobacco mosaic virus (Nilsson-Tillgren *et al.*, 1969; Nilsson-Tillgren, 1969) concluded that minus strands are formed rapidly at early stages of infection (Kielland-Brandt and Nilsson-Tillgren, 1973). After their rapid formation, the number of minus strands remains constant throughout a rapid phase of virus synthesis; at the end of this phase the ratio of plus to minus strands reaches about 100:1. Minus-strand concentration reaches a value of about 1 μg per mg cellular RNA, whereas plus-strand concentration is about 50–100 μg on the same basis. In the same study, it was determined that at early stages of infection the concentration of RI is somewhat greater than that of RF and that the ratio becomes reversed at later stages although the changes are not great. This study, although not definitive, is suggestive of asynchronous replication of the plus strand and is consistent with the concept that RI is the precursor of the viral plus strand (cf. Bishop and Levintow, 1971). The same suggestion could be drawn from data of an earlier study in which the kinetics of labeling of ribonuclease-resistant RNA was compared with that of tobacco mosaic virus RNA in shredded leaf tissue (Woolum *et al.*, 1967).

An investigation employing separated cells that had been previously infected with tobacco mosaic virus permitted the use of the pulse-chase technique (Jackson *et al.*, 1972). It was observed that, when cells were exposed to [^{3}H]-uridine for $\frac{1}{2}$ hour, considerably more label was incorporated into both RI and RF than into viral RNA. After incubation of these cells for an additional $3\frac{1}{2}$ hours in the presence of excess unlabeled uridine, it was found that all of the label had disappeared from RI and that much, but not all, of the label had disappeared from RF. Considerable label was incorporated into viral RNA as it disappeared from double-stranded forms during the chase period. It is clear from these experiments that RI turns over more rapidly than RF. Even after a considerably longer chase period (15 hours) most, but not all, of the label disappears from the RF component. These experiments suggest that RI is the more likely candidate than RF for a viral RNA precursor, although interpretation of the data suffers somewhat from the inherent difficulties of performing pulse-chase experiments with eukaryotic cells.

In summary, the results of *in vivo* experiments indicate that double-stranded forms of RNA are involved in RNA replication. It appears that at early stages of infection minus strands are preferentially synthesized, while the reverse is the case at later stages. RI seems to be the best candidate as source of virus RNA, but the roles of RF and RI in the replication process still remain to be clearly defined.

3.3.2. Evidence from *In Vitro* Studies

The *in vitro* studies of RNA replication mediated by replicase enzymes isolated from infected bacterial cells provide the model with which to compare experimental findings obtained with plant virus cell-free systems (Spiegelman *et al.*, 1968). Viral RNA (plus strand) provides a specific substrate for viral-induced polymerase in the bacterial system. Qβ polymerase, for instance, will recognize Qβ RNA and its complement to the exclusion of almost all other RNA species except for the homopolymer polycytidylic acid. The polymerase directs synthesis of minus strand in the $5' \rightarrow 3'$ direction using the plus strand as template to form the double-stranded intermediates, RF first and then RI. Upon completion of a minus strand, it in turn acts as a template for $5' \rightarrow 3'$ synthesis of plus strand, again via double-stranded intermediates. RI appears to act as the immediate precursor of plus strand. The involvement of RF in the replicative process is not clearly understood. Some regard it as "an end product or expended template" (Bishop and Levintow, 1971).

Virus-specific actinomycin D-resistant RNA polymerase activities have been detected in many extracts of infected plant tissues. The activity in most cases is associated with a rather large particle aggregate which sediments between 100 and $30,000 \times g$ and, in a few cases, the enzyme has been solubilized with mild detergent treatment and further characterized. None of the enzymes have as yet been purified to the extent where possible substructure organization could be examined.

Particulate cell-free replicases have been identified in extracts of tissues infected with turnip yellow mosaic virus (Bové *et al.*, 1967; Ralph and Wojcik, 1966), tobacco mosaic virus (Ralph and Wojcik, 1969), brome mosaic virus (Semal and Hamilton, 1968), broadbean mottle virus (Semal, 1970), tobacco ringspot virus (Peden *et al.*, 1972), and cucumber mosaic virus (May *et al.*, 1970). Enzyme activity is detected by incorporation of radioactive precursor nucleoside triphosphate into an acid-insoluble product and is dependent on the presence of all four ribonucleoside triphosphates. Except for one variant of cucumber mosaic virus particulate polymerase (May *et al.*, 1970), the reaction proceeds without the addition of exogenous RNA, indicating that the particulate system consists of a template–enzyme complex bound to or entrapped in a subcellular structure.

The product of the reaction is largely ribonuclease-resistant double-stranded RNA, indistinguishable in size and configuration from RF as extracted from infected tissue in the case of the single-component genome systems of turnip yellow mosaic virus and tobacco mosaic virus (Laflèche *et al.*, 1972; Bradley and Zaitlin, 1971). In the case of turnip yellow mosaic virus, at least 85% of incorporated label has been shown to be in plus strands. There is suggestive evidence that both plus and minus strands are synthesized in the tobacco mosaic virus system isolated from early infection and that only plus strand is synthesized by the particulate enzyme isolated from later infection. A component resembling RI is observed on occasion in the tobacco mosaic virus system, but in neither case is there evidence for release of single-stranded RNA from the double-stranded products. Failure to detect synthesis of single-stranded RNA may be due to nuclease activity in the crude preparations, but it is more likely either that the system is incomplete or that the incubation conditions so far employed are not optimal.

The particulate systems prepared from tissues infected with brome mosaic virus and broadbean mottle virus synthesize both double-stranded and single-stranded RNA with almost all incorporation of labeled precursor being into plus strand (Jacquemin, 1972; Semal and Kummert, 1971*b*.). In the early stages of the reaction (2–3 minutes), label is incorporated only into double-stranded RNA; the amount of this ribonuclease-resistant component thereafter stays constant while label is then incorporated into single-stranded RNA (Kummert and Semal, 1972; Jacquemin, 1972). The single-stranded product is composed of many components and has a size-range distribution which mimics that of the brome mosaic virus genome components (see Sect. 2). Pulse-chase experiments reveal that label which first appears as the plus-strand part of double-stranded RNA is displaced upon continued RNA synthesis, probably to appear in single-stranded RNA (Semal and Kummert, 1971*a*). The double-stranded RNA synthesized in the broadbean mottle system is composed of two components; one is insoluble in LiCl and acts as an intermediate in the generation of ribonuclease-sensitive plus strand, the other is soluble in LiCl and appears to be stable, once formed. The first component behaves in many respects like RI, the second like RF.

In summary, virus-specific RNA polymerase activity has been detected in a particulate fraction of leaf homogenates infected with a number of viruses. The enzyme activity does not require added template RNA and incorporates precursors into virus-specific RNA. The systems from tobacco mosaic virus and turnip yellow mosaic virus appear capable of completing the synthesis of RF-like double-stranded RNA. The enzymes from brome mosaic and broadbean mottle viruses also perform this function and, in addition, displace plus strand from double-stranded RNA to form what appears to be complete genomic RNA strands. Application of rapidly developing technology to the study of these particulate systems promises to yield valuable additional information concerning plant virus RNA biosynthesis.

Efforts have been made to solubilize and to purify further the virus-specific polymerase activity found in particulate fractions of infected cells in order to determine the properties of the enzyme(s) involved. These efforts have met with partial success in the case of activities found in tissues infected with brome mosaic virus (Hadidi and Fraenkel-Conrat, 1973), cucumber mosaic virus (May *et al.*, 1969), tobacco mosaic virus (Zaitlin *et al.*, 1973), tobacco ringspot virus (Peden *et al.*, 1972), and turnip yellow mosaic virus (Laflèche *et al.*, 1972).

The solubilized enzymes of all except that from turnip yellow mosaic virus have been found to have little activity in the absence of added RNA to serve as template. The soluble enzymes from tissues infected with cucumber mosaic virus, tobacco ringspot virus, and tobacco mosaic virus were found to have little template specificity; RNAs from diverse sources being almost equally effective in stimulating incorporation of labeled precursor into an acid-insoluble product. In contrast, the enzyme from brome mosaic virus-infected tissue exhibited partial specificity, being stimulated best by brome mosaic virus RNA and the closely related cowpea chlorotic mottle virus RNA, and, in decreasing efficiency, by $Q\beta$ RNA, tobacco necrosis satellite RNA, and broadbean mottle virus RNA. It was not stimulated by tobacco mosaic virus RNA, transfer RNA, or yeast RNA. The reason for low specificity of most solubilized plant virus RNA polymerases in comparison with that of the phage RNA polymerases is not known, but perhaps it may be attributed to insufficient purification of the enzyme or because factors imparting specificity to the enzyme have been lost during the purification.

The product synthesized by the solubilized enzymes of tobacco mosaic virus and cucumber mosaic virus is double-stranded; only the strand complementary to that used as template is synthesized. Of the BMV RNA components, the smallest appears to be the most effective template, and its double-stranded form is the predominant product (Hadidi *et al.*, 1973; Hadidi, 1974).

The soluble enzymes are large, with estimates of molecular

weights ranging from 120,000 to 160,000 daltons. Whether the plant virus polymerases prove to have a subunit structure similar to Qβ polymerase (Kamen, 1970; Weissmann *et al.*, 1973) remains to be determined, although the detection of a presumed subunit of the BMV enzyme suggests this possibility in some cases (Hariharasubramanian *et al.*, 1973).

During the course of study of plant virus-induced polymerase, it has been observed that extracts of healthy chinese cabbage (a host for turnip yellow mosaic virus) and tobacco (a host for tobacco mosaic virus) contain a DNA-independent RNA replicase (Astier-Manifacier and Cornuet, 1971; Duda *et al.*, 1973). Enzyme activity from both sources is found to be greater in infected than in healthy tissue but, otherwise, the enzymes have different properties, either intrinsically or because of different degrees of purification. The chinese cabbage enzyme is template dependent but has little specificity as to source of RNA and is even stimulated by denatured DNA and, to a lesser extent, native DNA. The product is 85% resistant to ribonuclease, and the synthesized RNA appears to be the complement of the template used to stimulate the reaction. The tobacco enzyme, prepared in a different manner and from a tissue fraction which, upon infection, does not contain the tobacco mosaic virus-induced polymerase, is template independent and produces a small, double-stranded product of about 5 S, as measured by polyacrylamide gel electrophoresis. Enzyme activity is stimulated by added RNA in a peculiar and not understood fashion, the added RNA having been shown to be neither template nor primer for the synthetic reaction. The functional signficance of the DNA-independent RNA replicase found in extracts of healthy plant tissue is unknown at the present time.

From the above description, it is clear that the study of plant virus-induced polymerase is in the early stages. Additional information should become available concerning RNA replication as progress is made in purifying and characterizing the involved replicase enzymes.

3.4. Site of RNA Replication

Several experimental approaches have been brought to bear on locating the intracellular site of plant virus RNA replication. Among these are high resolution autoradiography after [³H]-uridine incorporation by actinomycin D-treated plant tissues and identification of components related to viral RNA synthesis in plant cell macerates. The evidence to date indicates that the site of RNA replication is not the same for all viruses.

Labeled precursor taken up by actinomycin D-treated, turnip yellow mosaic virus-infected, chinese cabbage tissue is incorporated both into nucleoli- and chloroplast-associated vesicles. An extensive series of both *in vivo* and *in vitro* experiments have lead to the conclusion that the plastidial outer-membrane system is the site of active viral RNA synthesis (Laflèche *et al.*, 1972; Bové and Laflèche, 1972). This is supported by the work of other investigators (Gerola *et al.*, 1972; Ushiyama and Matthews, 1970), with the significance of nucleolar labeling remaining to be elucidated. Additional confirmation of the involvement of chloroplasts in turnip yellow mosaic virus biosynthesis comes from the finding that double-stranded virus-specific RNA is associated with chloroplasts following careful fractionation of infected cell extracts (Ralph *et al.*, 1971a).

The location of tobacco mosaic virus RNA synthesis is subject to conflicting evidence. Early cytological work suggested that the nuclei of infected cells were probably heavily involved in RNA synthesis (Bald, 1964; von Wettstein and Zech, 1962), but the nature of the RNA synthesized could not be determined. Radioautographic evidence and biochemical experiments in which parental viral RNA was traced to the nucleus tended to support the conclusion that the nucleus was the site of viral RNA synthesis (Schlegel *et al.*, 1967; Reddi, 1972). However, careful fractionation of extracts of infected tissue has revealed that neither double-stranded forms of RNA nor virus-related RNA polymerase is found in the nucleus. Both of these virus-related components are found to sediment with mitochondria (Ralph and Wojcik, 1969; Jackson *et al.*, 1971; Bradley and Zaitlin, 1971). Further fractionation of the "mitochondrial" pellet has revealed that double-stranded viral RNA is probably associated with cytoplasmic membranes (Ralph *et al.*, 1971b). Since the presumed intermediates in viral RNA synthesis and at least part of the presumptive enzymatic apparatus for RNA replication is found in a cytoplasmic particulate, it seems more reasonable to assume that the nucleus is not the site of RNA replication.

Cowpea mosaic virus double-stranded RNA has been found to sediment with the chloroplast fraction of an infected-cell homogenate, but whether it is associated with chloroplasts or with membranous or other material which sediments with chloroplasts has not been determined (Assink *et al.*, 1973).

Extracts of cucumber cotyledons infected with cucumber mosaic virus (May *et al.*, 1970), barley leaves infected with brome mosaic virus (Semal and Kummert, 1970), and broadbean leaves infected with broadbean mottle virus (Jacquemin, 1972) have virus-induced polymerase activity which is particulate and which sediments with chloroplasts and/or mitochondria.

The available evidence to date indicates that replication of turnip yellow mosaic virus RNA, cowpea mosaic virus RNA, and perhaps brome mosaic virus RNA (Hariharasubramanian *et al.*, 1973) is probably associated with chloroplasts and that the RNA of tobacco mosaic virus replicates in association with a cytoplasmic membrane or organelle. In none of the cases so far examined, however, has a complete RNA-replicating activity been demonstrated and, thus, conclusions concerning the intracellular site of replication of the several plant viral RNAs should be considered tentative.

4. TRANSLATION OF VIRAL NUCLEIC ACID

4.1. Virus-Related Proteins Found in Infected Tissue

The genome of the small RNA bacteriophages such as R17 and f2 is 1.2×10^6 daltons and in size it contains three cistrons, which code for capsid protein, an RNA synthetase subunit, and a maturation protein (Gussin *et al.*, 1966). Most plant virus genomes are larger than this and, thus, should contain at least as many cistrons. One would expect, therefore, that new proteins, in addition to capsid protein, would appear in virus-infected plant tissue. During the past few years a search has been underway for such proteins by comparing extracts of healthy and infected tissue for protein differences.

One method that has been used to detect new proteins in infected tissue has been to coelectrophorese sodium dodecyl sulfate and urea-treated differently labeled extracts of healthy and infected tissue. This technique, although moderately successful in the hands of some investigators, suffers from the inability to shut off normal host protein synthesis in infected cells. Although actinomycin D can be used to inhibit DNA-directed RNA synthesis in plant cells (Sänger and Knight, 1963), this inhibitor has little effect on protein synthesis in short-term experiments, presumably because of the presence of long-lived messenger RNA. Chloramphenicol has been used successfully to partially reduce host protein synthesis with particular virus infections (Zaitlin *et al.*, 1968). This inhibitor acts to suppress protein synthesis mediated by chloroplast ribosomes and, thus, can only be used where these ribosomes play no part in the infection process.

In spite of difficulties presented by a high background of host protein synthesis, several proteins, the synthesis of which is stimulated following virus infection, have been detected.

The synthesis of several proteins is found to be stimulated, while that of others is found to be depressed in tobacco mosaic virus-infected tissue. Among those showing stimulated synthesis are several large proteins in the molecular-weight range of $155-245 \times 10^6$ daltons (Zaitlin and Hariharasubramanian, 1970, 1972; Sakai and Takebe, 1972). Stimulation of synthesis of these large proteins could be demonstrated only under certain experimental conditions with the common strain of tobacco mosaic virus (Singer, 1971); more complex patterns of stimulated and inhibited synthesis were observed with other strains (Singer and Condit, 1974). The experimental procedure does not permit a conclusion to be drawn concerning whether protein whose synthesis is stimulated in infected tissue is coded for by the virus or the host genome. However, it seems likely at the present time that one of the high-molecular-weight proteins may be a virus-coded RNA synthetase with an independently estimated molecular weight of 160,000 daltons (Zaitlin *et al.*, 1973).

Six new virus-induced or virus-stimulated proteins were detected in extracts of tobacco necrosis virus-infected tissue. These had molecular weights of 64, 42, 32, 23, 15, and 12×10^3 daltons, with the 32,000-dalton component being capsid protein. No other new or stimulated proteins appeared in cells doubly infected with tobacco necrosis and satellite viruses except for the 20,000-dalton satellite capsid protein, thus providing additional evidence that the satellite genome contains only the cistron which codes for its capsid protein (Jones and Reichmann, 1973).

Brome mosaic virus-infected barley tissue extracts have been found to contain an apparently new protein of molecular weight 34,500 daltons. It is postulated that this protein may be an RNA replicase, or a portion of one, because the enzyme activity and the protein appear at the same time upon infection and they fractionate together (Hariharasubramanian *et al.*, 1973). An interesting and suggestive observation is the similarity in molecular weight between the new protein and the protein translated from brome mosaic virus RNA #3 in a wheat embryo-derived cell-free system (Shih and Kaesberg, 1973).

The difficulty in interpreting data from the double-label polyacrylamide gel procedure is exemplified by the work on tomato spotted wilt virus. This complex virus contains three major structural glycoproteins of molecular weights 84, 50, and 29×10^3 daltons and one large protein (220,000 daltons) present in small amount. However, only the

50,000-dalton protein is detected in extracts of infected cells (Mohamed *et al.*, 1973). An explanation for the failure to detect stimulation of synthesis of any of the other virus proteins in infected tissue awaits further experimentation.

4.2. Mapping of Cistrons in the Viral Genome

There are two aspects to the problem of the number and arrangement of genes in a plant virus genome; the arrangement of genes on single RNA molecules and the location of genes on the different RNA species of a split-genome virus.

4.2.1. The Number and Arrangement of Genes on Single RNA Molecules

Little is known of either the number or arrangement of genes on most plant virus RNAs, but some progress has been made in a number of instances. The exceptionally small plant viral RNAs are most likely monocistronic. These include the tobacco necrosis satellite virus RNA (Klein *et al.*, 1972; Rice and Fraenkel-Conrat, 1973), brome mosaic virus #4 (Shih and Kaesberg, 1973), and alfalfa mosaic virus top *a* (Van Ravenswaaij Classen *et al.*, 1967). About half of the length of these RNAs is accounted for by the respective gene for capsid protein; the rest is probably involved with other functions related to proper translation and encapsidation. In addition, as discussed in Sect. 3.1, satellite RNA probably contains a replicase recognition region. Brome mosaic virus #3 RNA has been shown to have two cistrons, one for capsid protein, the same as that on #4 RNA, and one for a protein of unknown function, but possibly a virus-specific subunit of the RNA polymerase (Hariharasubramanian *et al.*, 1973). The arrangement of these two genes on #3 RNA is not yet known. The number of genes on other viral RNAs remains to be determined.

An approximate location has been established for at least two of the gene functions contained on tobacco mosaic virus RNA. One of these genes determines whether tobacco mosaic virus induces systemic infection or hypersensitive, i.e., local necrotic, response in the differential host *Nicotiana sylvestris*. Kado and Knight (1966) took advantage of the facts that treatment with sodium dodecyl sulfate strips protein from RNA in a polar manner starting from the 3′ end of the RNA (May and Knight, 1965) and that free RNA is more sensitive to the mutagenic action of nitrous acid than is encapsidated RNA (Mundry and Gierer, 1958). By stripping the virus to various extents before treating it with nitrous acid, they determined that the gene controlling the differential response is located on the 5′ half of the viral RNA. Kado and Knight (1968) again took advantage of controlled polar stripping in an attempt to locate the capsid protein gene. In this case they digested the exposed nucleic acid with nuclease and inoculated the resultant viral fragments, together with helper virus of a serologically distinct strain. They reported that protein of the stripped strain was synthesized in the host when up to 50%, but no more than 72–90% of the protein was removed; thus the gene for coat protein was also located in the 5′ half of the viral RNA. Although this important observation has not yet been repeated, the conclusion drawn from it agreed with the results of Mandeles (1968), who determined that the coat protein cistron was not located near the 3′ terminus of viral RNA.

Another specialized region has been located on the tobacco mosaic virus RNA: that for recognition of a 20 S capsid-protein aggregate. This region, located at the 5′ terminus and estimated to be about 50 nucleotides long (Nazarova et al., 1973), combines with the 34-subunit, double-disc, coat protein aggregate in the first step of the assembly of the nucleoprotein virus rod from its components (Butler and Klug, 1971; Okada and Ohno, 1972; Thouvenal et al., 1971).

4.2.2. Location of Genes on the Components of Split Genomes

A number of studies have been performed with multicomponent viruses in which infection has been initiated with a mixture of components derived from different strains of the virus. The purpose of such experiments has been in large measure to determine gene assignments for the different RNA molecules of the split-genome viruses.

Tobacco rattle virus, as previously described, is composed of two nucleoprotein components, a long rod and a short rod (Harrison and Woods, 1966). These each have an RNA strand distinctive from that of the other in both length and nucleotide sequence (Minson and Darby, 1973), but both are encapsidated with identical protein subunits (Lister and Bracker, 1968). Infection can be initiated with both components or with the long rod alone. In the latter case no nucleoprotein is produced, only infectious nucleic acid, thus indicating that the gene for coat protein is located in the short-rod RNA and that the gene(s) for replicase is (are) located in long rod RNA (Lister, 1966, 1968; Frost *et al.*, 1967). This conclusion has been fortified by data obtained from experiments in which infection was initiated by a mixture of long rods and short rods derived from different virus strains (Sänger, 1968, 1969; Lister, 1969; Ghabrial and Lister, 1973). It has been found in such experiments that long and short progeny RNA molecules are both encapsidated with protein specified by the short RNA. Factors controlling the type of symptom induced in the host are located on both long and short rods.

Brome mosaic virus and cowpea chlorotic mottle virus are very similar multicomponent viruses with icosahedral symmetry that are closely related to each other on the basis of their serological cross-reactivity (Scott and Slack, 1971) and because their components can be substituted for each other (Bancroft, 1972). As detailed earlier, both of these viruses are composed of 4 RNA molecules, termed #1–4 in order of diminishing molecular weights, encapsidated in three nucleoprotein particles (Lane and Kaesberg, 1971, Bancroft and Flack, 1972). RNA species #4 is a monocistronic messenger for capsid protein and #3 also contains the cistron for capsid protein in addition to a cistron for a second protein (Shih and Kaesberg, 1973). Bancroft and Lane (1973) were able to assign functions to the different RNA species by an experimental approach which first involved isolating nitrous acid-induced mutant strains of the viruses. Following electrophoretic separation of the RNA components, infection was induced with mixtures containing combinations of the components from different mutants. Observation of the resultant infections permitted the following conclusions: The protein cistron is definitely located on #3, as is the gene controlling the nature of systemic symptoms, whereas control of local- and primary-lesion alterations is located on either #2 or #3. Control of temperature sensitivity of local-lesion formation is attributed to #1. As pointed out by Bancroft and Lane (1973), it is quite likely that many of the observed phenotypic characteristics are sometimes dependent on other changes in the virus. For instance, changes in capsid protein may result in a variety of effects on the nature of the infection, including ratio of the nucleoprotein components produced. It is of interest to note that both the cistron for coat protein and for the nature of systemic infection are located on the same piece of RNA.

Alfalfa mosaic virus, also characterized by four RNA components, has also been subjected to analysis by mixing components derived from different strains (Dingjan-Versteegh *et al.*, 1972). Thus it was found that both top *a* and top *b* contain the cistron for capsid protein (Bol *et al.*, 1971). In addition, top *b* determines serotype, the kind of symptom on tobacco, the relative proportion of components, and the sensitivity to cycloheximide. The middle component RNA determines the kind of symptoms on bean, and no marker has as yet been located on the bottom component RNA.

Cowpea mosaic and related viruses are two-component viruses, the capsids of which are composed of two proteins rather than a single protein, as is the case for most other small plant viruses (Wu and Bruening, 1971; Geelen *et al.*, 1972). It appears that the larger RNA component contains the cistron for one of the capsid proteins, whereas the smaller component contains the cistron for the other (Kassanis *et al.*, 1973). In addition, the amount of nucleic acid-free capsid produced is controlled by the smaller RNA component (Bruening, 1969; DeJager and Van Kammen, 1970), and the type of local lesion and the ratio of components is controlled by the larger RNA (Wood, 1972).

A number of other split-genome viruses has been analyzed to a greater or lesser extent by mixing components derived from different strains. Tobacco streak virus has most of its genetic determinants occuring in at least two of three particle types with the result that there appears to be much redundance in the genetic information carried by an infective set of particles (Fulton, 1972). Pea enation mosaic virus (Hull and Lane, 1973) differs from most other split-genome viruses in that the gene for its single capsid protein is located on the larger of two RNA species, rather than on the smaller. In contrast, raspberry ringspot virus has the gene for capsid protein located on the smaller RNA species (Harrison *et al.*, 1972).

4.3. Control Mechanisms for Translation

Plants contain two major groups of ribosomes: cytoplasmic 80 S and chloroplastic 70 S ribosomes. In only a few cases is it known which ribosomes mediate viral RNA translation. Tobacco mosaic virus, tobacco necrosis virus, and tobacco rattle virus RNAs appear to be translated by cytoplasmic 80 S ribosomes, as deduced by sensitivity of the translation process to cycloheximide but not to chloramphenicol (Zaitlin *et al.*, 1968; McCarthey *et al.*, 1972; Harrison and Crockatt, 1971).

The subject of RNA virus gene expression has been reviewed recently (Sugiyama *et al.*, 1972). There are at least two distinct translation mechanisms for small viral RNAs. Bacteriophage RNA contains three cistrons and behaves as a polycistronic messenger both *in vivo* and *in vitro*. A number of control mechanisms regulate the relative rate of translation of the three cistrons. One of these resides in the secondary and tertiary structure of the viral RNA and is such that ribosome attachment and translation initiation is favored for the coat protein cistron over that of the other two. In another control mechanism, translation of the replicase cistron is shut off as a consequence of specific attachment of capsid protein to viral RNA. In contrast to the independent translation of the individual cistrons of prokaryotic, polycistronic messengers, the entire animal picornavirus RNA is translated into a single large protein which is subsequently cleaved into functional peptides.

The evidence to date indicates that a variety of mechanisms may be employed to achieve proper translation of plant virus RNA. As indicated in the previous section, a number of plant virus RNAs are monocistronic in nature and act as efficient messengers for capsid protein. Such specialized single-protein messengers have been identified for the tobacco necrosis satellite and the smallest components of several split-genome viruses. The specialized monocistronic messengers found in split-genome viruses are probably not replicated and appear to arise from splitting of a larger, dicistronic RNA (Shih *et al.*, 1972). Although encapsidated, they are not required for infection. Given the limited number of known examples of specialized monocistronic messengers, one may inquire whether genome fracturing may be a general method for control of plant virus RNA translation. Are other monocistronic messengers produced during plant virus replication which do not become encapsidated and which, as a consequence, may have been overlooked? At the present time there is conflicting evidence on this point. Small pieces of viral RNA of about the same size as the known monocistronic messengers have been detected both in total RNA extracts of tobacco mosaic virus-infected tissue and in association with ribosomes (see Sect. 3.2). It remains to be determined however, whether these might be messengers for specific proteins.

When brome mosaic virus #3, the 7×10^5-dalton RNA species that most probably contains two cistrons, one for capsid protein and the other for a protein, 3a, of unknown function, is used as messenger for a wheat-embryo-derived cell-free system, the product is largely 3a, with only small amounts of capsid protein being synthesized (Shih and Kaesberg, 1973). This evidence suggests that control of translation of this polycistronic messenger is regulated, possibly by its tertiary structure. It has been postulated that animal ribosomes cannot serve in the translation of true polycistronic messenger (Jacobson and Baltimore, 1968); the above result suggests that animal and plant 80 S ribosomes may differ in this regard. There is uncertainty, however, as to whether brome mosaic virus #3 RNA is translated as such *in vivo* because it is suspected that #4 RNA arises by a splitting of component 3. Thus, it remains to be determined whether in the infected cell protein 3a is translated from #3 RNA or possibly from the other split product of #3.

It has been known for some time that the larger plant virus RNAs serve to stimulate *in vitro* protein-synthesizing systems without at the same time inducing the synthesis of recognizable specific protein products (Aach *et al.*, 1964). For instance, although tobacco mosaic virus RNA stimulates high incorporation of amino acids into acid-insoluble products in cell-free systems derived from *Eschericia coli* and wheat germ, at best only minimal synthesis of capsid protein or capsid protein peptides can be detected (Aach *et al.*, 1964; Efron and Marcus, 1973; Roberts *et al.*, 1973); this evidence indicates that unsplit viral RNA may not serve as an efficient polycistronic messenger. We have presented the available evidence for the hypothesis that *in vivo* translation of these larger RNAs may be controlled by fragmentation of the genome. However, there is also presumptive evidence that this does not happen, but that the viral RNAs serve directly as messenger. In the first instance, intact tobacco mosaic virus RNA has been found associated with ribosomes, thus suggesting a messenger function for large viral RNA (Van Kammen, 1963; Schuch, 1973); secondly, synthesis of very large proteins (245, 195, and 155 $\times$ 10³ daltons) is stimulated in tobacco mosaic virus-infected tissue (Zaitlin and Hariharasubramanian, 1972). This latter result suggests that, as with animal picornaviruses (Jacobson and Baltimore, 1968), the entire genome may be translated into a single polyprotein which is subsequently cleaved into functional peptides. However, appropriate pulse-chase experiments, utilizing separated infected cells, indicate that the very large proteins which are detected in infected-tissue extracts are not cleaved into smaller units (Zaitlin and Hariharasubramanian, 1972).

It is clear from the foregoing discussion that control mechanisms for translation of plant viral RNAs are not clearly understood at the present time. It is known that at least part of the RNA of some of the split-genome viruses is translated from monocistronic messenger, but how the larger plant RNAs are translated remains a mystery.

5. ASSEMBLY OF VIRIONS

The general principles of virus structure have been elucidated by the pioneering analysis of Caspar and Klug (1962) and it has been discovered that many of the rod-shaped and icosahedral, small RNA viruses can be both disassembled into their constituent components and reassembled into infectious units by appropriate manipulation of environmental conditions (Fraenkel-Conrat and Williams, 1955, Semancik and Reynolds, 1969; Bancroft, 1970). A variety of interactions are responsible for structural integrity of nucleoprotein virus structure. Kaper (1972) has recently reviewed this subject and has pointed out the importance of (1) interactions between the capsid protein subunits (protein–protein) interactions, (2) interactions between the protein subunits and RNA (protein–RNA interactions), and (3) intrachain interactions both in the RNA and protein components. A continuum of relative importance of these different types of interactions exists among the viruses; turnip yellow mosaic virus being an example of a stable structure where protein–protein interactions are relatively more important, and cucumber mosaic virus being an example toward the other end of the continuum, with a weak structure dependent primarily on protein–RNA interaction.

Although a start has been made in understanding virus structure and how to pull it apart and put it back together, little is known of the assembly process *in vivo*. The evidence is quite compelling for a number of viruses that biosynthesis of the RNA and protein components are quite independent processes and that one or another of the components can be present separately in the cell at different times of infection. Takahashi and Ishii (1953) were the first to observe that free tobacco mosaic virus protein (termed X protein) could be detected in extracts of infected tissue, and it was later observed that free viral RNA is present during early stages of infection (Engler and Schramm, 1959). Sarkar (1965) demonstrated quite clearly that the amount of ribonuclease-sensitive infectivity extractable from tobacco mosaic virus-infected leaf tissue reaches a maximum $1\frac{1}{2}$–2 days after initiation of infection, and is gone by 3 days, presumably because the synthesis of capsid protein reaches a level to favor virus assembly. To reinforce the hypothesis that protein and nucleic acid synthesis are indepent processes, mutant strains of tobacco mosaic virus and tobacco necrosis virus have been isolated which induce the synthesis of nonfunctional defective capsid protein so that infection is maintained by the nucleic acid component of the virus without production of nucleoprotein virus particles (Siegel *et al.*, 1962; Babos and Kassanis, 1962). In addition, it has been observed that infection with the long component of the split-genome tobacco rattle virus leads to a similar type of nucleoprotein-free infection (Lister, 1966). Other evidence for the independent synthesis of viral components lies in the observation that empty nucleic acid-free capsids, termed top components, are synthesized during infection of a number of plant viruses. Turnip yellow mosaic virus is an example of such a virus (Markham and Smith, 1949); it produces empty as well as full capsids during ordinary infection, and infected cells continue to produce empty capsids even when viral RNA synthesis is inhibited with the pyrimidine analogue 2-thiouracil (Francki and Matthews, 1962).

The conditions that have been established for successful *in vitro* assembly of many plant viruses are in many cases not likely to occur inside a living cell and, thus, the *in vivo* assembly of components into infectious nucleoprotein is a problem that requires independent analysis and about which little is known at the present time. Several considerations of the plant virus system that may be applicable to the problem of assembly are the following:

1.   Plant virus genomes appear to contain more information than required for specification of capsid protein and an RNA replicase. It may be, then, in analogy with bacteriophage coded maturation protein (Steitz, 1968), that additional proteins(s) may be specified which function in virus assembly. Presumptive evidence for such a hypothesis is provided by the temperature-sensitive tobacco mosaic virus mutant *ts*-II Ni 2519 (Bosch and Jockush, 1972), which continues to synthesize both viral RNA and unaltered coat protein at the nonpermissive temperature but fails to produce virus particles. Failure of assembly in this case may be due to production of a defective unidentified protein necessary for assembly, although other types of alterations leading to the same experimental observation are possible.

2.   The *in vivo* assembly of virions appears to be generally rather specific. The viral protein combines with viral nucleic acid and not with host nucleic acid, although the pseudovirions of tobacco mosaic virus constitute a known exception to this rule (Siegel, 1971). It is possible that in some instances the specificity of assembly may result from the intracellular compartmentalization of the assembly reaction such that no host RNA is available for encapsidation; on the other hand, it is known that the proteins of some viruses react quite specifically with their nucleic acids. Two recently studied examples are the affinity of double discs of tobacco mosaic virus for the 5′ end of tobacco mosaic virus RNA (Butler and Klug, 1971) and the specific reaction of alfalfa mosaic virus protein with its nucleic acid (Van Vloten-Doting and Jas-

pers, 1972). On the other hand, a variety of nucleic acids can participate in the *in vitro* reconstitution reaction with proteins from the brome mosaic virus group. Whether the reaction *in vivo* may be more specific remains to be determined. The reported *in vivo* encapsidation of barley stripe mosaic virus RNA by protein of the unrelated brome mosaic virus (Peterson and Brakke, 1973) is an observation which argues against absolute specificity of all assembly reactions.

3.   Little is known of the site of virus assembly within the plant cell. Matthews (1973) has postulated that assembly of turnip yellow mosaic virus occurs in the neck of the peripheral vesicles that are induced by infection to form on the surface of chloroplasts. The fact that tobacco mosaic virus pseudovirions which apparently contain chloroplast messenger RNA rather than viral RNA are formed preferentially during infection with the U2 strain suggests that this strain may be assembled in, or in the vicinity of, the chloroplast. This hypothesis is supported by the observation that particles of the U5 strain (a strain which is closely related to the U2 strain) are more likely to be found in chloroplasts than particles of other tobacco mosaic virus strains (Shalla, 1968). The studies by Singer (1972) suggest that wild-type TMV may be assembled in or on the chloroplasts, but other investigators come to a contrary conclusion on the basis of other types of evidence (cf. Matthews, 1970, pp. 204–207, Zaitlin *et al.*, 1968).*

6.   CONCLUDING REMARKS

Paucity of information turns the current attempt to describe replication of the small, RNA plant viruses into a progress report, containing little that is definitive. It is clear, however, that recent advances both in knowledge and technique permit the framing of questions and experimental approaches that are more meaningful than had previously been the case. Consequently, it is likely that the near future holds in store considerable improvement of our understanding of plant virus replication. Aspects of the problem that appear ripe for solution are definition of the enzymes involved in viral RNA replication and an understanding of the roles of the double-stranded forms in the replication process. It is also likely that additional information will soon be forthcoming concerning mechanisms of translation of viral RNA. A more complete description of the genetic content of plant virus RNA is needed and hopefully techniques will be devised to determine how

* See footnote on p. 71.

many genes exist and the nature and function of the gene products. The elucidation of the process by which infection is initiated and the mechanism by which the infecting virus is uncoated appears to be a recalcitrant problem, although perhaps the direction toward the solution lies in the recent type of experiment in which the adsorption of cowpea chlorotic mottle virus to protoplasts was studied, demonstrating the lowest number of particles (no more than 760) yet necessary for initiation of a plant virus infection (Motoyoshi *et al.*, 1973*a*). As pointed out elsewhere in this chapter, perhaps the technical advance that holds most promise for an enhanced understanding of plant virus replication is the plant protoplast system which has been developed in the past few years.

7. REFERENCES

Aach, H., Funatsu, G., Nirenberg, M., and Fraenkel-Conrat, H., 1964, Further attempts to characterize products of TMV-RNA directed protein synthesis, *Biochemistry* **3**, 1362.

Abou Haidar, M., Pfeiffer, P., Fritsch, C., and Hirth, L., 1973, Sequential reconstitution of tobacco rattle virus, *J. Gen. Virol.* **21**, 83.

Aoki, S., and Takebe, I., 1969, Infection of tobacco mesophyll protoplasts by tobacco mosaic virus ribonucleic acid, *Virology* **39**, 439.

Armstrong, J., Edmonds, M., Nakazato, H., Phillips, B., and Vaughn, M., 1972, Polyadenylic acid sequences in the virion RNA of poliovirus and eastern equine encephalitis virus, *Science (Wash., D.C.)* **176**, 526.

Assink, A-M., Swaans, H., and Van Kammen, A., 1973, The localization of virus-specific double-stranded RNA of cowpea mosaic virus in subcellular fractions of infected *Vigna* leaves, *Virology* **53**, 384.

Astier-Manifacier, S., and Cornuet, P., 1971, RNA-dependent RNA polymerase in chinese cabbage, *Biochim. Biophys. Acta* **232**, 484.

Babos, P., 1969, Rapidly labeled RNA associated with ribosomes of tobacco leaves infected with tobacco mosaic virus, *Virology* **39**, 893.

Babos, P., 1971, TMV-RNA associated with ribosomes of tobacco leaves infected with TMV, *Virology* **43**, 597.

Babos, P., and Kassanis, B., 1962, Unstable variants of tobacco necrosis virus, *Virology* **18**, 206.

Bald, J., 1964, Cytological evidence for the production of plant virus ribonucleic acid in the nucleus, *Virology* **22**, 377.

Baltimore, D., 1968, Structure of the poliovirus replicative intermediate RNA, *J. Mol. Biol.* **32**, 359.

Bancroft, J., 1970, The self-assembly of spherical plant viruses, *Adv. Virus Res.* **16**, 99.

Bancroft, J., 1971, The significance of the multicomponent nature of cowpea chlorotic mottle virus RNA, *Virology* **45**, 830.

Bancroft, J., 1972, A virus made from parts of the genomes of brome mosaic and cowpea chlorotic mottle viruses, *J. Gen. Virol.* **14**, 223.

Bancroft, J., and Flack, I., 1972, The behavior of cowpea chlorotic mottle virus in CsCl, *J. Gen. Virol.* **15**, 247.

Bancroft, J., and Lane, L., 1973, Genetic analysis of cowpea chlorotic mottle and brome mosaic viruses, *J. Gen. Virol.* **19**, 381.

Beijerinck, M., 1898, Over een contagium vivum fluidum als oorzaak van de vlekziekte der tabaksbladen, *Verhandl. Koninkl. Akad. Wetenschap. Afdel. Wiss.-Natuurk.* **7**, 229.

Bennett, C., 1967, Plant viruses: transmission by dodder, *In* "Methods in Virology," Vol. 1 (K. Maramorasch and H. Koprowski, eds.), pp. 393–401, Academic Press, New York.

Bennett, C., 1969, Seed transmission of plant viruses, *Adv. Virus Res.* **14**, 221.

Bishop, J., and Koch, G., 1967, Purification and characterization of poliovirus-induced infections double-stranded ribonucleic acid, *J. Biol. Chem.* **242**, 1736.

Bishop, J., and Levintow, L., 1971, Replicative forms of viral RNA; structure and function, *Progr. Med. Virol.* **13**, 1.

Black, L., and Markham, R., 1963, Base-pairing in ribonucleic acid of wound-tumor virus, *Neth. J. Plant Pathol.* **69**, 215.

Bol, J., and Van Vloten-Doting, L., 1973, Function of top component *a* RNA in the initiation of infection by alfalfa mosaic virus, *Virology* **51**, 102.

Bol, J., Van Vloten-Doting, L., and Jaspars, E., 1971, A functional equivalence of top component *a* RNA and coat protein in the initiation of infection by alfalfa mosaic virus, *Virology* **46**, 73.

Bosch, F., and Jockusch, H., 1972, Temperature-sensitive mutants of TMV: behaviour of a non-coat protein mutant in isolated tobacco cells, *Mol. Gen. Genet.* **116**, 95.

Bové, J., and Laflèche, D., 1972, The plastidial outer membrane as the site of turnip yellow mosaic virus replication, *in* "Proceedings of the Second International Congress for Virology, Budapest 1971" (J. Melnick, ed.), pp. 223–224, Karger Basle.

Bové, J., Bové, C., Rondot, M., and Morel, G., 1967, Chloroplasts and virus RNA synthesis, *in* "Biochemistry of Chloroplasts," Vol. II (T. Goodwin, ed.), pp. 329–339, Academic Press, New York.

Bové, J., Bové, C., and Mocquot, B., 1968, Turnip yellow mosaic virus-RNA synthesis *in vitro:* evidence for native double-stranded RNA, *Biochem. Biophys. Res. Commun.* **32**, 480.

Bradley, D., and Zaitlin, M., 1971, Replication of tobacco mosaic virus. II. The *in vitro* synthesis of high-molecular-weight virus-specific RNAs, *Virology* **45**, 192.

Brants, D., 1965, Relation between ectodesmata and infection of leaves by tobacco mosaic virus. *Virology* **26**, 554.

Brown, F., and Hull, R., 1973, Comparative virology of the small RNA viruses, *J. Gen. Virol.* **20**, 43.

Bruening, G., 1969, The inheritance of top component formation in cowpea mosaic virus, *Virology* **37**, 577.

Burdon, R., Billeter, M., Weissmann, C., Warner, R., Ochoa, S., and Knight, C., 1964, Replication of viral RNA. V. Presence of a virus-specific double-stranded RNA in leaves infected with tobacco mosaic virus, *Proc. Natl. Acad. Sci. USA* **52**, 768.

Butler, P. and Klug, A., 1971, Assembly of the particle of tobacco mosaic virus from RNA and disks of protein, *Nat. New Biol.* **299**, 47.

Caspar, D., and Klug, A., 1962, Physical principles in the construction of regular viruses, *Cold Spring Harbor Symp. Quant. Biol.* **27**, 1.

Cocking, E., 1966, An electron microscope study of the initial stages of infection of isolated tomato fruit protoplasts by TMV, *Planta (Berl.)* **68**, 206.

Coutts, R. H. A., Cocking, E. C., and Kassanis, B., 1972, Infection of tobacco mesophyll protoplasts with tobacco mosaic virus, *J. Gen. Virol.* **17**, 289.

DeJager, C., and Van Kammen, A., 1970, The relationship between the components of cowpea mosaic virus. III. Location of genetic information for two biological functions in the middle component of CPMV, *Virology* **41**, 281.

Diener, T., 1971, Potato spindle tuber "virus." IV. A replicating, low-molecular-weight RNA, *Virology* **45**, 411.

Diener, T., 1972, Viroids, *Adv. Virus Res.* **17**, 295.

Diener, T., and Lawson, R., 1973, Chrysanthemum stunt: a viroid disease, *Virology* **51**, 94.

Diener, T., and Raymer, W., 1969, Potato spindle tuber virus: A plant virus with properties of a free nucleic acid. II. Characterization and partial purification, *Virology* **37**, 351.

Diener, T., and Smith, D., 1973, Potato spindle tuber viroid. IX. Molecular-weight determination by gel electrophoresis of formylated RNA, *Virology* **53**, 359.

Dingjan-Versteegh, A., Van Vloten-Doting, L., and Jaspars, E., 1972, Alfalfa mosaic virus hybrids constructed by exchanging nucleoprotein components, *Virology* **49**, 716.

Duda, C., Zaitlin, M., and Siegel, A., 1973, *In vitro* synthesis of double-stranded RNA by an enzyme system isolated from tobacco leaves, *Biochim. Biophys. Acta* **319**, 62.

Edwardson, J., Purcifull, D., and Christie, R., 1968, Structure of cytoplasmic inclusions in plants infected with rod-shaped viruses, *Virology* **34**, 250.

Efron, D., and Marcus, A., 1973, Translation of TMV-RNA in a cell-free wheat embryo system, *Virology* **53**, 343.

El Manna, M., and Bruening, G., 1973, Polyadenylate sequences in the ribonucleic acids of cowpea mosaic virus, *Virology* **56**, 198.

Engler, R., and Schramm, G., 1959, Infectious ribonucleic acid as a precursor of tobacco mosaic virus, *Nature (Lond.)* **183**, 1277.

Esau, K., and Cronshaw, J., 1967, Relation of tobacco mosaic virus with host cells, *J. Cell Biol.* **33**, 665.

Fraenkel-Conrat, H., and Williams, R., 1955, Reconstitution of active tobacco mosaic virus from its inactive protein and nucleic acid components, *Proc. Natl. Acad. Sci. USA* **41**, 690.

Fraenkel-Conrat, H., Singer, B., and Williams, R., 1957, Infectivity of virus nucleic acid, *Biochim. Biophys Acta* **25**, 87.

Fraenkel-Conrat, H., Veldee, S., and Woo, J., 1964, The infectivity of tobacco mosaic virus, *Virology* **22**, 432.

Francke, B., and Hofschneider, P., 1966, Über infectiöse Substrukturen aus *Escherichia coli* Bakteriophagen. VII. Formation of a biologically intact replicative form in ribonucleic acid bacteriophage M12-infected cells, *J. Mol. Biol.* **16**, 544.

Francki, R., and Matthews, R., 1962, Some effect of 2-thiouracil on the multiplication of turnip yellow mosaic virus, *Virology* **17**, 367.

Franklin, R., 1966, Purification and properties of the replicative intermediate of the RNA bacteriophage R17, *Proc. Natl. Acad. Sci. USA* **55**, 1504.

Fraser, R., 1969, Effects of two TMV strains on the synthesis and stability of chloroplast ribosomal RNA in tobacco leaves, *Mol. Gen. Genet.* **106**, 73.

Fraser, R., 1973, TMV-RNA is not methylated and does not contain a polyadenylic acid sequence, *Virology* **56**, 379.

Frost, R., Harrison, B., and Woods, R., 1967, Apparent symbiotic interaction between particles of tobacco rattle virus, *J. Gen. Virol.* **1**, 57.

Fulton, R., 1962, The effect of dilution on necrotic ringspot·virus infectivity and the enhancement of infectivity by non-infective virus, *Virology* **18**, 477.

Fulton, R., 1972, Inheritance and recombination of strain-specific characters in tobacco streak virus, *Virology* **50**, 810.

Furumoto, W., and Mickey, R., 1967, A mathematical model for the infectivity-dilution curve of tobacco mosaic virus; theoretical considerations, *Virology* **32**, 216.

Furumoto, W., and Wildman, S., 1963, Studies on the mode of attachment of tobacco mosaic virus, *Virology* **20**, 45.

Geelen, J., Van Kammen, A., and Verduin, B., 1972, Structure of the capsid of cowpea mosaic virus, *Virology* **49**, 205.

Gerola, J., Bassi, M., and Favalli, M., 1972, Observations on the sites of virus synthesis in plant cells, *in* "Proceedings of the Second International Congress for Virology, Budapest 1971" (J. Melnick, ed.), pp. 225–226, Karger, Basle.

Ghabrial, S., and Lister, R., 1973, Coat protein and symptom specification in tobacco rattle virus, *Virology* **52**, 1.

Gibbs, A., 1969, Plant virus classification, *Adv. Virus Res.* **14**, 263.

Gibbs, A., Harrison, B., and Murant, A., ed., 1970–1971, "Descriptions of Plant Viruses, Sets 1–4," Commonwealth Mycological Institute and Association of Applied Biologists, London.

Green, M., and Cartas, M., 1972, The genome of RNA tumor viruses contains polyadenylic acid sequences, *Proc. Natl. Acad. Sci. USA* **69**, 791.

Gussin, G., Capecchi, M., Adams, J., Argetsinger, J., Tooze, J., Weber, K., and Watson, J., 1966, Protein synthesis directed by RNA phage messengers, *Cold Spring Harbor Symp. Quant. Biol.* **31**, 257.

Hadidi, A., 1974, The nature of the products of BMV-RNA polymerase, *Virology*, **58**, 536.

Hadidi, A., and Fraenkel-Conrat, H., 1973, Characterization and specificity of soluble RNA polymerase of brome mosaic virus, *Virology* **52**, 363.

Hadidi, A., Hariharasubramanian, V., and Fraenkel-Conrat, H., 1973, Template activity of brome mosaic virus-RNA components with soluble brome mosaic virus RNA polymerase, *Intervirology* **1**, 201.

Hall, T., Shih, D., and Kaesberg, P., 1972, Enzyme mediated binding of tyrosine to brome mosaic virus ribonucleic acid, *Biochem. J.* **129**, 969.

Hariharasubramanian, V., Hadidi, A., Singer, B., and Fraenkel-Conrat, H., 1973, Possible identification of a protein in brome mosaic virus infected barley as a component of viral RNA polymerase, *Virology* **54**, 190.

Harrison, B., and Crockatt, A., 1971, Effects of cycloheximide on the accumulation of tobacco rattle virus in leaf discs of *Nicotiana clevelandii, J. Gen. Virol.* **12**, 183.

Harrison, B., and Murant, A., ed. 1972–1973, "Descriptions of Plant Viruses, Sets 5–7," Commonwealth Mycological Institute and Association of Applied Biologists, London.

Harrison, B., and Woods, R., 1966, Serotypes and particle dimensions of tobacco rattle virus from Europe and America, *Virology* **28**, 610.

Harrison, B., Finch, J., Gibbs, A., Hollings, M., Shepherd, R., Valenta, V., and Wetter, C., 1971, Sixteen groups of plant viruses, *Virology* **45**, 356.

Harrison, B., Murant, A., and Mayo, M., 1972, Two properties of raspberry ringspot virus determined by its smaller RNA, *J. Gen. Virol.* **17**, 137.

Hiebert, E., and McDonald, J., 1973, Characterization of some proteins associated with viruses in the Potato Y group, *Virology* **56**, 349.

Hitchborn, J., and Hills, G., 1968, A study of tubes produced in plants infected with a strain of turnip yellow mosaic virus, *Virology* **35**, 50.

Hohn, T., and Hohn, B., 1970, Structure and assembly of simple RNA bacteriophages, *Adv. Virus Res.* **16**, 43.

Howatson, A., 1970, Vesicular stomatitis and related viruses, *Adv. Virus Res.* **16**, 195.

Hull, R., 1972, The multicomponent nature of broad bean mottle virus, and its nucleic acid, *J. Gen. Virol.* **17**, 111.

Hull, R., and Lane, L., 1973, The unusual nature of the components of a strain of pea enation mosaic virus, *Virology* **55**, 1.

Iwanowski, D., 1892, Über die Mosaikkrankheit der Tabakspflanze, *Bull. Acad. Imp. Sci. St. Petersburg N.S. III* **35**, 65.

Jackson, A., and Brakke, M., 1973, Multicomponent properties of barley stripe mosaic virus ribonucleic acid, *Virology* **55**, 483.

Jackson, A., Mitchell, D., and Siegel, A., 1971, Replication of tobacco mosaic virus, I. Isolation and characterization of double-stranded forms of ribonucleic acid, *Virology* **45**, 182.

Jackson, A., Zaitlin, M., Siegel, A., and Francki, R., 1972, Replication of tobacco mosaic virus. III. Viral RNA metabolism in separated leaf cells, *Virology* **48**, 655.

Jacobson, M., and Baltimore, D., 1968, Polypeptide cleavages in the formation of poliovirus proteins, *Proc. Natl. Acad. Sci. USA* **61**, 77.

Jacquemin, J., 1972, *In vitro* product of an RNA polymerase induced in broadbean by infection with broadbean mottle virus, *Virology* **49**, 379.

Jedlinski, H., 1956, Plant virus.infection in relation to the interval between wounding and inoculation, *Phytopathology* **46**, 673.

Johnston, R., and Bose, H., 1972, Correlation of messenger RNA function with adenylate-rich segments in the genomes of single-stranded RNA viruses, *Proc. Natl. Acad. Sci. USA* **69**, 1514.

Jones, I., and Reichmann, M., 1973, The proteins synthesized in tobacco leaves infected with tobacco necrosis virus and satellite tobacco necrosis virus, *Virology* **52**, 49.

Joubert, J., Hahn, J., von Wechmar, M., and van Regemmortal, M., 1974, Purification and properties of tomato spotted wilt virus, *Virology* **57**, 11.

Kado, C., 1972, Mechanical and biological inoculation principles, *in* "Principles and Techniques in Plant Virology" (C. Kado and H. Agrawal, eds.), pp. 3–31, Van Nostrand Reinhold, New York.

Kado, C., and Agrawal, H., eds., 1972, "Principles and Techniques in Plant Virology," Van Nostrand Reinhold, New York.

Kado, C., and Knight, C. A., 1966, Location of a local lesion gene in tobacco mosaic virus RNA, *Proc. Natl. Acad. Sci. USA* **55**, 1276.

Kado, C., and Knight, C. A., 1968, The coat protein genes of tobacco mosaic virus. I. Location of the gene by mixed infection, *J. Mol. Biol.* **36**, 15.

Kamen, R., 1970, Characterization of the sub-units of Qβ replicase, *Nature (Lond.)* **228**, 527.

Kaper, J., 1972 Experimental analysis of the stabilizing interactions of simple RNA viruses: a systematic approach, *in* "RNA Viruses: Ribosomes" (H. Bloemendal, E. Jaspars, A. Van Kammen, and R. Plants, eds.), pp. 19–41, North-Holland, Amsterdam.

Kaper, J., and Waterworth, H., 1973, Comparison of molecular weights of single-stranded viral RNAs by two empirical methods, *Virology* **51**, 183.

Kassanis, B., 1960, Comparison of the early stages of infection by intact and phenol-disrupted tobacco necrosis virus, *Virology* **10**, 353.

Kassanis, B., 1962, Properties and behavior of a virus depending for its multiplication on another, *J. Gen. Microbiol.* **27**, 477.

Kassanis, B., and Nixon, H., 1961, Activation of one tobacco necrosis virus by another, *J. Gen. Microbiol.* **25**, 459.

Kassanis, B., and Welkie, G., 1963, The nature and behaviour of unstable variants of tobacco necrosis virus, *Virology* **21**, 540.

Kassanis, B., White, R., and Woods, R., 1973, Genetic complementation between middle and bottom components of two strains of radish mosaic virus, *J. Gen. Virol.* **20**, 277.

Kielland-Brandt, M., and Nilsson-Tillgren, T., 1973, Studies on the biosynthesis of TMV RNA and its complementary RNA at different times after infection, *Mol. Gen. Genet.* **121**, 229.

Kleczkowski, A., 1950, Interpreting relationships between the concentrations of plant viruses and numbers of local lesions, *J. Gen. Microbiol.* **4**, 53.

Klein, W., Nolan, C., Lazar, J., and Clark, J., 1972, Translation of satellite tobacco necrosis virus ribonucleic acid. I. Characterization of *in vitro* procaryotic and eucaryotic translation products, *Biochemistry* **11**, 2009.

Kummert, J., and Semal, J., 1972, Properties of single-stranded RNA synthesized by a crude RNA polymerase fraction from barley leaves infected with brome mosaic virus. *J. Gen. Virol.* **16**, 11.

Lafleche, D., Bové, C., DuPont, G. Mouches, C., Astier, T., Garnier, M., and Bové, J., 1972, Site of viral RNA replication in the cells of higher plants: TYMV-RNA synthesis on the chloroplast outer membrane system, *in* "RNA Viruses; Ribosomes" (H. Bloemendal, E. Jaspars, A. Van Kammen, and R. Planta, eds.), pp. 43–65, North-Holland, Amsterdam.

Lane, L., and Kaesberg, P., 1972, Multiple genetic components in bromegrass mosaic virus, *Nat. New Biol.* **232**, 40.

Lauffer, M., and Price, W., 1945, Infection by viruses, *Arch. Biochem.* **8**, 449.

Lister, R., 1966 Possible relationships of virus specific products of tobacco rattle virus infections, *Virology* **28**, 350.

Lister, R., 1968, Functional relationships between virus-specific products of infection by viruses of the tobacco rattle type, *J. Gen. Virol.* **2**, 43.

Lister, R., 1969, Tobacco rattle, NETU, viruses in relation to functional heterogeneity in plant viruses, *Fed. Proc.* **28**, 1875.

Lister, R., and Bracker, C., 1968, Defectiveness and dependence in three related strains of tobacco rattle virus, *Virology* **37**, 262.

Litvak, S., Tarrago, A., Tarrago-Litvak, L. and Allende, J., 1973, Elongation factor-viral genome interaction dependent on the amino-acylation of TYMV and TMV RNAs, *Nat. New Biol.* **241**, 88.

McCarthy, D., Lander, D., Hawkes, S., and Ketteridge, S., 1972, Effects of cycloheximide and chloramphenicol on the multiplication of tobacco necrosis virus, *J. Gen. Virol.* **17**, 91.

Macleod, R., Black, L., and Moyer, F., 1966, The fine structure and intracellular localization of potato yellow dwarf virus, *Virology* **29**, 540.

Mandel, H., Matthews, R., Matus, A., and Ralph, R., 1964, Replicative form of plant viral RNA, *Biochem. Biophys. Res. Commun.* **16**, 604.

Mandeles, S., 1968, Location of unique sequences in tobacco mosaic virus ribonucleic acid, *J. Biol. Chem.* **243**, 3671.

Markham, R., and Smith, K., 1949, Studies on the virus of turnip yellow mosaic, *Parasitology* **39**, 330.

Matthews, R., 1970, "Plant Virology," Academic Press, New York.

Matthews, R., 1973, Induction of disease by viruses, with special reference to turnip yellow mosaic virus, *Annu. Rev. Phytopathol.* **11**, 147.

May, D., and Knight, C. A., 1965, Polar stripping of protein subunits from tobacco mosaic virus, *Virology* **25**, 502.

May, J., Gilliland, J., and Symons, R., 1969, Plant virus-induced RNA polymerase: properties of the enzyme partly purified from cucumber cotyledons infected with cucumber mosaic virus, *Virology* **39**, 54.

May, J., Gilliland, J., and Symons, R., 1970, Properties of a plant virus-induced RNA polymerase in particulate fractions of cucumber infected with cucumber mosaic virus, *Virology* **41**, 653.

Merkens, W., de Zoeten, G., and Gaard, G., 1972, Observations on ectodesmata and the virus infection process, *J. Ultrastr. Res.* **41**, 397.

Mills, D., Kramer, F., and Spiegelman, S., 1973, Complete nucleotide sequence of a replicating RNA molecule, *Science (Wash., D.C.)* **180**, 916.

Minson, A., and Darby, G., 1973, A study of sequence homology between tobacco rattle virus ribonucleic acids, *J. Gen. Virol.* **19**, 253.

Mohamed, N., Randles, J., and Francki, R., 1973, Protein composition of tomato spotted wilt virus, *Virology* **56**, 12.

Montagnier, L., and Sanders, F., 1963, Replicative form of encephalomyocarditis virus ribonucleic acid, *Nature (Lond.)* **199**, 664.

Motoyoshi, F., Bancroft, J., and Watts, J., 1973*a*, A direct estimate of the number of cowpea chlorotic mottle virus particles absorbed by tobacco protoplasts that become infected, *J. Gen. Virol.* **21**, 159.

Motoyoshi, F., Bancroft, J., Watts, J., and Burgess, J., 1973*b*, The infection of tobacco protoplasts with cowpea chlorotic mottle virus and its RNA, *J. Gen. Virol.* **20**, 177.

Mundry, K., and Gierer, A., 1958, Die Erzeugung von Mutationen des Tabakmosaikvirus durch chemische Behandlung seiner Nucleinsäure *in vitro, Z. Vererbungsl.* **89**, 614.

Nazarova, G., Tynl'kina, L., Rodionova, N., Kaftanova, A., and Atabekov, I., 1973, Interaction of disc-like aggregates of virus protein with short fragments of TMV RNA, *Dok. Akad. Nauk SSSR* (Eng. translation) **208**, 969.

Nilsson-Tillgren, T., 1969, Studies on the biosynthesis of TMV. II. On the RNA synthesis of infected cells, *Mol. Gen. Genet.* **105**, 191.

Nilsson-Tillgren, T., 1970, Studies on the biosynthesis of TMV. III. Isolation and characterization of the replicative form and the replicative intermediate RNA, *Mol. Gen. Genet.* **109**, 246.

Nilsson-Tillgren, T., Kolehmainen-Seveus, L., and von Wettstein, D., 1969, Studies on the biosynthesis of TMV. I. A system approaching a synchronized virus synthesis in tobacco leaf, *Mol. Gen. Genet.* **104**, 124.

Ohno, T., Nozu, Y., and Okada, Y., 1971, Polar reconstitution of tobacco mosaic virus, *Virology* **44**, 510.

Okada, Y., and Ohno, T., 1972, Assembly mechanism of tobacco mosaic virus particle from its ribonucleic acid and protein, *Mol. Gen. Genet.* **114**, 205.

Paul, H., and Bode, O., 1955, Elektronemikroskopische Untersuchungen über Kartof-felviren. II. Vermessung der Teilchen von drei Stämmen des Rattle-Virus, *Phy-topathol. Z.* **24**, 341.

Peden, K., and Symons, R., 1973, Cucumber mosaic virus contains a functionally divided genome, *Virology* **53**, 487.

Peden, K., May, J., and Symons, R., 1972, A comparison of two plant virus induced RNA polymerases, *Virology* **47**, 498.

Peterson, J., and Brakke, M., 1973, Genomic masking in mixed infections with brome mosaic and barley stripe mosaic viruses, *Virology* **51**, 174.

Pinck, L., and Hirth, L., 1972, The replicative RNA and viral RNA synthesis rate in tobacco infected with alfalfa mosaic virus, *Virology* **49**, 413.

Pinck, M., Yot, P., Chappeville, F., and Duranton, H., 1970, Enzymatic binding of valine to the 3′ end of TYMV RNA, *Nature (Lond.)* **226**, 954.

Pinck, M., Chan, S., Genevaux, M., Hirth, L., and Duranton, H., 1972, Valine specific tRNA-like structure in RNAs of two viruses of turnip yellow mosaic virus group, 1972, *Biochimie* **54**, 1093.

Pons, M., 1964, Infectious double-stranded poliovirus RNA, *Virology* **24**, 467.

Pring, D., 1972, Barley stripe mosaic virus replicative form RNA: preparation and characterization, *Virology* **48**, 22.

Ralph, R., 1969, Double-stranded viral RNA, *Adv. Virus Res.* **15**, 61.

Ralph, R., and Wojcik, S., 1966, Synthesis of double-stranded RNA by cell-free ex-tracts from turnip yellow mosaic virus-infected leaves, *Biochim. Biophys. Acta* **119**, 347.

Ralph, R. and Wojcik, S., 1969, Double-stranded tobacco mosaic virus RNA, *Virology* **37**, 276.

Ralph, R., Bullivant, S., and Wojcik, S., 1971a, Evidence for the intracellular site of double-stranded turnip yellow mosaic virus, *Virology* **44**, 473.

Ralph, R., Bullivant, S., and Wojcik, S., 1971b, Cytoplasmic membranes a possible site of tobacco mosaic virus RNA replication, *Virology* **43**, 713.

Ralph, R., Matthews, R., Matus, A., and Mandel, H., 1965, Isolation and properties of double-stranded RNA from virus infected plants, *J. Mol. Biol.* **11**, 202.

Rappaport, I., and Wu, J.-H., 1962, Releawe of inhibited virus infection following ir-radiation with ultraviolet light, *Virology* **20**, 472.

Rappaport, I., and Wu, J.-H., 1963, Activation of latent virus infection by heat, *Virology* **20**, 472.

Reddi, K., 1972, Tobacco mosaic virus with emphasis on the events within the host cell following infection, *Adv. Virus Res.* **17**, 51.

Reddy, D., and Black, L., 1973, Electrophoretic separation of all components of double-stranded RNA of wound tumor virus, *Virology* **54**, 557.

Reichmann, M., 1964, The satellite tobacco necrosis virus; a single protein and its genetic code, *Proc. Natl. Acad. Sci. USA* **52**, 1009.

Rezaian, M., and Francki, R., 1973, Replication of tobacco ringspot virus. I. De-tection of a low molecular weight double-stranded RNA from infected plants, *Virology* **56**, 238.

Rice, R., and Fraenkel-Conrat, H., 1973, Fidelity of translation of satellite tobacco ne-crosis virus ribonucleic acid in a cell-free *Escherichia coli* system, *Biochemistry* **12**, 181.

Roberts, B., Mathews, M., and Bruton, C., 1973, Tobacco mosaic virus RNA directs the synthesis of a coat protein peptide in a cell-free system from wheat, *J. Mol. Biol.* **80**, 733.

Romero, J., 1972, RNA synthesis in broadbean leaves infected with broadbean mottle virus, *Virology* **48**, 591.

Rubio-Huertos, M., 1972, Inclusion bodies, *in* "Principles and Techniques in Plant Virology" (C. Kado and H. Agrawal, eds.), pp. 62–75, Van Nostrand Reinhold, New York.

Sakai, F., and Takebe, I., 1972, A non-coat protein synthesized in tobacco mesophyll protoplasts infected by tobacco mosaic virus, *Mol. Gen. Genet.* **118**, 93.

Sänger, H., 1966, Characteristics of tobacco rattle virus. I. Evidence that its two particles are functionally defective and mutually complementary, *Mol. Gen. Genet.* **101**, 346.

Sänger, H., 1969, Functions of the two particles of tobacco rattle virus, *J. Gen. Virol.* **3**, 304.

Sänger, H., and Knight, C. A., 1963, Action of actinomycin D on RNA synthesis in healthy and virus infected tobacco leaves, *Biochem. Biophys. Res. Commun.* **13**, 455.

Sarkar, S., 1965, The amount and nature of ribonuclease sensitive infectious material during biogenesis of tobacco mosaic virus, *Z. Vererbungsl.* **97**, 166.

Schlegel, D., Smith, S., and de Zoeten, G., 1967, Site of virus synthesis within cells, *Annu. Rev. Phytopathol.* **5**, 223.

Schneider, I., Hull, R., and Markham, R., 1972, Multidense satellite of tobacco ringspot virus: a regular series of components of different densities, *Virology* **47**, 320.

Schuch, W., 1973, Association of TMV-RNA with cytoplasmic ribosomes of tobacco leaves, *Virology* **56**, 636.

Scott, H., and Slack, S., 1971, Serological relationship of brome mosaic and cowpea chlorotic mottle viruses, *Virology* **46**, 490.

Sego, J. M., Schneider, I. R., and Koller, Th., 1974, Size determination by electron microscopy of the RNA of tobacco ringspot satellite virus, *Virology* **57**, 459.

Sela, I., 1972, Tobacco enzyme-cleaved fragments of TMV-RNA specifically accepting serine and methionine, *Virology* **49**, 90.

Semal, J., 1970, Properties of the products of UTP incorporation by cell-free extracts of leaves infected with bromegrass mosaic virus or with broadbean mottle virus, *Virology* **40**, 244.

Semal, J., and Hamilton, R., 1968, RNA synthesis in cell-free extracts of barley leaves infected with bromegrass mosaic virus, *Virology* **36**, 293.

Semal, J., and Kummert, J., 1970, Virus-induced polymerase and synthesis of bromegrass mosaic virus in barley, *J. Gen. Virol.* **7**, 173.

Semal, J., and Kummert, J., 1971*a*, Sequential synthesis of double-stranded and single-stranded RNA by cell-free extracts of barley leaves infected with brome mosaic virus, *J. Gen. Virol.* **10**, 79.

Semal, J., and Kummert, J., 1971*b*, *In vitro* synthesis of a segment of bromegrass mosaic virus ribonucleic acid, *J. Gen Virol.* **11**, 189.

Semancik, J., and Reynolds, D., 1969, Assembly of protein and nucleoprotein particles from extracted tobacco rattle virus protein and RNA, *Science (Wash., D.C.)* **164**, 559.

Semancik, J., and Weathers, L., 1972, Exocortis disease: Evidence for a new species of "infectious" low-molecular-weight RNA in plants, *Nat. New Biol.* **237**, 242.

Semancik, J., Morris, T., and Weathers, L., 1973, Structure and conformation of low molecular weight pathogenic RNA from exocortis disease, *Virology* **53**, 448.

Shalla, T., 1968, Virus particles in chloroplasts of plants infected with the U5 strain of tobacco mosaic virus, *Virology* **35**, 194.

Shatkin, A., Sipe, J., and Loh, P., 1968, Separation of ten reovirus genome segments by polyacrylamide gel electrophoresis, *J. Virol.* **2**, 986.

Sheffield, F., 1939, Micrurgical studies on virus-infected plants, *Proc. Roy. Soc. Lond. Ser. B* **126**, 529.

Shepherd, R., 1972, Transmission of viruses through seed and pollen, *in* "Principles and Techniques in Plant Virology" (C. Kado and H. Agrawal, eds.), pp. 267–292, Van Nostrand Reinhold, New York.

Shepherd, R., Wakeman, R., and Romanko, R., 1968, DNA in cauliflower mosaic virus, *Virology* **36**, 150.

Shih, D., and Kaesberg, P., 1973, Translation of brome mosaic viral ribonucleic acid in a cell-free system derived from wheat embryo, *Proc. Natl. Acad. Sci. USA* **70**, 1799.

Shih, D., Lane, L., and Kaesberg, P., 1972, Origin of the small component of brome mosaic virus RNA, *J. Mol. Biol.* **64**, 353.

Shipp, W., and Haselkorn, R., 1964, Double-stranded RNA from tobacco leaves infected with TMV. *Proc. Natl. Acad. Sci. USA* **52**, 401.

Siegel, A., 1959, Mutual exclusion of strains of tobacco mosaic virus, *Virology* **8**, 470.

Siegel, A., 1966, The first stages of infection, *in* "Viruses of Plants" (A. Beemster and J. Dijkstra, eds.), pp. 3–18, North-Holland, Amsterdam.

Siegel, A., 1971, Pseudovirions of tobacco mosaic virus, *Virology* **46**, 50.

Siegel, A., Ginoza, W., and Wildman, S., 1957, The early events of infection with tobacco mosaic virus nucleic acid, *Virology* **3**, 554.

Siegel, A., Zaitlin, M., and Sehgal, O., 1962, The isolation of defective tobacco mosaic virus strains, *Proc. Natl. Acad. Sci. USA* **48**, 1845.

Siegel, A., Zaitlin, M., and Duda, C., 1973, Replication of tobacco mosaic virus. IV. Further characterization of viral related RNAs, *Virology* **53**, 75.

Singer, B., 1971, Protein synthesis in virus-infected plants. I. The number and nature of TMV-directed proteins detected on polyacrylamide gels, *Virology* **46**, 247.

Singer, B., 1972, Protein synthesis in virus-infected plants. II. The synthesis and accumulation of TMV and TMV coat protein in subcellular fractions of TMV-infected tobacco, *Virology* **47**, 397.

Singer, B., and Condit, C., 1974, Protein synthesis in virus-infected plants. III. Effects of tobacco mosaic virus mutants on protein synthesis in *Nicotiana tabacum*, *Virology* **57**, 42.

Slykhuis, J., 1972, Transmission of plant viruses by eriophyid mites, *in* "Principles and Techniques in Plant Virology" (C. Kado and H. Agrawal, eds.), pp. 204–225, Van Nostrand Reinhold, New York.

Spiegelman, S., Pace, N., Mills, D., Levisohn, R., Eikhow, T., Taylor, M., Peterson, R., and Bishop, D., 1968, The mechanism of RNA replication, *Cold Spring Harbor Symp. Quant. Biol.* **33**, 101.

Steere, R., 1955, Concepts and problems concerning the assay of plant viruses, *Phytopathology* **45**, 196.

Steere, R., and Williams, R., 1953, Identification of crystalline inclusion bodies extracted intact from plant cells infected with tobacco mosaic virus, *Am. J. Bot.* **40**, 81.

Steitz, J., 1968, Identification of the A protein as a structural component of bacteriophage R17, *J. Mol. Biol.* **33**, 923.

Sugiyama, T.; Korant, B., and Lonberg-Holm, K., 1972, RNA virus gene expression and its control, *Annu. Rev. Microbiol.* **26**, 467.

Takahashi, W., and Ishii, M., 1953, An abnormal protein associated with tobacco mosaic virus infection, *Nature (Lond.)* **169**, 419.

Takebe, I., and Otsuki, Y., 1969, Infection of tobacco mesophyll protoplasts by tobacco mosaic virus, *Proc. Natl. Acad. Sci. USA* **64**, 843.

Taylor, C., 1972, Transmission of viruses by nematodes, *in* "Principles and Techniques in Plant Virology" (C. Kado and H. Agrawal, eds.), pp. 226–247. Van Nostrand Reinhold, New York.

Teakle, D., 1972, Transmission of plant viruses by fungi, *in* "Principles and Techniques in Plant Virology" (C. Kado and H. Agrawal, eds.), pp. 248–266, Van Nostrand Reinhold, New York.

Thouvenal, J., Guilley, H., Stussi, C., and Hirth, L., 1971, Evidence for polar reconstitution of TMV, *FEBS (Fed. Eur. Biochem. Soc.) Lett.* **16**, 204.

Tollin, P., and Wilson, H., 1971, Some observations on the structure of compinas strain of tobacco rattle virus, *J. Gen. Virol.* **13**, 433.

Ushiyama, R. and Matthews, R., 1970, The significance of chloroplast abnormalities associated with infection by turnip yellow mosaic virus, *Virology* **42**, 293.

Van Griensven, L., and Van Kammen, A., 1969, The isolation of ribonuclease-resistant RNA induced by cowpea mosaic virus: evidence for two double-stranded RNA components, *J. Gen. Virol.* **4**, 423.

Van Kammen, A., 1963, The occurrence of infectious virus ribonucleic acid in the ribosomal fraction from tobacco mosaic virus infected tobacco leaves, *Mededeel. Landbouwhogeschool Wageningen* **63**, 1.

Van Kammen, A., 1968, The relationship between the components of cowpea mosaic virus. I. Two ribonucleoprotein particles necessary for the infectivity of CPMV, *Virology* **34**, 312.

Van Kammen, A., 1972, Plant viruses with a divided genome, *Annu. Rev. Phytopathol.* **10**, 125.

Van Ravenswaaij Claasen, J. C., Van Leeuwen, J. C. J., Duyts, G. A. H., and Bosch, L., 1967, *In vitro* translation of alfalfa mosaic virus RNA, *J. Mol. Biol.* **23**, 535.

Van Vloten-Doting, L. and Jaspars, E., 1972, The uncoating of alfalfa mosaic virus by its own RNA, *Virology* **48**, 699.

Van Vloten-Doting, L., Kruseman, J., and Jaspars, E., 1968, The biological function and mutual dependence of bottom component and top component *a* of alfalfa mosaic virus, *Virology* **34**, 728.

Van Vloten-Doting, L., Dingjan-Versteegh, A., and Jaspars, E., 1970, Three nucleoprotein components of alfalfa mosaic virus necessary for infectivity, *Virology* **40**, 419.

von Wettstein, D., and Zech, H., 1962, The structure of nucleus and cytoplasm in hair cells during tobacco mosaic virus reproduction, *Z. Naturforsch.* **17b**, 376.

Watson, M., 1972, Transmission of plant viruses by aphids, *in* "Principles and Techniques in Plant Virology" (C. Kado and H. Agrawal, eds.), pp. 131–167, Van Nostrand Reinhold, New York.

Weissmann, C., Feix, G., and Slor, H., 1968, *In vitro* synthesis of phage RNA: the nature of the intermediates, *Cold Spring Harbor Symp. Quant. Biol.* **33**, 83.

Weissmann, C., Billeter, M., Goodman, H., Hindley, J., and Weber, H., 1973, Structure and function of phage RNA, *Annu. Rev. Biochem.* **42**, 303.

Whitcomb, R., 1972, Transmission of viruses and mycoplasma by the auchenorrhynchous homoptera, *in* "Principles and Techniques in Plant Virology" (C. Kado and H. Agrawal, eds.), pp. 168–203, Van Nostrand Reinhold, New York.

Wolanski, B., Francki, R., and Chambers, T., 1967, Structure of lettuce necrotic yellow virus. 1. Electron microscopy of negatively stained preparations, *Virology* **33**, 287.

Wood, H., 1972, Genetic complementation between two nucleoprotein components of cowpea mosaic virus, *Virology* **49**, 592.

Woolum, J., Shearer, G., and Commoner, B., 1967, The biosynthesis of tobacco mosaic virus RNA: relationships to the biosynthesis of virus-specific ribonuclease resistant RNA, *Proc. Natl. Acad. Sci. USA* **58**, 1197.

Wu, G., and Bruening, G., 1971, Two proteins from cowpea mosaic virus, *Virology* **46**, 596.

Wu, J.-H., 1963, Extension of the host-range of tobacco mosaic virus by heat activation of latent infections, *Nature (Lond.)* **200**, 610.

Yarwood, C., 1961, Heat activation of plant virus infections, *Virology* **14**, 312.

Zaitlin, M., and Beachy, R., 1974, The use of protoplasts and separated cells in plant virus research, *Adv. Virus Res.* **19**, in press.

Zaitlin, M., and Hariharasubramanian, V., 1970, Proteins in tobacco mosaic virus-infected tobacco plants, *Biochem. Biophys. Res. Commun.* **39**, 1031.

Zaitlin, M., and Hariharasubramanian, V., 1972, A gel electrophoretic analysis of proteins from plants infected with tobacco mosaic and potato spindle tuber viruses, *Virology* **47**, 296.

Zaitlin, M., Spencer, D., and Whitfeld, P., 1968, Studies on the intracellular site of tobacco mosaic virus assembly, *in* "Proceedings of the International Symposium on Plant Biochemical Regulation in Viral and Other Disease or Injury" (T. Hirai, Z. Hidaka, and I. Uritani, eds.), pp. 91–103, Phytopathological Society of Japan, Tokyo.

Zaitlin, M., Duda, C., and Petti, M., 1973, Replication of tobacco mosaic virus. V. Properties of the bound and the soluble replicase, *Virology* **53**, 300.

CHAPTER 3

The Reproduction of Picornaviruses

Leon Levintow

Department of Microbiology
University of California
San Francisco, California 94143

1. INTRODUCTION

The term picornavirus, i.e., small RNA virus, was proposed in 1963 (International Enterovirus Study Group, 1963) as a category encompassing the small, ether-resistant, polyhedral, RNA-containing viruses of man and animals. Having survived for more than a decade in the face of numerous new proposals for the classification of viruses (Lwoff and Tournier, 1971), the term appears to have become firmly rooted in the vocabulary of virology.

Picornaviruses include two main subdivisions which are differentiated on the basis of their stability under mildly acidic conditions. Those which retain their structural integrity and infectivity at pH 3 include the enteroviruses and cardioviruses; those unstable at pH 3 include the rhinoviruses and foot-and-mouth disease virus. The latter subdivision is further distinguished by relatively higher buoyant density of the virion in CsCl solutions (Rueckert, 1971). Additional subdivisions, based on more subtle physicochemical distinctions, have been proposed (Newman *et al.,* 1973).

The distinctive properties of the various subdivisions presumably reflect significant differences between them, at least with respect to the forces which govern the interaction of the structural elements, but no corresponding important differences in their mode of replication are yet apparent. Picornavirus replication has accordingly been considered as a whole in the present discussion, with incidental comment concerning special features pertinent to particular viruses.

The experimental study of picornaviruses from the biochemical point of view became possible with the development by Enders, Weller, and Robbins (1949) of a practical method for the propagation of poliovirus in cultured cells. Other important advances which facilitated subsequent investigation include the development of a plaque assay for infectivity (Dulbecco and Vogt, 1954); the definition in chemical terms of the essential nutrients of cultured cells (Eagle, 1955), making possible the synchronous infection of mass cultures under chemically defined conditions; and the purification, crystallization, and physicochemical characterization of poliovirus (Schaffer and Schwerdt, 1955).

Darnell and Eagle (1960) reviewed the initial decade of the quantitative study of poliovirus replication in cultured cells, and pointed out that it was both the most extensively studied and best understood animal virus system at that time. At least the broad outlines of many important aspects of the interaction of picornaviruses with cells had already been established, or were in the process of being established.

The sequence of events during a one-step growth cycle had been delineated, including the course of synthesis of viral RNA and protein, and the formation and ultimate release of mature progeny (Fig. 1) (Darnell, 1958; Darnell and Levintow, 1960; Darnell et al., 1961). The susceptibility of cells to infection had been shown to be correlated with the presence of specific receptors, and the kinetics of the adsorption of viruses to cells had been studied (Holland and McLaren, 1959; Darnell and Sawyer, 1960). The intrinsic infectivity of isolated picornavirus RNA had been demonstrated (Colter et al., 1957; Alexander et al., 1958), and the early inhibition of the synthesis of cellular RNA, DNA, and protein had been shown to be a characteristic feature of picornavirus infection (Salzman et al., 1959). Experiments with various inhibitors pointed to the independence of viral replication from cellular growth (E. H. Simon, cited in Darnell and Eagle, 1960; Simon, 1961), and the fact that picornaviruses are able to replicate normally in the absence either of DNA synthesis (Salzman, 1960) or of DNA-directed RNA synthesis (Reich et al., 1961) was shortly established.

During the succeeding decade, at least three discoveries with important implications for molecular biology as a whole were first reported for picornavirus systems: the induction of virus-specific, RNA-dependent RNA polymerase (Baltimore and Franklin, 1963a),

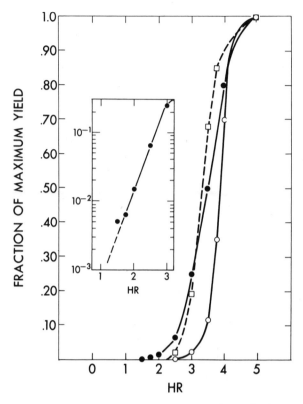

Fig. 1. Time course of appearance in poliovirus-infected HeLa cells of infectious virus (O——O); viral protein, measured as the sum of detectable soluble and particulate antigens (□---□); and viral RNA, measured as uridine incorporated into RNA in the presence of actinomycin D (●——●). The initial portion of the last curve is re-plotted on semilogarithmic coordinates in the inset. Data from Levintow *et al.* (1962), Scharff *et al.* (1963*b*, 1964), and Baltimore *et al.* (1966).

the identification of a base-paired, double-helical replicative form of viral RNA (Montagnier and Sanders, 1963*b*), and the demonstration of the translation of a polycistronic gene product and its subsequent cleavage into functional polypeptide units (Summers and Maizel, 1968; Holland and Kiehn, 1968; Jacobson and Baltimore, 1968*b*).

The foregoing outline of the features of picornavirus replication will be amplified in the present chapter, making use of experimental evidence reported up to about mid-1973.

2. SOME ASPECTS OF THE STRUCTURE AND CHEMISTRY OF PICORNAVIRUSES

2.1. General Considerations

The architecture and physicochemical characteristics of picornaviruses have been reviewed elsewhere (Rueckert, 1971), and a comprehensive treatment of these topics may be found in the chapter on the morphogenesis and *in vitro* assembly of picornaviruses in a later volume of this work; the following brief summary deals only with matters of more or less immediate relevance to replication. Picornaviruses are comprised of a molecule of RNA enclosed in a roughly spherical protein coat about 28–30 nm in diameter. There is no evidence for the presence of lipid as an integral component of the virion, or for the essential presence of any carbohydrate other than the ribose moiety of the RNA. A value around 8×10^6 daltons probably represents the best estimate for the particle weight of the virion, about 30% of which represents RNA. No polyamines or other substances of low molecular weight are specifically associated with the virion.

Pure preparations of picornaviruses are free of detectable cellular material, and the viral nucleic acid and protein are synthesized *de novo* from precursors in the intracellular pool of metabolites (Darnell and Levintow, 1960; Levintow and Darnell, 1960).

2.2. Nature and Organization of Structural Proteins

The capsids of mature virions of all classes of picornaviruses contain equal or nearly equal numbers of four species of polypeptide chains, with molecular weights of 32,000–35,000, 28,000–30,000, 23,000–27,000, and around 7000 daltons, respectively (Rueckert, 1971; Stoltzfus and Rueckert, 1972). In certain cases, at least, a particular "species" may actually be composed of similar, but not identical, polypeptides (Cooper *et al.*, 1970*b*; Vanden Berghe and Boeyé, 1972). In accordance with the nomenclature employed for poliovirus (Summers *et al.*, 1965), the major polypeptides are here designated VP1, VP2, VP3, and VP4, in order of decreasing molecular weight. Analysis of intermediate structures in the morphogenesis of the virion, including the empty capsid or procapsid, make it clear, however, that VP2 and VP4 are not primary building blocks in the assembly process, but are formed by cleavage *in situ* of another polypeptide (designated VP0) at a late stage in the course of morphogenesis (Phillips *et al.*, 1968;

Jacobson and Baltimore, 1968a). In the case of the cardioviruses, approximately one molecule equivalent to VP0 may necessarily persist in each mature virion (Rueckert, 1971).

A reasonable model (Rueckert, 1971) for the structure of the picornavirus capsid postulates that it is built up of 60 identical structural elements, or protomers, originally composed of one copy each of VP1, VP3, and VP0, the last largely replaced by VP2 and VP4 in the mature virion. The 60 protomers are joined by two types of bonding, one holding groups of 5 protomers together to form pentamers, the other holding 12 pentamers together to form a shell with icosahedral symmetry. Although X-ray diffraction patterns and electron micrographs of poliovirus were originally interpreted as evidence for the presence of 60 identical capsomers or morphologic subunits, it is now clear that the number of morphologic units is less, possibly 32 or 42, the uncertainty arising from difficulties in the interpretation of electron micrographs of negatively stained virus preparations. Capsids with both 32 and 42 capsomers, as well as other configurations, are compatible with the postulated model, assuming different modes of grouping juxtaposed polypeptide chains to form the features distinguishable in electron micrographs (Rueckert, 1971).

2.3. Correlations between Structural Organization and Immunological Reactivity

The process of infection gives rise not only to mature virions, but to several other distinguishable virus-specific entities. The mature virion has a sedimentation coefficient on the order of 150 S and a characteristic immunological reactivity, called N or D, different from that of any of the subviral structures (Roizman et al., 1958). Empty capsids, which sediment at about 75 S, are also produced in infected cells, most probably comprising in part precursors of the virion, or procapsids, and in part abortive end products of the infective process (Scharff and Levintow, 1963; Jacobson and Baltimore, 1968a). As indicated above, naturally occurring empty capsids, in distinction to mature virions, include VP0 rather than VP2 and VP4. The immunological reactivity of empty capsids, called H or C, is different from that of mature virions, but is identical to that of virions inactivated by heat or by treatment with various chemical or physical agents (LeBouvier, 1959). The conversion of N-reactive virions to H-reactive particles is typically accompanied by the loss of VP4 (Maizel et al., 1967; Breindl, 1971, Korant et al., 1972).

Purified poliovirus, disrupted into its constituent polypeptides by treatment with 6.5 M guanidine hydrochloride, exhibits an antigenic specificity called S, distinct from that of either virions or empty capsids. Antibodies elicited by guanidine-disrupted poliovirus react with polysome-associated nascent viral protein (Scharff *et al.*, 1963*a*) and with a soluble precursor of the virion in the cytoplasm of the infected cell (Scharff *et al.*, 1964). In addition to the intracellular S-reactive protein, which has a sedimentation coefficient around 5 S, a soluble antigen with a sedimentation coefficient of 14 S is also found in the cytoplasm (Watanabe *et al.*, 1962, 1965; Kerr *et al.*, 1965; Phillips *et al.*, 1968); there is some evidence that the 14 S structure has a distinct antigenic specificity (Ghendon *et al.*, 1968). The significance of the 5 S and 14 S structures is considered further in the discussion of the morphogenesis of the virion (see p. 142).

2.4. Viral RNA

Among the properties which indicate the single-strandedness of the RNA of the virion are asymmetric base composition (Schaffer *et al.*, 1960), sensitivity to ribonuclease (Montagnier and Sanders, 1963*b*), and dependence of sedimentation behavior upon the ionic strength of the solvent (Warner *et al.*, 1963; Montagnier and Sanders, 1963*a*). The inability to form double-stranded structures by annealing (Watanabe, 1965) argues against the presence of any extensive complementary base sequences either within individual molecules or between different molecules.

Measurement of the length of the poliovirus RNA molecule by electron microscopy (Granboulan and Girard, 1969), yields a molecular weight about 2.6×10^6 daltons, corresponding to roughly 7500 nucleotides, a value consistent with the sedimentation coefficient and electrophoretic mobility of the molecule (Tannock *et al.*, 1970). The size of rhinovirus RNA is similar (Brown *et al.*, 1970; Nair and Lonberg-Holm, 1971). Consideration of the molecular weight of the RNA and the mass and composition of the virion indicates that each virion contains a single molecule of RNA.

The poliovirus RNA molecule is linear, possessing unique 5′ and 3′ termini; both terminal residues are adenosine, as the monophosphate at the 5′ end, and unesterified at the 3′ end (Wimmer, 1972; Yogo and Wimmer, 1972). A sequence of adenylic acid residues of variable length occurs immediately adjacent to the 3′-terminal adenosine; different determinations of the average length of the polyadenylic acid sequence are at variance, ranging from about 15 residues in the case of mengovirus (Miller and Plagemann, 1972) to about 90 residues for poliovirus (Yogo and Wimmer, 1972). Methylated bases are apparently absent from picornavirus RNA (Grado et al., 1968).

RNA extracted from picornaviruses can function as mRNA in vitro, specifying the synthesis of virus-specific peptides (Warner et al., 1963; Smith et al., 1970), and RNA similar to the viral RNA in size (Penman et al., 1964) and base composition (Summers and Levintow, 1965) can be extracted from the virus-specific polyribosomes of infected cells. The genomic RNA, being equivalent to mRNA, is designated as the plus strand, according to convention (Baltimore, 1971a).

3. FEATURES OF THE INTERACTION BETWEEN PICORNAVIRUSES AND CELLS

3.1. Ratio of Physical Particles to Infectious Units

The ratio between physical particles and infective units is typically, but not invariably, much greater than unity, even when care is taken to exclude defective or inactivated particles from consideration. Although a wide range of values has been reported, typically about 1000 particles correspond to one plaque-forming unit (PFU) (Schwerdt and Schaffer, 1955). The linear relationship between titer of infectivity and quantity of virus (Dulbecco and Vogt, 1954) rules out the possibility that a number of particles must cooperate to initiate infection; the most reasonable explanation for the disparity is that a given potentially infectious particle is most likely to be wasted in an abortive virus–cell interaction (see p. 120). Since a high multiplicity of infecting virus particles is necessary to insure the simultaneous infection of cells in a mass culture, the consequent presence of many nonparticipating particles makes it difficult to study the fate of the parental genome in the infectious cycle.

3.2. Intracellular Site of Replication

The synthesis of viral protein and RNA, as well as the subsequent steps leading to the formation of mature virus, take place in the cytoplasm of the cell. A cytoplasmic site for viral RNA synthesis was first demonstrated by autoradiography (Franklin and Rosner, 1962; Hausen, 1962), and a membrane-associated "replication complex," including template and nascent RNA and the virus-specific RNA polymerase, was subsequently identified (Girard et al., 1967). Newly synthesized viral protein is associated with viral "plus strand" RNA in specific polyribosomes (Scharff et al., 1963a; Summers and Levintow, 1965). Morphogenesis of virions takes place in the cytoplasmic matrix, and the virions aggregate into crystalline arrays (Dales et al., 1965). In keeping with the independence of virus replication from the genetic apparatus of the cell, enucleated fragments are capable of supporting picornavirus replication (Crocker et al., 1964). Although the infectious cycle may be interrupted at almost any point by a variety of means, there is no indication for the development of any temperate virus–cell interaction in the strict sense. Chronically infected carrier cultures have been described, but virus is produced in such cases by a small fraction of the cells which undergo productive cytocidal infection (Vogt and Dulbecco, 1958).

3.3. Role of Cellular Functions

A number of observations point to a role for cellular functions in picornavirus replication, although available information is fragmentary and inconclusive. Virus multiplication may be more or less sensitive to actinomycin D as a function of the strain of virus (Schaffer and Gordon, 1966), type of host cell (Grado et al., 1965), or various nutritional or physiological factors (Cooper, 1966), suggesting that actinomycin blocks the formation of a necessary cellular product which is limiting under certain circumstances.

A role for some cyclical cell function is suggested by several reports which indicate that the capacity to support virus multiplication may vary during the course of the cellular life cycle. For example, cells arrested in metaphase may (Marcus and Robbins, 1963) [but may not (Johnson and Holland, 1965)] be relatively incapable of supporting the production of poliovirus RNA, and lymphocytes become susceptible to infection only after they have been induced to divide by treatment with phytohemagglutinin (Willems et al., 1969). Finally, marked differences in the kinetics of viral RNA synthesis have been observed in synchronized cells infected at different times in the life cycle, with maximal production in cells infected toward the end of the S phase (Eremenko et al., 1972).

In the case of the RNA-containing bacteriophages, the enzyme responsible for RNA replication includes subunits derived from the host (Eikhom *et al.*, 1968; Blumenthal *et al.*, 1972), but it has not been possible to determine whether the analogous enzyme of picornaviruses is similarly constituted. The only clear indication of the participation of a cellular function in the replication of picornaviruses is provided by the evidence, discussed below, for a critical role of membranes.

4. INFECTIVITY OF PICORNAVIRUS RNA

Isolated picornavirus RNA is infectious, i.e., it is capable under appropriate conditions of initiating the infectious cycle and giving rise to complete, infectious progeny. The extremely low efficiency of infection can be raised by sensitizing the cells and/or inhibiting nucleases by the use of osmotic shock (Koch *et al.*, 1960), polycations (Vaheri and Pagano, 1965), or dimethylsulfoxide (Amstey and Parkman, 1966), thus facilitating effective uptake of the RNA. Even with these agents, however, the infectivity titer of isolated RNA is at least 100-fold, and typically more than 1000-fold, lower than that of the equivalent amount of intact virus. The course of viral growth following infection with isolated RNA is distinctive only in being displaced about 30 minutes earlier than usual (Oppermann and Koch, 1973).

Free complementary or minus strands have been shown to be noninfectious (Roy and Bishop, 1970; Bechet, 1972), but both the double- and multistranded replicative structures possess inherent infectivity, differing in this respect from the corresponding structures of bacteriophages (Montagnier and Sanders, 1963b; Bishop *et al.*, 1969). A number of characteristics of the infectivity of double-stranded RNA are distinctive, including its relative resistance to RNase, formaldehyde, and ultraviolet light (Montagnier and Sanders, 1963b; Pons, 1964; Bishop and Koch, 1967; Bishop *et al.*, 1967). The infectivity of multistranded RNA is partly resistant, and partly sensitive, to such treatment (Bishop and Koch, 1969; Bishop *et al.*, 1969).

The means by which the information inherent in the double-stranded molecules of RNA is expressed in the cell is not clear. The fact that actinomycin D has a differential inhibitory effect on the establishment of infective centers by double-stranded poliovirus RNA (Koch *et al.*, 1967) suggests that an unstable host cell function may be necessary. Presumably, initiation of the infectious cycle would require translation or transcription of the duplex molecule, or separation of its strands, but no close analogy for any of these reactions is known. The phenotype of artificially produced, "heterozygous," double-stranded poliovirus RNA corresponds to the plus strand of the hybrid molecule; in view of the fact that the minus strand is incapable of initiating infection, it is therefore unlikely that transcription of the double-stranded RNA is the initial step in the expression of the information (Best *et al.,* 1972).

5. THE ROLE OF MEMBRANES IN PICORNAVIRUS REPLICATION

Various lines of evidence point to an important, if not indispensable role of membranous structures in the infective process. In distinction to the inhibition of protein, RNA, and DNA synthesis in infected cells, the incorporation of choline into phospholipid is stimulated, in conjunction with the proliferation of smooth membranous vesicles (Penman, 1965; Amako and Dales, 1967; Plagemann *et al.,* 1970). At least the early phases of this phenomenon appear to be dependent on the production of some virus-specific product(s), but the process can continue in the absence of concomitant protein synthesis (Plagemann *et al.,* 1970). The extent to which the stimulation of lipid synthesis is a specific manifestation of the infective process is uncertain, however, since a response of similar character can be elicited by other viruses and by various nonviral noxious agents (King *et al.,* 1959). Particularly in the case of the alterations of lipid metabolism late in the infectious cycle (e.g., Cornatzer *et al.,* 1961), it is not unlikely that the nonspecific cellular response to injury is a major factor.

Electron micrographs of negatively stained sections of poliovirus-infected cells (Horne and Nagington, 1969) suggested that maturation takes place within membrane-bound cytoplasmic structures, and biochemical evidence was obtained for the existence of a membranous entity with which virus-specific polyribosomes and nascent viral protein and RNA are associated (Penman *et al.,* 1964). The foregoing results, in conjunction with evidence for a special class of membrane-bound polyribosomes in infected cells (Penman *et al.,* 1964; Dalgarno *et al.,* 1967), prompted the concept that the sequence of events leading to the production of mature virions occurs within discrete, membrane-bound, "virus-synthesizing bodies."

The literal existence of such structures may be doubted in view of subsequent evidence that (1) the fraction of membrane-bound ribosomes in picornavirus-infected cells is the same as that in corresponding uninfected cells (Roumiatzeff *et al.,* 1971*a*); (2) viral morphogenesis can take place not only in proximity to membranes, but also in the cytoplasmic matrix proper (Dales et al., 1965); and (3) virus-specific polyribosomes can readily be separated from structures concerned with RNA synthesis by a variety of straightforward procedures (e.g., Girard et al., 1967), with each structure retaining its capacity for functional activity in vitro.

Membrane-bound polyribosomes comprise only about 25% of the total in poliovirus-infected and uninfected HeLa cells (Roumiatzeff et al., 1971a), but they are about 5-fold more active in protein synthesis per unit mass than the free polyribosomes, at least as judged by their capacity to incorporate amino acids in vitro (Roumiantzeff et al., 1971b). In the infected cell, the membrane-bound polyribosomes are predominately associated with the more dense, rough fraction of the cellular membranes (Caliguiri and Tamm, 1970a,b).

The intracellular site of viral RNA synthesis can be isolated in the form of a "replication complex," which appears to include one or more RNA polymerase molecules together with template and progeny RNA, associated, in this case, with the less dense, smooth cytoplasmic membranes (Caliguiri and Tamm, 1970b). The functional capacity of the replication complex is dependent on the association with membranes; the membrane-bound complex is capable of labeling all the forms of viral RNA, including single-stranded RNA, in vitro, but detergent-treated soluble preparations generally are functionally impaired and produce little single-stranded RNA (e.g., Plagemann and Swim, 1968). However, as discussed below (p. 133), the manner in which the membranes affect enzymatic function is by no means clear.

In summary, the weight of available evidence suggests that viral RNA synthesis and viral protein synthesis are distinct processes, both geographically and functionally, with membranes playing important, albeit incompletely defined roles in each case.

6. EARLY EVENTS IN THE INFECTIOUS CYCLE

The adsorption of picornaviruses to susceptible cells is mediated by the interaction of the viral capsid with specific receptors on the cell membrane. No morphologically distinct viral structures have been implicated in the process, but the involvement of VP4, one of the capsid polypeptides, is suggested by its absence from virions which have reacted with cells (Crowell and Philipson, 1971; Lonberg-Holm and Korant, 1972). The precise role of VP4, however, is uncertain in view of the evidence that the isolated polypeptide is unreactive, and at least

certain particles which lack VP4 as a distinct polypeptide are
nevertheless able to adsorb to cells (Noble and Lonberg-Holm, 1973).
In any case, the active site does not include glycoprotein, which is apparently absent from picornaviruses (Burness *et al.*, 1973).

Characterization of the cellular receptors is likewise incomplete.
The capacity of cells to adsorb virus is generally unaffected by
treatment with neuraminidase (Zajac and Crowell, 1965; Lonberg-
Holm and Korant, 1972); encephalomyocarditis virus, and presumably
other cardioviruses, may represent exceptions to the rule (Kozda and
Jungeblut, 1958). This generalization also may not apply in the case of
bovine enterovirus, the receptors for which are sensitive to neuraminidase (Stoner *et al.*, 1973); this property may be related to the selective
affinity of bovine enterovirus for malignant cells (Taylor *et al.*, 1971;
Sedmak *et al.*, 1972). Receptors for different classes of picornaviruses
are functionally independent and geographically distinct, and differ in
their susceptibility to proteolytic enzymes (Zajac and Crowell, 1965;
Lonberg-Holm and Korant, 1972). Membrane preparations from susceptible cells and soluble lipoprotein fractions derived from such
preparations are capable of interacting with virions and altering them
in a more or less specific manner (Philipson and Lind, 1964; Chan and
Black, 1970).

The initial virus–cell interaction has generally been reported to be
independent of temperature (e.g., Mak *et al.*, 1970), but apparently this
conclusion is not universally valid, since the rate of attachment of at
least some picornaviruses to cells has been shown to vary with the
temperature (Lonberg-Holm and Korant, 1972). The reason for this
discrepancy is not evident.

Two alternate fates may befall an adsorbed virion: it may be
released into the medium in altered form (elution), or it may enter the
cell (penetration). As indicated above, eluted virus lacks VP4, one of
the structural polypeptides; it is not capable of reattaching to cells, and
its structural integrity, depending on the type of virus, is more or less
compromised (Joklik and Darnell, 1961; Fenwick and Cooper, 1962;
Hall and Rueckert, 1971). Comparatively little elution is observed
when the particle: infectious unit ratio is low (Homma and Graham,
1965); presumably, greater likelihood of penetration is correlated with
higher efficiency of infection.

Penetration of adsorbed virus may be equated with the disappearance or eclipse of the infecting virus as a biological entity, with the
establishment of an infective center not neutralizable with antiviral
serum, or, in biochemical terms, with the release of the viral RNA in a
form accessible to nucleolytic enzymes. It is not clear whether

uncoating in the sense of separation of the capsid from the RNA takes place on the cell surface or intracellularly; possibly, different picornaviruses differ in this respect (Mandel, 1967; Hall and Rueckert, 1971). In any event, a considerable portion of the cell-associated viral RNA is promptly degraded to acid-soluble products, and only a small fraction of the input RNA persists as such in the cell (Joklik and Darnell, 1961).

Surprisingly little morphological evidence is at hand concerning the process of penetration and uncoating of the infecting virus. It has been proposed that the virus enters the cell by engulfment into a vacuole (Mandel, 1962; Dales, 1973), but micrographs which illustrate a direct penetration of the plasma membrane also have been published (Dunnebacke et al., 1969).

The specificity of the initial virus–cell interaction plays an important role in the determination of the host range of picornaviruses. For example, the distinctive susceptibility of primate cells to infection with poliovirus is correlated with the presence of specific receptors (McLaren et al., 1959). However, naturally insusceptible nonprimate cells, which lack the receptors, are capable of supporting a single cycle of poliovirus replication after infection by viral RNA (Holland et al., 1959). Susceptibility of a cell is not entirely or invariably a function of the receptors; the restriction of picornavirus replication in certain cells with fully functional receptors has been shown to be correlated with deranged production of viral RNA at a later point in the infectious cycle (Wall and Taylor, 1970).

7. INHIBITION OF THE BIOSYNTHETIC PROCESSES OF THE HOST CELL

7.1. General Considerations

A characteristic early feature of picornavirus infection is the inhibition of cellular protein, RNA, and DNA synthesis. The rapidity and extent of the shutoff varies widely with different viruses, and is also dependent on the species of the host, e.g., the inhibitory effect of mengovirus infection is more rapid and profound in mouse than in human cells (McCormick and Penman, 1967).

7.2. Effects of Infection on the Synthesis of Cellular Protein

The virus-induced inhibition of cellular protein synthesis is paralleled by progressive disaggregation of the polyribosomes; the

remaining fraction of polyribosomes at a given time, however, appears
to be at the most only slightly altered with respect to size, constitution,
and functional capacity (Summers and Maizel, 1967; Leibowitz and
Penman, 1971). The ribosomes themselves are apparently unaltered
and remain capable of being recruited into virus-specific
polyribosomes. No gross qualitative or quantitative changes in tRNA
have been observed. The inhibition of protein synthesis can take place
when the formation of mRNA is relatively unaffected (see below), and,
in any case, the inhibition typically occurs too rapidly to be ascribed
simply to decay of mRNA.

The foregoing considerations lead to the hypothesis that a
substance is produced in infected cells which selectively interferes with
the attachment of cellular mRNA to ribosomes. The substance in
question is presumably virus-specific, since inhibition of protein synthesis not only requires the integrity of the viral genome but can take
place when the synthesis of cellular mRNA is blocked by actinomycin
(Penman and Summers, 1965). Blockade of at least the bulk of virus-
specific RNA and protein synthesis by guanidine (Penman and Summers, 1965) also does not prevent the shutoff of host protein synthesis,
but, in this case, appreciable amounts of at least certain species of viral
RNA continue to be made (Noble and Levintow, 1970). The interference by poliovirus, in doubly infected cells, with the growth of
herpes simplex virus (Saxton and Stevens, 1972) or vesicular stomatitis
virus (Doyle and Holland, 1972) resembles the inhibition of cellular
protein synthesis in a number of respects and may be effected by a
similar mechanism. The identity of the substance which mediates the
shutoff is unknown, as is the means by which it presumably is able to
discriminate between host and viral mRNA. Of possible relevance to
this question is the fact that poliovirus double-stranded RNA (Ehrenfeld and Hunt, 1971), as well as other species of double-stranded RNA
(Robertson and Mathews, 1973), have the property of inhibiting the
translation of endogenous or exogenous mRNA in cell-free systems,
probably by interfering with the binding of mRNA to ribosomes
(Kaempfer and Kaufman, 1973). The translation of viral and nonviral
mRNA however, at least in the systems which have been studied, is inhibited indiscriminately.

Perhaps coincidentally, double-stranded RNA is also a potent inducer of interferon, and may even be a common denominator of interferon induction (Colby and Duesberg, 1969). Interferon, in a sense,
may be considered the converse of the hypothetical virus-induced inhibitory substance since it inhibits the synthesis of viral, but not

cellular, protein. In this case also, the means by which viral and cellular processes are differentiated is poorly understood.

7.3. Inhibition of Cellular RNA Synthesis

The pattern of virus-induced inhibition of RNA synthesis is qualitatively as well as quantitatively different in different cells, e.g., both ribosomal RNA and mRNA are rapidly and profoundly affected in mengovirus-infected L cells, but HeLa cells infected by the same virus manifest only a relatively slow decline in the rate of appearance of ribosomal RNA (McCormick and Penman, 1967). The inhibition of the formation of ribosomal RNA appears to be the resultant of several phenomena: depression of synthesis of the 45 S precursor of ribosomal RNA and interference with one or more of the subsequent steps leading to the formation of mature ribosomes (Darnell *et al.*, 1967). The disturbances of ribosome maturation are unlike those caused by cycloheximide, implying that the effect is not simply secondary to the inhibition of protein synthesis (Darnell *et al.*, 1967). Inhibition of RNA methylation has been observed after infection by foot-and-mouth disease virus (Vande Woude *et al.*, 1970), but extensive interference with ribosome production in poliovirus-infected HeLa cells takes place without any appreciable effect on the methylation of the precursors of ribosomal RNA (Darnell *et al.*, 1967).

The inhibition of cellular RNA synthesis is paralleled by a reduction of the activity of the crude nuclear DNA-dependent RNA polymerase, which cannot be ascribed to loss, degradation, or impaired template activity of the cellular DNA (Baltimore and Franklin, 1962a; Holland and Peterson, 1964). Inhibition of the RNA polymerase from uninfected cells by a cytoplasmic extract of infected cells has been reported (Balandin and Franklin, 1964), but the specificity and significance of this phenomenon has been questioned (Martin and Kerr, 1968). The fact that the inhibition of RNA synthesis is prevented by irradiation of the infecting virus (Franklin and Baltimore, 1962) or by agents which interfere with protein synthesis (Baltimore *et al.*, 1963b) implies that the inhibition is mediated by a virus-specific protein, but the identity and site of action of the postulated inhibitory protein have not been established.

7.4. Inhibition of DNA Synthesis

The inhibition of DNA synthesis in picornavirus-infected cells takes place without appreciable effect on the activities of several enzymes related to DNA replication, and the rate of elongation of DNA chains is unaltered. The effects of infection on DNA synthesis can be reproduced by treating uninfected cells with inhibitors of protein synthesis, and it is supposed that in both cases the initiation of DNA synthesis is limited by the availability of a putative regulatory protein (Ensminger and Tamm, 1970; Hand *et al.*, 1971; Hand and Tamm, 1972). In any event, available evidence is consistent with the view that the inhibition of DNA synthesis and mitosis in infected cells is probably secondary to virus-induced inhibition of protein synthesis.

7.5.   Degeneration and Death of the Infected Cell

It is uncertain whether the characteristic degeneration and ultimate death of the picornavirus-infected cell simply represent further manifestations of the same processes which bring about inhibition of the synthesis of cellular macromolecules. Some of the uncertainty may arise from the difficulty in defining cell degeneration in precise terms. Apart from various descriptive criteria (Lwoff *et al.*, 1955; Dales and Franklin, 1962), degeneration has been equated with loss of ability to bind vital stains (Cordell-Stewart and Taylor, 1971), stimulation of the incorporation of choline into cell membranes (Amako and Dales, 1967; Collins and Roberts, 1972), and the release of lysosomal enzymes (Wolff and Bubel, 1964). The degenerative changes are not the simple consequence of the inhibition of protein, RNA, or DNA synthesis; experiments with various inhibitors of virus replication (e.g., Bablanian *et al.*, 1965) make it clear that although the phenomenon is not dependent on the completion of the full replicative cycle, the production of some virus-specific product(s) is necessary. Double-stranded viral RNA, extracted from cells infected with a bovine enterovirus, rapidly kills uninfected cells (Cordell-Stewart and Taylor, 1971, 1973), but degeneration can occur in mengovirus-infected cells even when the production of double-stranded RNA is almost completely inhibited (Collins and Roberts, 1972). A substance with properties of a lipid, which both inhibits RNA synthesis and is cytotoxic, has been extracted from poliovirus-infected cells (Ho and Washington, 1971), but its nature and possible role in the infectious process remain to be clarified.

8.   SYNTHESIS OF VIRAL PROTEIN

8.1.   Formation and Function of Virus-Specific Polyribosomes

The site of viral protein synthesis is a polyribosome with a sedimentation coefficient of about 350 S, apparently comprised of the entire plus strand of viral RNA associated with approximately 35 ribosomes (Summers *et al.*, 1967). Presumably, the association of the incoming parental RNA with ribosomes is a prerequisite for the subsequent events in the infectious cycle, and in fact such an association is demonstrable if steps are taken to minimize the contribution of the nonparticipating fraction of the inoculum (Levy and Carter, 1968). However, formulation of a mechanism which would enable the incoming RNA molecule to act first as messenger directing the synthesis of RNA polymerase and subsequently as template for the synthesis of the first minus strand of RNA presents difficulties which have not been satisfactorily resolved. In brief, either the RNA would have to be cleared of ribosomes to permit the progress of the polymerase in the opposite direction, or the polymerase would have to be able to displace the ribosomes.

As discussed below (p. 131), much of the single-stranded viral RNA which is produced early in the infectious cycle is destined for incorporation into polyribosomes. Evidence has been obtained (Huang and Baltimore, 1970) that a newly synthesized RNA molecule is released from its site of synthesis in free form, and that it associates with a ribosome or ribosomal subunit within a few minutes. A polyribosome is formed by the progression of the initial ribosome down the mRNA and the attachment of additional ribosomes, the entire process of assembly requiring about 10 minutes.

As discussed in a previous section (p. 119), the association of virus-specific polyribosomes with membranes may be critical or essential for their functional activity. It has been reported (Fenwick and Wall, 1972), the the membrane-bound poliovirus-specific polyribosomes contain a species of cellular protein not found either in free polyribosomes or in single ribosomes, but the significance of this finding is unclear.

8.2. Kinetics of Synthesis of Viral Protein

It has been estimated that the time required for a ribosome to traverse a molecule of picornavirus RNA is of the order of five minutes (Huang and Baltimore, 1970). Late in the infectious cycle, the average size of virus-specific polyribosomes decreases as a consequence of the reduction of the number of ribosomes from 35 to about 20, and the time required for the translation of the message is increased (Summers *et al.*, 1967).

Protein which is immunologically virus-specific can first be detected in the infected cell about half an hour in advance of the onset of maturation (Scharff *et al.*, 1964), and the course of synthesis of structural protein, as determined by measuring the incorporation of labeled amino acid into virions, proceeds somewhat faster than maturation (Darnell and Levintow, 1960). The existence, at mid-cycle, of a sizable pool of precursors of structural protein is indicated by the fact that there is a lag of 20 minutes between the addition of isotopically labeled amino acid and the appearance of isotope in virions (Penman *et al.*, 1964), but the composition of the pool, which presumably contains a series of intermediate polypeptides and subviral structures, has not been defined.

8.3. Initiation of Protein Synthesis

The translation of picornavirus RNA is most probably initiated at a single point on the molecule, not far from the 5′ end. One persuasive argument for this model is the fact that a primary gene product, representing virtually all of the information in the RNA, can be demonstrated under appropriate conditions (Jacobson *et al.*, 1970; Kiehn and Holland, 1970). Confirmation is provided by various lines of evidence discussed below, including the analysis of the effects of pactamycin on viral protein synthesis, and by the demonstration that a single N-terminal peptide is specified by picornavirus RNA *in vitro* with mammalian ribosomes and factors (Öberg and Shatkin, 1972; Smith, 1973). As discussed more fully below, there is no apparent difference between the initiation of viral protein synthesis and that of cellular protein in general (Chatterjee *et al.*, 1973). In both cases, the N-terminal amino acid of nascent peptides is methionine, donated in unacylated form by Met–tRNA$_f^{Met}$, a specific "initiator" species of tRNA (Öberg and Shatkin, 1972; Smith, 1973).

The apparent similarity between cellular and viral initiation signals makes it more difficult to formulate a model for the selective inhibitory effect of interferon on viral protein synthesis. It has been reported that ribosomes prepared from cells previously treated with interferon are relatively unresponsive to added mRNA, whether of viral origin or not; this evidence leads to the suggestion that interferon acts by virtue of its recognition of exogenous RNA in general rather than viral mRNA *per se* (Falcoff *et al.*, 1972). Whether the sequence of polyadenylate at the 3′ end of the viral RNA serves a function in protein synthesis is unsettled; in any case, it is difficult to envisage any specific role for it in the initiation of translation.

8.4 Polypeptide Synthesis and Cleavage

Analysis of extracts of infected cells by gel electrophoresis resolves a wide spectrum of virus-specific polypeptides, the sum of whose molecular weights exceeds by several times the theoretical coding capacity of the viral RNA (Maizel and Summers, 1968). Moreover, certain peptides are preferentially labeled during a short pulse of radioactive amino acids, and certain larger species lose and other smaller species gain label during a "chase" of unlabeled amino acids. These considerations led to the concept that various viral peptides arise by the cleavage of larger primary products (Summers and Maizel, 1968; Holland and Kiehn, 1968; Jacobson and Baltimore, 1968b).

A polypeptide corresponding approximately to the entire coding capacity of the RNA was subsequently identified when infection was carried out in the presence of amino acid analogues (Jacobson et al., 1970) or when infection was initiated at 43°C (Baltimore, 1971b). A similar "giant polypeptide" has been observed in at least one case without the use of some special maneuver (Kiehn and Holland, 1970), but generally no product larger than 100,000 daltons is formed in the infected cell unless cleavage is inhibited in some manner. Three major primary products are typically observed, and it is supposed that these peptides arise by cleavage of the ultimate precursor before (or simultaneously with) its release from the polyribosome.

Figure 2 depicts an example of the electrophoretic analysis of the peptides in cardiovirus-infected cells labeled by a brief pulse of radioactive amino acids, followed by a "chase" of unlabeled amino acids. The three panels represent the patterns obtained with a 5-minute pulse of label followed by chases of 1, 10, and 90 minutes, and illustrate the transfer of label from primary products to polypeptides formed secondarily by cleavage.

Analysis of the effects of the drug pactamycin on the pattern of labeling of virus-specific peptides has provided, on the one hand, independent validation of the concept of a single initiation site for the translation of picornavirus RNA, and, on the other hand, a means for ordering the gene products and constructing a genetic map. At appropriate concentrations, the addition of pactamycin to infected cells prevents the initiation of protein synthesis but has comparatively little effect on the completion of peptide chains already initiated (Taber et al., 1971; Summers and Maizel, 1971). Therefore, the farther a nucleotide sequence is from the initiation site, the more likely it is to be translated during the "run-off" after the addition of the drug. In other words, the amount of a particular gene product formed in the presence

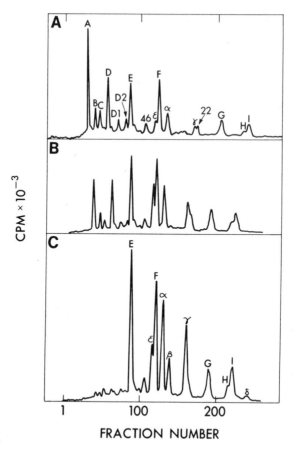

Fig. 2. Distribution of radioactivity among encephalomyocarditis virus-specific polypeptides after a 5-
minute exposure to radioactive amino acids, followed
by a "chase" of unlabeled amino acids for 1 minute
(A); 10 minutes (B); and 90 minutes (C) (analysis by
polyacrylamide gel electrophoresis). The peaks labeled
α, β, γ, and δ are equivalent to the poliovirus-specific
peptides VP1, VP2, VP3, and VP4, respectively; ϵ corresponds to VP0; and A is the precursor of the structural proteins. See Fig. 3 for identification of other
peaks. From Butterworth and Rueckert (1972*b*) with the
kind permission of the authors.

of the drug, relative to the amount formed in its absence, should be a
direct measure of the distance of the corresponding gene from the 5′
end of the RNA.

Genetic maps for picornaviruses of several subgroups have been
constructed in this manner. The results with the different viruses are
closely analogous, and in each case the genes can be ordered in a single

linear array (Rekosh, 1972; Butterworth and Rueckert, 1972*a,b*;
McLean and Rueckert, 1973). The gene for the precursor which gives
rise to the structural proteins is found closest to the origin of the
genetic map, and the order of the individual capsid proteins (in the
poliovirus nomenclature) is VP4–VP2–VP3–VP1. Study of genetic
interactions between temperature-sensitive mutants of poliovirus (p.
150) also suggests that the coat protein genes are clustered near one
end of the genetic map.

Analysis of the pattern of virus-specific polypeptides labeled under
various conditions, with and without pactamycin, permits the construction of a model for the synthesis and processing of the viral protein, an
example of which is shown in Fig. 3. The precursor of the structural
proteins, plus two other major primary products, account for most of
the information encoded in the viral RNA. One of the other primary
polypeptides is stable, and the other is apparently cleaved to yield at
least two distinct products. The functional roles of the nonstructural
peptides are unknown.

It is clear that peptide cleavage is an enzymatic process, but the
identity of the putative enzyme(s) is unknown. Generally similar pat-

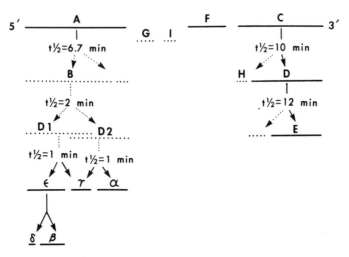

Fig. 3. Model for the synthesis and cleavage of encephalomyocarditis virus-specific proteins based on data such as those shown
in Fig. 2, and based on the gene order determined with the aid of the
drug pactamycin (p. 127). Translation proceeds from left to right;
dotted arrows and lines indicate tentatively identified reactions and
products. The half-life ($t^{1/2}$) of each intermediate is indicated for
all except ϵ, which cleaves at a constant rate. Modified from Butterworth and Rueckert (1972*b*) by permission of the authors.

terns of cleavage are observed with the same virus in different host cells (Kiehn and Holland, 1970), but various inhibitors of proteolytic enzymes affect the process of cleavage differently in different cells (Korant, 1972; Summers *et al.*, 1972). Although viral proteins synthesized *in vitro* do not ordinarily undergo typical cleavage (Öberg and Shatkin, 1972; Roumiantzeff *et al.*, 1971*b*), capsid proteins can be produced *in vitro* by incubation of their precursor with extracts of infected cells (Korant, 1972). These results, among others, suggest that proteolytic cleavage is catalyzed by preexisting cellular enzymes, possibly activated or released in the course of infection, and that the specificity of cleavage, i.e., the susceptibility of particular peptide bonds, is probably determined by the structure of the substrate. The fact that defective or "ambiguous" cleavage is observed with certain mutant virus strains (Cooper *et al.*, 1970*b*; Garfinkle and Tershak, 1971) is consistent with this view.

8.5. Synthesis of Viral Protein *In Vitro*

Early attempts to translate picornavirus RNA *in vitro* with homologous or heterologous ribosomes and soluble factors met with only limited success (e.g., Warner *et al.*, 1963; Summers and Levintow, 1965), but extensive, faithful translation has subsequently been obtained with more refined techniques. A system comprised of ribosomes, tRNA, and soluble factors from *Escherichia coli* faithfully translates relatively short sequences of poliovirus RNA with the production of a number of peptides initiated by N-formylmethionine, and it has been concluded that eight or more unnatural internal initiation signals are recognized by the bacterial system (Rekosh *et al.*, 1970). With mammalian ribosomes and factors under optimal conditions, on the other hand, translation of cardiovirus RNA is initiated at a single site, and peptides up to about 100,000 daltons are formed (Öberg and Shatkin, 1972; Smith, 1973). For unexplained reasons, cardiovirus RNA is more efficient than poliovirus RNA in this system. N-terminal N-formylmethionine is incorporated with the mammalian system when the correspondingly charged tRNA is provided, but the absence of this amino acid from animal cells indicates that synthesis is normally initiated by the transfer of unblocked methionine from the non-formylated "initiator" species of tRNA, Met–tRNA$_t^{Met}$. A similar mode of initiation has been proposed for globin synthesis (Housman *et al.*, 1970). In both cases, the N-terminal methionine is rapidly removed from the nascent protein, but the removal is prevented when the methionine is formylated. In the case of encephalomyocarditis virus, the N-terminal sequence of amino acids specified *in vitro* does not correspond to any known sequence in the coat protein; this suggests either the loss of additional amino acids or the initiation of synthesis with a nonstructural "lead in" protein (Smith, 1973).

9. SYNTHESIS OF VIRAL RNA

9.1. Time Course of Synthesis of Viral RNA

The course of synthesis of viral RNA has been followed in several ways: by determining the titer of infectious RNA in a culture during the course of the infectious cycle (Darnell *et al.*, 1961), by measuring the incorporation of isotopically labeled uridine into virus-specific RNA in a culture infected in the presence of actinomycin D (Scharff *et al.*, 1963b), and by adding a labeled precursor at different times and measuring the specific activity of the RNA incorporated into mature virions (Darnell *et al.*, 1961). In each instance, the course of formation of the bulk of the RNA was found to precede the course of appearance of infectious virus by no more than half an hour (cf. Fig. 1). This relationship suggests that the pool of RNA destined to be incorporated into virions is small, a conclusion which is borne out by the fact that labeled RNA can be detected in mature virions within 5 minutes of its synthesis (Baltimore *et al.*, 1966). The latter result, in conjunction with the fact that the amount of viral RNA in polyribosomes at mid-cycle is comparatively large, indicates that pathways by which RNA is incorporated into polyribosomes and into mature virions are largely separate.

A relatively small amount of viral RNA can be detected in infected cultures considerably in advance of the appearance of infectious virus. This early RNA accumulates exponentially between 90 minutes (or earlier) and 3 hours after infection (Fig. 1, inset) and is largely destined for incorporation into polyribosomes (Baltimore *et al.*, 1966). The major portion of the RNA, which is formed between 3 and 5 hours after infection, accumulates in linear fashion at a rate of about 2000–3000 molecules per cell per minute. It has been suggested (Baltimore, 1969) that the apparently exponential increase in infectious virus during part of the same period is a consequence of the availability of a progressively expanding pool of viral protein. The time necessary for the synthesis of a molecule of viral RNA has been estimated to be about 45 seconds (Baltimore, 1969).

9.2. Induction of RNA-Dependent RNA Polymerase or Replicase

Implicit in the finding that picornaviruses replicate independently of the synthesis or template activity of DNA is the existence of an enzyme capable of polymerizing ribonucleotides under the direction of an RNA template. The first evidence for an enzyme of this description was obtained with mengovirus-infected cells: all four ribonucleoside triphosphates are required, the product is a heteropolymer, and in distinction to the cellular DNA-dependent RNA polymerases, the activity is found in the cytoplasm and is insensitive to actinomycin D (Baltimore and Franklin, 1962b, 1963a; Franklin and Baltimore, 1962; Baltimore et al., 1963a).

The course of appearance of polymerase activity in the infected cell generally parallels the course of viral RNA synthesis. The induction of the enzyme is prevented by general inhibitors of protein synthesis and by agents, such as guanidine, which specifically block virus replication; the activity rapidly falls if ongoing production of the enzyme is interrupted by the addition of either a general or specific inhibitor (Eggers et al., 1963). The apparent instability of the enzyme is in accord with the observation that viral RNA synthesis is dependent on concurrent protein synthesis (Scharff et al., 1963b).

In view of the foregoing considerations, and by analogy with the case of bacteriophage Qβ, it seems likely that the polymerase is, or includes, a product of the viral genome, but it has not been possible to assign this role to any of the known virus-specific peptides.

As isolated from cytoplasmic extracts, enzymatic activity is associated with the "replication complex," including protein, nucleic acids, and smooth cytoplasmic membranes. Such crude membrane-bound enzyme preparations carry out reactions which appear to be a valid reflection of the processes by which viral RNA is duplicated in the cell; the three characteristic species of viral RNA are labeled in vitro, and the sequence of labeling is similar, albeit on a compressed time scale, to the pattern observed in the intact cell. Moreover, it is possible to demonstrate the transfer of label from the multistranded replicative intermediate to single-stranded RNA, thus confirming a precursor–product relationship which cannot, for technical reasons, be clearly demonstrated in the intact cell. (Girard, 1969; McDonnell and Levintow, 1970).

The function in vitro of membrane-bound polymerase preparations is apparently limited, however, to the completion, against pre-existing template strands, of "plus" strands previously initiated in the cell (Girard, 1969; Dietzschold and Ahl, 1970). Dissociation of the membranous complex with detergents yields a soluble enzyme–template complex, but such preparations generally produce little or no single-stranded RNA and exhibit other evidence of functional impairment (e.g., Plagemann and Swim, 1968). In explanation of this effect, it has been proposed (McDonnell and Levintow, 1970) that the template and products of the enzyme are sequestered in the membrane-bound enzyme complex, and that dissolution of the membranes renders the single-stranded portion of the RNA accessible to adventitious nucleases. If this view is correct, the association of the enzyme with membranes may be neither specific nor essential.

Be that as it may, attempts to obtain soluble, purified, fully active preparations of picornavirus-induced RNA polymerase have not been notably successful. Purification to the point of template dependence has not thus far been possible, and the best soluble preparations (Arlinghaus and Polatnick, 1968; Ehrenfeld et al., 1970) exhibit no greater functional capacity than the crude membrane-bound complex. An enzyme which catalyzes the polymerization of guanylate residues in response to added polycytidylate has been obtained from cells infected with encephalomyocarditis virus, but it is not clear that this activity is in fact a manifestation of the virus-specific RNA polymerase (Rosenberg et al., 1972).

9.3. Multistranded Species of RNA: Replicative Form (RF) and Replicative Intermediate (RI)

Proceeding from the example of the double-stranded replicative form of the single-stranded DNA bacteriophage ϕX174, Montagnier and Sanders (1963b) sought and found an analogous RNase-resistant species of RNA in extracts of picornavirus-infected cells. As summarized below, the properties of this structure, termed replicative form or RF, indicate that it is a double-helical molecule made up of a strand of viral RNA base-paired to a complementary strand.

Another class of virus-specific RNA, distinct from both single- and double-stranded RNA but sharing some properties of each, can also be extracted from picornavirus-infected cells. Analogous to the replicative intermediate or RI of bacteriophage R17 (Fenwick et al., 1964), this species of RNA is heterogeneous, partly RNase-resistant, and preferentially labeled by brief pulses of radioactive precursor (Baltimore and Girard, 1966). The properties of picornavirus RI, discussed in some detail below, lead to its formulation as a double-stranded "core" with several attached single-stranded "tails" of variable length. Electron micrographs of structures corresponding to this model have been obtained; the cores correspond to the viral genome in length, and there are, on the average, 4–5 tails per core (Savage *et al.*, 1971).

Both RF and RI have been prepared separately in purified form, taking advantage of various properties including differential solubility in *ca.* 1M salt and affinity for various chromatographic adsorbents (see Bishop and Levintow, 1971).

9.4. Relationship of Extracted RF and RI to Intracellular Structures

It has been proposed in the case of RNA-containing bacteriophages that RF and RI assume their base-paired RNase-resistant character only upon deproteinization and that their actual intracellular counterparts are loosely associated complexes of enzyme, template, and nascent RNA (Weissmann *et al.*, 1968). This view is based on the observation that much of the nascent RNA in an untreated enzymatic reaction mixture has the properties of single-stranded RNA, including sensitivity to RNase, and also that double-stranded RNA is inactive as a template for phage polymerase. On the other hand, treatment of a mixture of plus and minus strands under conditions used for extraction of RI and RF does not produce any detectable multistranded RNA, and the observed properties of the nascent RNA in the reaction mixture do not necessarily indicate the presence of free single-stranded RNA.

The existence of loosely associated replicative structures in poliovirus-infected cells has also been proposed on the basis of the finding that treatment of the cells with diethyl pyrocarbonate prior to extraction of the RNA reduces the yield of RF and RI and permits the detection of a small amount of free minus strands (Öberg and Philipson, 1971).

In any case, however, in view of the characteristic physicochemical and biological properties of the extracted multistranded forms of RNA described below, it appears certain that the complementary strands of RNA within the cell, if not literally hydrogen-bonded to each other, must at least be extensively aligned in a specific configuration. In other words, there is little reason to doubt that the extracted structures are accurate reflections of their native intracellular counterparts and, hence, valid objects for the study of the replication of viral RNA.

9.5.   Formation and Fate of RF and RI

The distinctive properties of RF, RI, and single-stranded (SS) RNA, including electrophoretic mobility (Noble *et al.*, 1969; Öberg and Philipson, 1969), make it possible to follow the course of incorporation of labeled precursor into each species during the infectious cycle. As depicted in Fig. 4, labeled RF accumulates in the infected cell at a constant rate during most of the course of the cycle, thus suggesting that RF may not be immediately relevant to the production of SS RNA. On the other hand, although RI is the most rapidly labeled species at all times, its accumulation in the cell reaches a plateau at

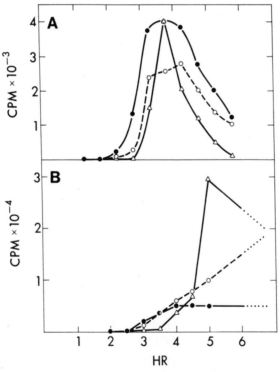

Fig. 4.   A comparison of (A) rates of labeling of poliovirus-specific RNA species during successive 30-minute intervals after infection and (B) accumulation of these three species in the infected cell: RI (●——●), RF (O---O), and SS RNA (△——△). RNA synthesis measured by incorporation of uridine in the presence of actinomycin D; species of RNA separated by gel electrophoresis. Modified from Noble and Levintow (1970).

mid-cycle. Labeled SS RNA appears later than either RF or RI, but it becomes the predominant species at mid-cycle. Late in the cycle, there is a decline in the amount of SS RNA, presumably as a result of the loss or degradation of molecules not incorporated into virions, and RF becomes the predominant species (Noble and Levintow, 1970).

It is difficult to demonstrate a precursor–product relationship between one species of RNA and another in intact animal cells because of the sluggish response of the intracellular pool of precursors of RNA to changes in the medium, i.e., incorporation of labeled compounds cannot be abruptly terminated (Darnell, 1968). However, experiments *in vitro* with membrane-bound enzyme preparations confirm the conclusion that RI is a functional intermediate in the synthesis of SS RNA, and they indicate further that RF is largely a collateral by-product (Girard, 1969; McDonnell and Levintow, 1970). However, there is some evidence that, at least under certain circumstances, RF is able to give rise to functional RI (Noble and Levintow, 1970).

9.6.   Properties of RF

The base composition of RF is in accord with a structure composed of a strand of viral RNA plus a complementary strand. It differs from SS RNA in its relative resistance to RNase in solutions of moderate ionic strength, its solubility in *ca.* 1 M salt solutions, its relatively low sedimentation coefficient, and its relatively low density in Cs_2SO_4 (Montagnier and Sanders, 1963*b*; Bishop and Koch, 1967). RF undergoes a sharp, reversible, thermal transition which is apparent not only by a hyperchromic shift, but also by a transition from RNase resistance to RNase sensitivity (Bishop and Koch, 1967). Denaturation of the molecule with dimethyl sulfoxide (Katz and Penman, 1966; Bishop *et al.*, 1969) yields intact plus and minus strands.

As discussed in a preceding section, native RF is inherently infectious, and the infectivity, which is determined by the plus strand, is resistant to exposure to RNase, formaldehyde, or ultraviolet light. A covalently linked 3′-terminal sequence of polyadenylate is present in the plus strand of RF; a complementary sequence of polyuridylate is present at the 5′ terminus of the minus strand (E. Wimmer, personal communication; see p. 140).

9.7.   Properties of RI

Unlike RF, preparations of RI are insoluble in 1 M NaCl, an indication of the presence of a substantial single-stranded component.

The sedimentation coefficient of RI ranges between 20 and 70 S, and its buoyant density is intermediate between those of RF and SS RNA (Baltimore, 1968a; Bishop et al., 1969).

The course of thermal denaturation of RI is biphasic—a gradual rise in optical density at relatively low temperatures, representing denaturation of the single-stranded tails being followed by a sharp increase in the optical density, representing denaturation of the base-paired portion of the molecule. The products of denaturation include (1) a fraction indistinguishable from the viral genome in size and comprised of both plus and minus strands and (2) a heterogeneous population of smaller material, largely segments of the plus strand.

Partial digestion of RI with RNase yields a double-stranded "core" which resembles RF in sedimentation coefficient, buoyant density, and electrophoretic mobility. Unlike RF, cores yield not only intact single strands on denaturation, but a collection of shorter fragments as well. About 90% of the intact single strands derived from cores are minus, and 10% are plus; conversely, the shorter pieces are predominantly, if not exclusively, fragments of plus strands (Bishop et al., 1969; Bishop and Levintow, 1971; Savage et al., 1971).

Some 10% of the infectivity of purified preparations of RI is resistant to treatment with formaldehyde or RNase, and the remainder is sensitive to both reagents (Bishop et al., 1969). The infectivity which survives RNase treatment is associated with the cores; this evidence suggests the presence of intact, hydrogen-bonded, plus strands, and, in fact, infectious single-stranded RNA can be recovered by denaturing cores with dimethyl sulfoxide (Bishop et al., 1969). These results suggest that purified RI preparations include two classes of molecules: (1) a minor class in which an intact plus strand is fully complexed to a minus strand and (2) a major class in which no intact plus strand is hydrogen-bonded to an extent sufficient to protect it from attack by RNase or formaldehyde.

9.8. Mechanism of Replication of RNA

Granting the relevance of extracted RI to elucidation of the mechanism by which RNA is duplicated in the cell, consideration of its physicochemical and biological properties provides certain insights into the process. The fact that a great majority of full-length, fully base-paired strands of RNA in RI are minus strands suggests that the mechanism of replication is largely semiconservative, i.e., plus strands are transcribed against a conserved minus strand and displace the

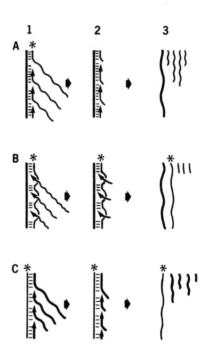

Fig. 5.   Alternative formulations of the structure of RI: (A) "semiconservative" RI; (B) "conservative" RI; and (C) "semiconservative, negative" RI. Column 1 illustrates the structures as isolated from the cell; column 2, "cores" produced by treatment with RNase; and column 3, treatment of "cores" with dimethyl sulfoxide. In each case, light lines signify plus strands or fragments thereof; heavy lines, minus strands; and short dashes, forces holding complementary strands together. Asterisks indicate full-length, infectious, plus strands.

existing plus strand of the duplex in the process (Fig. 5). This con-clusion is supported by the finding that a large proportion of the ra-dioactivity in pulse-labeled RI is found in RNase-resistant plus strands, i.e., the nascent RNA is largely hydrogen-bounded to the tem-plate (Girard, 1969).

The significance of the minor fraction of RI which contains intact, infectious, fully based-paired, plus strands is less clear. One possible in-terpretation of this finding is that a conservative mechanism of replication, i.e., production of plus strands from a conserved duplex template, is also utilized, albeit to a minor extent.

It is also possible that this finding is indicative of the existence of "negative RI." Some 5–10% of RNA produced during the course of the infectious cycle consists of minus strands in one form or another (Baltimore and Girard, 1966). The generation of minus strands by a semiconservative mechanism converse to that involved in the production of plus strands would give rise to cores containing intact plus strands. However, this explanation for the presence of some intact plus strands in cores requires that a corresponding fraction of the shorter segments be incomplete minus strands. There are published data which suggest the possibility that this may be the case (Savage et al., 1971), but a careful search for small segments of minus strands among the products of denatured cores was unsuccessful (J. M. Bishop, personal communication). The question of the existence of negative RI, and the question of the origin of negative strands as well, accordingly remain in doubt.

A final explanation for the presence of full-length plus strands in cores follows from the concept that the intracellular counterparts of RF and RI are loosely associated structures which assume their base-paired character only upon extraction (Weissmann et al., 1968). According to this view, the complexes of template, nascent strands, and enzyme "collapse" upon deproteinization to form either "conservative" or "semiconservative" RI, "positive" or "negative" as the case may be. This view leads to a "symmetrical" model of RNA replication which obviates need for any distinction between conservative and semiconservative mechanisms (Fig. 6). The process cannot be strictly symmetrical, however, in view of the 10-fold disparity between the rates of production of plus and minus strands. Also, the observed properties of the extracted RI are not in accord with completely random "collapse" of the putative, loose, replicative complexes.

In distinction to the foregoing models, all of which involve the participation of linear molecules no longer than unit length, a mechanism of RNA replication involving a circular template has been proposed, in analogy to the model for the replication of DNA (Gilbert and Dressler, 1968). The basis for this model was the identification of virus-specific, single-stranded, linear RNA longer than the viral genome in foot-and-mouth disease virus-infected cells (Brown and Martin, 1965; Wild et al., 1968); a similar observation has been reported with at least one other picornavirus (Clements and Martin, 1971), but such reports are isolated exceptions to the usual findings with picornaviruses in general.

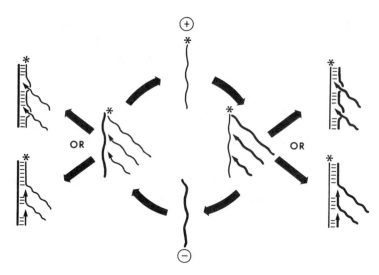

Fig. 6. "Symmetrical" model of RNA replication (symbols as in Fig. 5).The putative loosely associated replicative structures are indicated in the center of the figure; the alternative base-paired structures derived from them are shown at the left and right. Simplified after Weissmann *et al.* (1968).

Several other observations, if not fully explained, are at least compatible with the existence of circular intermediates, e.g., the sensitivity of virus replication to ethidium bromide (Semmel *et al.,* 1973) and the presence, in electron micrographs of preparations of RF, of a minor fraction of circular structures (Agol *et al.,* 1972). An RNA ligase presumably capable of cyclizing a molecule of RF has been detected in mammalian cells (Cranston *et al.,* 1973). The presence of a sequence of polyadenylate at the 3′ end of the plus strand of poliovirus RF, in conjunction with the supposed presence of a complementary sequence of polyuridylate at the 3′ end of the minus strand, was originally interpreted as evidence for the transient existence of a cyclic molecule (Yogo and Wimmer, 1973); the subsequent determination that the polyuridylate is actually located at the 5′ end of the minus strand, however, makes this observation irrelevant to the question of possible circular intermediates (E. Wimmer, personal communication). In summary, a variety of observations suggest the possible involvement of circular intermediates in RNA replication, but direct evidence of a functional role for such structures is lacking.

10. REGULATION OF THE VIRAL GROWTH CYCLE

In the case of the RNA-containing bacteriophages, it is probable that specific interactions between viral macromolecules play an important part in the growth cycle, e.g., capsid protein can form a complex with single-stranded RNA and thereby repress the translation of the polymerase cistron, or, alternatively, it can bind to RI and interrupt transcription (see Stavis and August, 1970; also, pp. 22, 23). Whether or not analogous control mechanisms operate during the replicative cycle of picornaviruses is uncertain. It has been proposed that the complex of VP0, VP1, and VP3 can bind both to the larger ribosomal subunit and to single-stranded viral RNA, thereby exercising variable control over the production of viral RNA and protein; experimental support for this scheme, however, is provided only by some evidence for the existence of structures with the properties of the putative regulatory complexes (Caliguiri and Mosser, 1971; Cooper et al., 1973).

A contrary view holds that the sequence of events in the infectious cycle can be accounted for without recourse to any specific regulatory mechanisms (Baltimore, 1969). According to this view, the switch from exponential to linear accumulation of single-stranded RNA, for example, is explicable by supposing that it simply reflects the attainment of a balance between the rates of formation and decay of RI. Further, it is supposed that assembly of virions begins only when the intracellular concentration of precursors of the capsid reaches a certain level, and the initiation or termination of other steps in the replicative cycle is similarly determined by the concentration of critical reactants. The fact that there is no difference in the relative amounts of the various virus-specific polypeptides produced at widely different times after infection (Summers et al., 1967) has been adduced as an argument against the operation of specific controls. Also, cells infected with defective-interfering particles of poliovirus (see p. 153) produce viral RNA despite the fact that the defective capsid protein is rapidly degraded; this evidence argues against a necessary role for capsid protein in the events prior to assembly (Cole and Baltimore, 1973a).

In summary, the question of the operation of specific regulatory interactions in the replication of picornaviruses is unsettled, but no persuasive evidence in favor of mechanisms of this sort has yet been obtained.

11. ASPECTS OF THE MORPHOGENESIS OF PICORNAVIRUSES

In view of their comprehensive treatment elsewhere in this work, matters relating to morphogenesis of the virion are only briefly considered here. Although the virion can be dissociated by 6.5 M guanidine into polypeptides with a sedimentation coefficient of about 2 S, the smallest recognizable virus-specific entity in the infected cell sediments at 5-6 S and probably corresponds to the "immature protomer," i.e., a complex of VP0, VP1, and VP3 (Scharff *et al.*, 1964; Phillips *et al.*, 1968). Presumably, the protomer arises immediately upon cleavage of the precursor of the capsid proteins, and the individual dissociated polypeptides do not exist independently as such.

The next recognizable stage in the course of morphogenesis is represented by a structure which sediments at 14 S (Watanabe *et al.*, 1962, 1965; Kerr *et al.*, 1965; Phillips *et al.*, 1968), the size and composition of which is consistent with its formulation as an aggregate of five of the 5-6 S units, i.e., it is equivalent to the proposed pentameric subunit of the capsid (Rueckert, 1971). The 14 S units are capable under certain conditions of aggregating spontaneously to form a particle with a sedimentation coefficient of 73 S, indistinguishable in this and other respects from the naturally occurring empty capsid (Phillips, 1971). The formation of empty capsids from 14 S units is promoted by crude extracts of infected, but not uninfected, cells (Phillips *et al.*, 1968; Phillips, 1969); this activity has been ascribed to the rough membranes of the cell (Perlin and Phillips, 1973). A role for membranes in the earlier stages of morphogenesis has also been proposed; possibly, the membranes serve to promote the assembly process by adsorbing and concentrating the reactants (Perlin and Phillips, 1973).

The empty capsid appears to be a usual, if not obligatory, precursor of the complete virion. Empty capsids of poliovirus which accumulate in the presence of guanidine are converted to virions upon removal of the inhibitor, and the pattern of labeling of virus-specific structures in the cell is consistent with the sequence: 14 S particle → empty capsid → virion (Jacobson and Baltimore, 1968a).

The mechanism by which the empty capsid, or procapsid, interacts with RNA to form the virion is unknown and difficult to picture. The process requires not only the insertion or enwrapment of the RNA, but also the cleavage of all the VP0 molecules to VP2 and VP4. There is a report suggesting that, at least in certain host cells, procapsids may not necessarily be involved in the process of morphogenesis (Ghendon *et al.*, 1972).

12. INHIBITION OF MULTIPLICATION OF PICORNAVIRUSES

12.1. General Considerations

A number of agents prevent, interrupt, or otherwise modify the replication of picornaviruses *in vitro*; these include general inhibitors such as puromycin and cycloheximide which do not discriminate between viral and cellular processes and compounds such as guanidine and 2-(α-hydroxybenzyl)-benzimidazole (HBB) which in one manner or another specifically block the replicative cycle. Furthermore, the multiplication of picornaviruses is sensitive to the environment of the infected cell, i.e., ionic strength of the medium, temperature, etc. Also, picornavirus multiplication is subject to interference by homologous or heterologous viruses, mediated both by interferon and by other mechanisms. Apart from their interest as possible chemotherapeutic agents, inhibitors have served as probes for the elucidation of various steps in the growth cycle; some instances of the latter use of inhibitors have already been mentioned, and other examples are discussed below.

12.2. Agents Which Interfere with Protein Synthesis

Puromycin and cycloheximide, which inhibit protein synthesis by dissimilar mechanisms, have similar inhibitory effects on the replication of picornaviruses. In brief, these inhibitors prevent the initiation of, or promptly interrupt the progress of, the synthesis of both viral protein and viral RNA (Levintow *et al.*, 1962; Baltimore and Franklin, 1963*b*; Scharff *et al.*, 1963*b*). The production of mature virions proceeds, but only to the extent permitted by existing pools of building blocks. As mentioned in the discussion of the properties of the virus-induced RNA polymerase, the rapid inhibition of RNA synthesis is paralleled by a corresponding decline in the activity of the polymerase; enzymatic activity, however, is unaffected by the addition of either inhibitor to a reaction mixture *in vitro*. The decline in the production of RNA takes place with relatively little alteration of the relative amounts of RI, RF, and single-stranded RNA, and the latter is release from the replication complex in normal fashion (Baltimore, 1968b; Noble and Levintow, 1970). In summary, the inhibitory effects of cycloheximide and puromycin on viral RNA synthesis appear to be a reflection of the rapid turnover or decay of RNA polymerase following the block of its formation. It is likely that two other agents which inhibit growth of picornaviruses, phenethyl alcohol (Plagemann, 1968) and diphtheria toxin (Duncan and Groman, 1967), also act by virtue of their general inhibitory effect on protein synthesis.

Rather than inhibiting protein synthesis, p-fluorophenylalanine (FPA) exerts its effects primarily by being incorporated in place of phenylalanine and giving rise to more or less defective proteins. The effects of FPA on picornavirus multiplication are variable, depending on the degree to which it replaces phenylalanine in viral proteins. With relatively little substitution, determined by a low ratio of FPA to phenylalanine in the medium, nearly normal amounts of viral RNA and virus-specific antigens are formed, but the titer of infectious virus is sharply reduced. With increasing degrees of substitution, the formation both of RNA and of recognizable viral antigens is progressively inhibited. With maximum substitution, the effects of FPA resemble those of puromycin (Scharff et al., 1965). These observations suggest that there is progressive functional impairment of viral proteins with increasing replacement of phenylalanine by FPA, and that various viral functions vary in their sensitivity to the presence of FPA. As discussed in another section, at least one effect of the presence of FPA and other amino acid analogues is impairment of the cleavage of the precursors of the functional viral proteins.

Other inhibitors of protein synthesis have been exploited in the experimental study of picornaviruses. A noteworthy example, described in the discussion of viral protein synthesis, is the use of pactamycin to determine the order of the viral genes. Sparsomycin, which selectively inhibits peptide chain elongation vis à vis initiation, has been used to identify the N-terminal peptide formed in vitro under the direction of encephalomyocarditis virus RNA (Smith, 1973).

12.3. Agents Which Affect RNA Synthesis

As already discussed, interference with DNA-directed RNA synthesis affects the growth of picornaviruses only under exceptional circumstances. Cordycepin, which blocks the post-transcriptional addition of polyadenylate to cellular mRNA, either does not affect viral replication (Penman et al., 1970), or causes only moderate inhibition

(E. Wimmer, personal communication); in the latter case, viral RNA formed in the presence of the drug contains the normal complement of polyadenylate.

In the presence of 5-fluorouracil, the yield of poliovirus is only moderately reduced, but up to 35% of the uracil residues in the viral RNA may be replaced by the analogue (Munyon and Salzman, 1962). Virus which contains fluorouracil is fully infectious, but the analogue is mutagenic and it confers increased sensitivity to ultraviolet light (Cooper, 1964; Tershak, 1964, 1966). The inhibitory effect of 2,6-diaminopurine on the growth of poliovirus is reversed by adenine, suggesting that this inhibitor may also act at the level of RNA synthesis (Munyon, 1964).

At least one inhibitor of viral RNA synthesis, N-methylisatin-β-4′:4′-dibutylthiosemicarbazone, has a demonstrable inhibitory effect on the activity *in vitro* of the virus-induced RNA polymerase (Pearson and Zimmerman, 1969). Addition of the fungal metabolite gliotoxin at the appropriate time in the growth cycle immediately interrupts the synthesis of viral RNA with little effect on the production of viral protein; no information is available on the mode of action or the basis of the selectivity (Miller *et al.*, 1968).

Infectious virus is produced in the presence of acridine dyes such as proflavine when the growth cycle takes place in the dark; the dye is presumably bound to RNA of the newly formed virus, which is thereby rendered sensitive to visible light (Crowther and Melnick, 1961; Wilson and Cooper, 1962; Schaffer, 1962). The inhibitory effects of pyronine and ethidium bromide on the growth of picornaviruses have been explained in terms of the affinity of these compounds for the double-stranded species of viral RNA (Semmel and Huppert, 1970; Semmel *et al.*, 1973).

12.4. Specific Inhibitors of Picornaviruses

A group of compounds, of which guanidine is by far the best-studied example, selectively inhibits the replication of certain picornaviruses with minimal effects on the host cell. Only certain strains of certain enteroviruses (and of foot-and-mouth disease virus) are sensitive to guanidine, other strains of the same viruses are resistant to the effects of the drug, and still other strains multiply only in its presence (Loddo *et al.*, 1962; Dixon *et al.*, 1965). The inhibitory effect of guanidine can be reversed by a variety of compounds, e.g., choline, and a number of amino acids (Lwoff and Lwoff, 1964b; Dinter and

Bengtsson, 1964). Many characteristics of the antiviral properties of guanidine are shared by certain other compounds, particularly-2-(α-hydroxybenzyl)-benzimidazole (HBB) (Eggers and Tamm, 1961) and D-penicillamine (Gessa *et al.,* 1966); to what extent the analogies indicate similarity in mode of action, however, is not clear.

In any case, despite intensive study for more than a decade, many questions concerning the effects of guanidine remain unanswered. With sensitive strains of virus, 1–2 mM guanidine prevents the formation of infectious virus, or promptly interrupts ongoing maturation. The early steps in the growth cycle, up to and including at least the switch-off of cellular protein synthesis, proceed in the presence of the drug (Penman and Summers, 1965).

Guanidine has a prompt and striking effect on ongoing viral RNA synthesis, but it does not completely suppress it (Baltimore, 1968*b*; Noble and Levintow, 1970). Of the three species of virus-specific RNA, single-stranded RNA is inhibited to the greatest degree, and RF to the least degree. The labeling and turnover of RI continues at a reduced rate, and it appears to have fewer tails or growing points. The molecules of RF which accumulate in the presence of guanidine apparently include inactive templates; on removal of the drug, there is an immediate resumption of synthesis of all three species of RNA at an enhanced rate. The activity of virus-induced RNA polymerase in infected cells falls with time after the addition of guanidine, but the drug has no effect on enzyme activity *in vitro* (Baltimore *et al.,* 1963*a*).

The rate of synthesis of viral protein diminishes relatively slowly after the addition of guanidine, and the normal spectrum of proteins continues to be formed during this interval (Jacobson and Baltimore, 1968*a*). Despite the continued synthesis of viral protein and at least some single-stranded viral RNA, the formation of mature virions is abruptly interrupted (Baltimore, 1968*b*). The RNA remains associated with an aberrant form of the replication complex (Baltimore, 1968*b*), and the protein is organized into either empty capsids (Halperen *et al.,* 1964; Jacobson and Baltimore, 1968*a*) or smaller precursors of the virion (Ghendon *et al.,* 1972). Empty capsids which accumulate in the presence of guanidine are converted into mature virus upon removal of the drug (Jacobson and Baltimore, 1968*a*).

The effects of guanidine differ in a number of respects from those of agents which primarily inhibit protein synthesis (Noble and Levintow, 1970), and the effects likewise cannot be explained by postulating a specific block in the formation of functional RNA polymerase. The continued formation and turnover of RI is incompatible with a primary block of initiation of synthesis of single-stranded RNA. It has been proposed that guanidine acts in some manner to prevent release of single-stranded RNA from the replication complex, thereby blocking entry of RNA into polyribosomes and virions (Baltimore, 1968*b*, 1969).

In any case, the locus at which guanidine acts and the structural basis for its activity are unknown. Likewise, little is known concerning the means by which certain amino acids and sundry other compounds antagonize its inhibitory effect. The definition of guanidine dependence in molecular terms is even less clear.

13. GENETICS OF PICORNAVIRUSES

13.1. General Comments

It may be said that this entire chapter, concerned with the ways and means by which picornaviruses are reproduced, deals with genetics in the broad sense of the word; the present section, however, deals with matters germane to genetics in a narrower sense—induced and naturally occurring variation of picornaviruses, the interactions between variant forms which may take place in the course of the growth cycle, and related topics. The impetus for much of the early study of picornaviruses from this point of view was provided by the search for attenuated or avirulent strains of poliovirus suitable for use as live vaccines (e.g., Sabin *et al.,* 1954). A large number of strains with various mutant characters, associated in some instances with reduced neurovirulence, were isolated by serial passage under more or less selective conditions; the first evidence for genetic interaction between dissimilar strains was reported in 1962 (Hirst, 1962; Ledinko, 1962). Mutagenic agents have been employed to increase the number and variety of mutants (Dulbecco and Vogt, 1958), and conditionally lethal mutants, particularly mutants which fail to grow at a certain temperature (Lwoff, 1958) have been exploited for genetic analysis.

Study of the genetics of picornaviruses and similar small RNA-containing viruses has been hindered by a number of inherent problems; these problems have been discussed at length by Cooper (1969). Briefly, these problems include a high rate of spontaneous occurrence (and reversion) of mutation, and "leakiness," i.e., partial expression of the character of the wild type. Also, in comparison with the T-even bacteriophages, for example, the scope of complementation between mutants is sharply restricted and the frequency of apparent genetic recombination is low. The low rate of recombination may simply be a consequence of the small size of the genome, but several technical problems further complicate the task of genetic analysis, including the necessity for high multiplicities of virus to initiate infection and the possibility of aggregation of the infecting virus particles. Further problems arise from the covariation of many of the observed mutant characteristics, due perhaps to double mutations or to dual expression of the same mutation. Although some of these problems may be minimized by various measures, the genetic analysis of picornaviruses by the classical techniques of bacteriophage genetics has been both difficult and of limited value.

13.2.   Isolation and Characterization of Mutants

A variety of mutant characters of poliovirus were identified in the search for markers correlated with reduced neurovirulence; these include sensitivity or resistance to various inhibitors, sensitivity or resistance to thermal inactivation, small plaque size, and many others [see Cooper (1969) for a comprehensive list]. Many of the strains which have been described were isolated by serial passage of standard viral stocks under altered conditions of growth, and thus probably bear multiple mutations. Strains selected for reduced neurovirulence generally are also unable to grow at elevated temperature; this correlation will be considered further in the course of the following discussion of temperature-sensitive mutants.

The various mutagenic agents which have been employed in the attempt to obtain mutants suitable for genetic analysis include proflavine (Dulbecco and Vogt, 1958), nitrous acid (Boeyé, 1959), and 5-fluorouracil (Cooper, 1964). Strains selected by a single passage under selective conditions after treatment with a mutagenic agent are more likely to bear mutations at a single locus, but many such mutants are unsuitable for study because of intolerably high rates of reversion.

13.3.   Effects of Temperature on the Growth of Picornaviruses; Properties of Temperature-Sensitive Mutants

In general, optimal growth of picornaviruses takes place within a relatively narrow temperature range. The optimal zone for the multiplication of a virulent strain of poliovirus may be $37° \pm 2°C$; attenuated strains of poliovirus, and rhinoviruses in general, typically grow best in a range several degrees lower.

The disturbances of viral growth at supraoptimal temperatures are both general and specific. The general effects of elevated temperature operate to the detriment of all viruses and include such phenomena as disturbed function of polyribosomes (Shea and Plagemann, 1971), enhanced activation of lysosomes, and enhanced release of nucleases (Fiszman *et al.,* 1970; Adler *et al.,* 1973). In HeLa cells, for example, single-stranded viral RNA not enclosed in virions is rapidly degraded late in the infectious cycle; this process is exaggerated at higher temperatures. In such cells, presumably, successful replication at elevated temperatures is a function of prompt enclosure of the viral RNA; conversely, any block in the assembly of virions would lead to a secondary loss of RNA.

In addition to being susceptible to the general detrimental effects of elevated temperature, certain mutant viral strains bear one or more specific temperature-sensitive lesions. As mentioned above, attenuated vaccine strains of poliovirus are generally unable to grow at elevated temperatures, and a wide variety of other temperature-sensitive mutants have been isolated after the use of mutagenic agents.

The Sabin vaccine strain of poliovirus Type 1, designated LSc, 2ab, is a particularly well-studied and illustrative example of an attenuated strain which is also temperature-sensitive. Replication is normal at 36°C, but the formation of both the infectious virus and viral RNA is sharply restricted at 40°C (Tershak, 1969). The amount of RNA polymerase induced by the mutant virus at 40°C is diminished, but once induced, the enzyme is fully active at 40°C (Priess and Eggers, 1968). In contrast to the foregoing observations, however, the formation of mature infectious virus is inhibited by 90% at 38.5°C, with only moderate interference with the formation of viral RNA (Fiszman *et al.,* 1972). At the lower restrictive temperature it is possible to demonstrate a block in the morphogenesis of the virion at a point between the cleavage of the primary gene product and the assembly of the 14 S subunit of the capsid. The absence of viral RNA at high temperatures, therefore, may represent either its degradation secondary to the defect in maturation, or, possibly, a second temperature-sensitive lesion. The possibility of yet an additional lesion is suggested by the fact that a block at an earlier stage in the processing of viral protein is demonstrable with nominally the same strain under somewhat different conditions (Garfinkle and Tershak, 1971). Finally, the probability of an alteration of a structural component of the virion is suggested by its altered chromatographic behavior (Hodes *et al.,* 1960). It should be noted that the strain was originally isolated under conditions favorable for the accumulation of multiple mutations; whether the reduced virulence is necessarily correlated with any or all of the temperature-sensitive functions is not clear.

Many of the temperature-sensitive mutants which can be isolated after the use of mutagenic agents revert with high frequency, but others are reasonably stable and exhibit functional incapacities of various sorts at nonpermissive temperatures (McCahon and Cooper, 1970; Cooper et al., 1970a,b; Shea and Plagemann, 1971). Such mutants may be considered to bear "structural" or "nonstructural" defects on the basis of several criteria. Structural mutants generally produce some antigenically recognizable protein (Wentworth et al., 1968) and at least some species of RNA under nonpermissive conditions, but no mature virus is formed; the virions in many cases are unusually labile to heat (McCahon and Cooper, 1970). Virions with structural defects may also be more susceptible to disruption by high concentrations of urea (Cooper, 1963). On the other hand, mutants with nonstructural defects generally exhibit normal stability to heat, but they produce neither mature virus nor viral RNA under nonpermissive conditions.

Disturbances of viral maturation at infraoptimal temperatures have not been extensively studied, but in this case too the observed effects may be a resultant of general depression of metabolic processes and specific interference with some step of replication (Ageeva et al., 1971). Cold-sensitive viral strains have been described from which cold-resistant mutants can be selected (Lwoff, 1965).

13.4. Genetic Recombination

Study of recombination in picornaviruses is subject to the various difficulties, technical and otherwise, which have been enumerated at the beginning of this section. The phenomenon has been observed with foot-and-mouth disease virus (Pringle, 1965) and poliovirus (Hirst, 1962; Ledinko, 1963b; Bengtsson, 1968; Sergiescu et al., 1969), but in only one instance (Cooper, 1968) has the frequency of recombination between a selected group of temperature-sensitive mutants been utilized to construct an internally consistent, linear genetic map of any extent. With appropriate pairs of mutants under favorable conditions, the occurrence of wild-type recombinants is on the order of 0.02–0.85%, 5–30 times the background due to leakiness or reversion. The map derived from recombination frequencies is consistent with the structure of the genome deduced from other evidence (cf. Fig. 3) to the extent that the genes for structural proteins are grouped at one end. The mutants with defects of RNA synthesis are largely grouped at the other end of the recombination map, but there are several unexplained exceptions to the latter generalization (Cooper *et al.*, 1970*a*). It generally has not been possible to correlate positions on the map with specific viral products or functions, and no satisfactory description of the mechanism of recombination in molecular terms has yet been proposed.

13.5. Complementation

Complementation in the strict sense, e.g., the production of viral progeny through the cooperative interaction of pairs of temperature-sensitive mutants under nonpermissive conditions, is at best only barely demonstrable with picornaviruses (Cooper, 1965, 1969; Ghendon, 1966). Moreover, the observed complementation is not reciprocal, i.e., only one of the pair of parental viruses appears in the progeny.

On the other hand, the utilization by one of a pair of infecting viruses of a product produced by the other can occur under certain circumstances. Generally, the exchange of capsid proteins between related picornaviruses takes place with reasonable efficiency, leading to the production of phenotypically mixed or phenotypically masked particles (Ledinko and Hirst, 1961). Also, a guanidine-dependent or guanidine-resistant strain multiplying in the presence of guanidine is able to provide product(s) which permit the concurrent multiplication of a guanidine-sensitive strain, and a guanidine-dependent strain may similarly be "rescued" in the absence of guanidine. In each case, most of the rescued virus is phenotypically masked by the heterologous capsid (Wecker and Lederhilger, 1964*a,b*; Cords and Holland, 1964*b*; Holland and Cords, 1964; Agol and Shirman, 1965). Appreciable rescue takes place, however, only under conditions which permit the replication of one of the strains; different guanidine-dependent strains, for example, are unable to complement one another to any extent in the absence of guanidine (Ikegami *et al.*, 1964). It was formerly supposed that the rescue phenomenon between strains with different sensitivities to guanidine implied that one strain could utilize the RNA polymerase of another, but the validity of this conclusion is now doubtful in view of the uncertainty concerning the mode of action of the drug.

The reason for the general inefficiency of complementation between picornaviruses, except for the special instances noted above, is not presently apparent. In any event, it has not been possible to use a complementation test to differentiate separate genes or cistrons, and the phenomenon has consequently been of little or no use for genetic analysis.

14. OTHER TOPICS

14.1. Interference

Picornaviruses, by a variety of mechanisms, may either interfere with the growth of other viruses or be subject to interference by other viruses; the following discussion deals only with certain instances of this phenomenon relevant to questions concerning viral replication. The scope of the discussion has been further restricted by the exclusion from consideration of interference caused by interferon and diffusable interfering substances in general.

In cells doubly infected with a picornavirus and a heterologous virus, the picornavirus generally (Freda and Buck, 1971; Doyle and Holland, 1972; Saxton and Stevens, 1972), but not invariably (Choppin and Holmes, 1967), is dominant. As mentioned earlier, it is supposed that the selective inhibition of the growth of certain other viruses may be brought about by a mechanism similar to the switch-off of cellular protein synthesis.

Interference is also demonstrable between different picornaviruses, different serotypes of a particular virus, and different variants or strains of the same serotype. Such homologous interference may contribute to the general inefficiency of genetic interaction between different strains discussed in the preceding section.

Interference is minimal when cells are simultaneously infected with two serotypes of poliovirus (Ledinko and Hirst, 1961), but the second virus is excluded if the times of infection are offset by 30–60 minutes (Ledinko, 1963a; Cords and Holland, 1964a). The multiplicities of the interfering and challenge viruses also influence the rapidity and degree of development of interference. Prevention of the multiplication of a virus may increase its capacity to interfere under certain circumstances (Pohjanpelto and Cooper, 1965), but in other cases the interference is abolished (McCormick and Penman, 1968); moreover, interruption of the multiplication of the interfering virus $1-2\frac{1}{2}$ hours after infection reverses the interference (Cords and Holland, 1964a). The exclusion of the challenge virus occurs at a point subsequent to adsorption and penetration, and soluble interfering substances play no role in the phenomenon (Lediniko, 1963a).

It is difficult to formulate a single mechanism to account for all the foregoing features of interference between picornaviruses; it has been proposed that interference between multiplying strains is a reflection of competition for limited intracellular sites or resources (Cords and Holland, 1964a) or for the cell's limited capacity to synthesize viral RNA (Baltimore, 1969); interference without multiplication may reflect a different, earlier event (Pohjanpelto and Cooper, 1965).

14.2. Defective-Interfering Particles

In addition to virions and empty capsids, the products formed in the poliovirus-infected cell include a class of virions which contain about 15% less RNA than normal and which are incapable of initiating a productive infectious cycle (Cole *et al.*, 1971; Cole and Baltimore, 1973a,b). The production of these defective-interfering (DI) particles, initially identified as a contaminant in a viral stock, is favored by serial passage at a high multiplicity of infection. Infection by purified DI particles alone leads to the production of virus-specific RNA and protein, but no particles of any sort. Apparently, the information coding for a portion of the precursor of the capsid protein is deleted, and the altered protein is nonfunctional and unstable. In coinfection with standard virions, DI particles interfere with the production of standard progeny to varying degrees, depending on the respective multiplicities. In doubly infected cells, the standard viral RNA and the RNA of DI particles appear to replicate with about equal efficiency, and the two species of RNA compete on equal terms for the limited supply of functional capsid protein.

14.3. Effects of Various Environmental Factors on the Multiplication of Picornaviruses

The effects of high or low temperature on virus development have already been discussed. The process of maturation is also affected by other factors in the environment of the infected cell; for example, the production of mature poliovirus is inhibited in a hypotonic environment although formation of viral RNA continues and morphogenesis proceeds up to the point of production of empty capsids. Mutants which are able to multiply in hypotonic medium can be isolated under selective conditions (Tolskaya *et al.,* 1966; Agol *et al.,* 1970). The presence of heavy water in the medium of the cell generally inhibits maturation; mutants resistant to heavy water have been described, and the effect of supraoptimal temperature on certain thermosensitive mutants is ameliorated by heavy water (Carp and Koprowski, 1962; Lwoff and Lwoff, 1964*a*; Lwoff, 1965).

14.4. Homologies in Nucleotide Sequences among Picornaviruses

Homologies in nucleotide sequence, determined by RNA–RNA hybridization between denatured RF and an excess of single-stranded viral RNA, have been utilized to provide a quantitative measure of the degree of genetic relatedness between various picornaviruses. Despite their lack of antigenic cross-reactivity, the three types of poliovirus hold on the order of 30–50% of their nucleotide sequences in common; the shared sequences are short and presumably scattered throughout the genome (Young *et al.,* 1968; Young, 1973*a,b*). A similar degree of relatedness was also observed within other classes of human enteroviruses, but the degree of homology between members of different classes, e.g., between poliovirus and echovirus, is considerably less. Different serological types of foot-and-mouth disease virus, which share minor antigenic cross-reactivity, have major nucleotide homologies (Dietzschold *et al.,* 1971), but three representative types of human rhinoviruses are only distantly related to each other by this criterion (Yin *et al.,* 1973). The latter viruses also differ in their buoyant density; this evidence raises the possibility of divergent origins of the viruses despite many common physicochemical and biological properties.

15.   CONCLUDING COMMENTS

The pace of research on the molecular biology of picornaviruses has declined from a peak in the mid-1960's; this probably reflects the virtual eradication of paralytic poliomyelitis by mass vaccination on the one hand, and the discovery and experimental exploitation of the RNA-containing bacteriophages on the other. Despite a number of impressive parallels, however, it is clear that picornaviruses differ from the RNA-containing phages in a number of important respects, particularly in the manner by which the events of the growth cycle are regulated. Also, picornaviruses are the agents of a number of other important diseases of man and animals which remain to be controlled, including the common cold.

In any event, there would appear to be ample justification for further investigation of a number of significant questions concerning the multiplication of picornaviruses which remain unresolved. For example, no functional role has yet been assigned to any of the nonstructural virus-specific peptides, some of which may be effectors of the inhibition of cellular biosynthetic processes. Also, the virus-induced RNA-dependent RNA polymerase has not yet been obtained in fully functional purified form, and the significance of the association of the crude enzyme with cellular membranes remains to be clarified. A number of questions concerning viral morphogenesis are unanswered, including the mechanism by which empty capsids and RNA interact to form infectious virions. Another unresolved matter is the means by which the asymmetry of viral RNA synthesis is maintained, i.e., the production of a tenfold excess of plus over minus strands. As a final example, the basis for the selective antiviral action of agents such as guanidine is incompletely understood, and it remains to be seen whether practical antiviral agents can be developed which are effective *in vivo* as well as *in vitro*.

ACKNOWLEDGMENTS

I am grateful to J. Michael Bishop for valuable discussion and criticism. This work was supported in part by USPHS Grant AI 06862.

16. REFERENCES

Adler, R., Garfinkle, B. D., Mitchell, W., and Tershak, D. R., 1973, Degradation of poliovirus RNA *in vivo, Can. J. Microbiol.* **19,** 539.

Ageeva, O. N., Gutkina, A. V., Ghendon, Y. Z., 1971, Synthesis of ribonucleic acid and protein of poliomyelitis virus at low temperature, *Vop. Virus.* **2,** 164.

Agol, V. I. and Shirman, G. A., 1965, Formation of virus particles by means of enzyme systems and structural proteins induced by another "helper" virus, *Vop. Virus* **10,** 8.

Agol, V. I., Lipskaya, G. Y., Tolskaya, E. A., Voroshilova, M. K., and Romanova, L. I., 1970, Defect in poliovirus maturation under hypotonic conditions, *Virology* **41,** 533.

Agol, V. I., Romanova, L. I., Čumakov, I. M., Dunaevskaya, L. D., and Bogdanov, A. A., 1972, Circularity and cross-linking in preparations of replicative form of encephalomyocarditis virus RNA, *J. Mol. Biol.* 72:77.

Alexander, H. E., Koch, G., Mountain, I. M., Sprunt, K., and Van Damme, O., 1958,

Infectivity of ribonucleic acid of poliovirus on HeLa cell monolayers, *Virology* **6**, 172.

Amako, K., and Dales, S., 1967, Cytopathology of mengovirus infection. II. Proliferation of membranous cisternae, *Virology* **32**, 201.

Amstey, M. S. and Parkman, P. D., 1966, Enhancement of polio-RNA infectivity by dimethyl sulfoxide, *Proc. Soc. Exp. Biol. Med.* **123**, 438.

Arlinghaus, R. B. and Polatnick, J., 1969, The isolation of two enzyme–ribonucleic acid complexes involved in the synthesis of foot-and-mouth disease virus ribonucleic acid, *Proc. Natl. Acad. Sci. USA* **62**, 821.

Bablanian, R., Eggers, H. J., and Tamm, I., 1965, Studies on the mechanism of poliovirus-induced cell damage, II. The relation between poliovirus growth and virus-induced morphological changes in cells, *Virology* **26**, 114.

Balandin, I. G., and Franklin, R. M., 1964, The effect of mengovirus infection on the activity of the DNA-dependent RNA polymerase of L-cells, II. Preliminary data on the inhibitory factor, *Biochem. Biophys. Res. Commun.* **15**, 27.

Baltimore, D., 1968a, Structure of the poliovirus replicative intermediate RNA, *J. Mol. Biol.* **32**, 359.

Baltimore, D., 1968b, Inhibition of poliovirus replication by guanidine, *in* "Medical and Applied Virology," (M. Sanders and E. H. Lennette, eds.), pp. 340–347, Warren H. Green, St. Louis.

Baltimore, D., 1969, The replication of picornaviruses, *in* "The Biochemistry of Viruses" (H. B. Levy, ed.), pp. 101–176, Marcel Dekker, New York.

Baltimore, D., 1971a, Expression of animal virus genomes, *Bacteriol. Rev.* **35**, 235.

Baltimore, D., 1971b, Is poliovirus dead? *in* "Perspectives in Virology," Vol. VII (M. Pollard, ed.) pp. 1–14, Academic Press, New York.

Baltimore, D., and Franklin, R. M., 1962a, The effect of mengovirus infection on the activity of the DNA-dependent RNA polymerase of L-cells, *Proc. Natl. Acad. Sci. USA* **48**, 1383.

Baltimore, D. and Franklin, R. M., 1962b, Preliminary data on a virus-specific enzyme system responsible for the synthesis of viral RNA, *Biochem. Biophys. Res. Commun.* **9**, 388.

Baltimore, D., and Franklin, R. M., 1963a, A new ribonucleic acid polymerase appearing after mengovirus infection of L-cells, *J. Biol. Chem.* **238**, 3395.

Baltimore, D. and Franklin, R. M., 1963b, Effects of puromycin and *p*-fluorophenylalanine on mengovirus ribonucleic acid and protein synthesis, *Biochim. Biophys. Acta* **76**, 431.

Baltimore, D., and Girard, M., 1966, An intermediate in the synthesis of poliovirus RNA, *Proc. Natl. Acad. Sci. USA* **56**, 741.

Baltimore, D., Eggers, H. J., Franklin, R. M., and Tamm, I., 1963a, Poliovirus-induced RNA polymerase and the effects of virus-specific inhibitors on its production, *Proc. Natl. Acad. Sci. USA* **49**, 843.

Baltimore, D., Franklin, R. M., and Callender, J., 1963b, Mengovirus-induced inhibition of host ribonucleic acid and protein synthesis, *Biochim. Biophys. Acta* **76**, 425.

Baltimore, D., Girard, M., and Darnell, J. E., Jr., 1966, Aspects of the synthesis of poliovirus RNA and the formation of virus particles, *Virology* **29**, 179.

Bechet, J. M., 1972, Isolation of the minus strand of encephalomyocarditis virus RNA, *Virology* **48**, 855.

Bengtsson, S., 1968, Attempts to map the poliovirus genome by analysis of selected recombinants, *Acta Pathol. Microbiol. Scand.* **73**, 592.

Best, M., Evans, B., and Bishop, J. M., 1972, Double-stranded replicative form of poliovirus RNA: Phenotype of heterozygous molecules, *Virology* **47**, 592.

Bishop, J. M., and Koch, G., 1967, Purification and characterization of poliovirus-induced infectious double-stranded RNA, *J. Biol. Chem.* **242**, 1736.

Bishop, J. M. and Koch, G., 1969, Infectious replicative intermediate of poliovirus: purification and characterization, *Virology* **37**, 521.

Bishop, J. M., and Levintow, L., 1971, Replicative forms of viral RNA. Structure and function, *Prog. Med. Virol.* **13**, 1.

Bishop, J. M., Quintrell, N., and Koch, G., 1967, Poliovirus double-stranded RNA: Inactivation by ultraviolet light, *J. Mol. Biol.* **24**, 125.

Bishop, J. M., Koch, G., Evans, B., and Merriman, M., 1969, Poliovirus replicative intermediate: Structural basis of infectivity, *J. Mol. Biol.* **46**, 235.

Blumenthal, T., Landers, T. A., and Weber, K., 1972, Bacteriophage Qβ replicase contains the protein biosynthesis elongation factors EF Tu and EF Ts. *Proc. Natl. Acad. Sci. USA* **69**, 1313.

Boeyé, A., 1959, Induction of a mutant in poliovirus by nitrous acid, *Virology* **9**, 691.

Breindl, M., 1971, VP4, the D-reactive part of poliovirus, *Virology* **46**, 962.

Brown, F. and Martin, S. J., 1965, A new model for virus ribonucleic acid replication, *Nature (Lond.)* **208**, 861.

Brown, F., Newman, J. F. E., and Stott, E. J., 1970, Molecular weight of rhinovirus ribonucleic acid, *J. Gen. Virol.* **8**, 145.

Burness, A. T. H., Pardoe, I. U., and Fox, S. M., 1973, Evidence for lack of glycoprotein in the encephalomyocarditis virus particle, *J. Gen. Virol.* **18**, 33.

Butterworth, B. E. and Rueckert, R. R., 1972a, Gene order of encephalomyocarditis virus as determined by studies with pactamycin, *J. Virol.* **9**, 823.

Butterworth, B. E. and Rueckert, R. R., 1972b, Kinetics of synthesis and cleavage of encephalomyocarditis virus-specific proteins, *Virology* **50**, 535.

Caliguiri, L. A., and Mosser, A. G., 1971, Proteins associated with the poliovirus RNA replication complex, *Virology* **46**, 375.

Caliguiri, L. A. and Tamm, I., 1970a, The role of cytoplasmic membranes in poliovirus biosynthesis, *Virology* **42**, 100.

Caliguiri, L. A. and Tamm, I., 1970b, Characterization of poliovirus-specific structures associated with cytoplasmic membranes, *Virology* **42**, 112.

Carp, R. I. and Koprowski, H., 1962, Investigations of the reproductive capacity temperature marker of poliovirus, *Virology* **16**, 371.

Chan, V. F. and Black, F. L., 1970, Uncoating of poliovirus by isolated plasma membranes, *J. Virol.* **5**, 309.

Chatterjee, N. K., Koch, G., and Weissbach, H., 1973, Initiator of protein synthesis *in vivo* in poliovirus-infected HeLa cells, *Arch. Biochem. Biophys.* **154**, 431.

Choppin, P. W., and Holmes, K. V., 1967, Replication of SV5 RNA and the effects of super-infection with poliovirus, *Virology* **33**, 442.

Clements, J. B. and Martin, S. J., 1971, Evidence for large strands of ribonucleic acid induced by a bovine enterovirus, *J. Gen. Virol.* **12**, 221.

Colby, C. and Duesberg, P. H., 1969, Double-stranded RNA in vaccinia virus-infected cells, *Nature* 222:940.

Cole, C. N., and Baltimore, D., 1973a, Defective interfering particles of poliovirus, II. Nature of defect, *J. Mol. Biol.* **76**, 325.

Cole, C. N. and Baltimore, D., 1973*b*, Defective interfering particles of poliovirus, III. Interference and enrichment, *J. Mol. Biol.* **76**, 345.

Cole, C. N., Smoler, D., Wimmer, E., and Baltimore, D., 1971, Defective interfering particles of poliovirus. I. Isolation and physical properties, *J. Virol.* **7**, 478.

Collins, F. D. and Roberts, W. K., 1972, Mechanism of mengovirus-induced cell injury in L-cells: use of inhibitors of protein synthesis to dissociate virus-specific events, *J. Virol.* **10**, 969.

Colter, J. S., Bird, H. H. and Brown, R. A., 1957, Infectivity of ribonucleic acid from Ehrlich ascites tumor cells infected with mengo encephalitis, *Nature (Lond.)* **179**, 859.

Cooper, P. D., 1963, The effect of concentrated urea solutions on poliovirus strains adapted to different growth temperatures, *Virology* **21**, 322.

Cooper, P. D., 1964, The mutation of poliovirus by 5-fluorouracil, *Virology* **22**, 186.

Cooper, P. D., 1965, Rescue of one phenotype in mixed infections with heat-defective mutants of Type 1 poliovirus, *Virology* **25**, 431.

Cooper, P. D., 1966, The inhibition of poliovirus growth by actinomycin D and the prevention of the inhibition by pretreatment of the cells with serum or insulin, *Virology* **28**, 663.

Cooper, P. D., 1968, A genetic map of poliovirus temperature-sensitive mutants, *Virology* **35**, 584.

Cooper, P. D., 1969, The genetic analysis of poliovirus, *in* "The Biochemistry of Viruses," (H. B. Levy, ed.), pp. 117–218, Marcel Dekker, New York.

Cooper, P. D., Stancek, D., and Summers, D. F., 1970*a*, Synthesis of double-stranded RNA by poliovirus temperature-sensitive mutants, *Virology* **40**, 971.

Cooper, P. D., Summers, D. F., and Maizel, J. V., Jr., 1970*b*, Evidence for ambiguity in the posttranslational cleavage of poliovirus proteins, *Virology* **41**, 408.

Cooper, P. D., Steiner-Pryor, A., and Wright, P. J., 1973, A proposed regulator for poliovirus: The equestron, *Intervirology* 1:1.

Cordell-Stewart, B., and Taylor, M. W., 1971, Effect of double-stranded viral RNA on mammalian cells in culture, *Proc. Natl. Acad. Sci. USA* **68**, 1326.

Cordell-Stewart, B., and Taylor, M. W., 1973, Effect of double-stranded RNA on mammalian cells in culture: Cytotoxicity under conditions preventing viral replication and protein synthesis, *J. Virol.* **12**, 360.

Cords, C. E., and Holland, J. J., 1964*a*, Interference between enteroviruses and conditions effecting its reversal, *Virology* **22**, 226.

Cords, C. E., and Holland, J. J., 1964*b*, Replication of poliovirus RNA induced by heterologous virus, *Proc. Natl. Acad. Sci. USA* **51**, 1080.

Cornatzer, W. E., Sandstrom, W., and Fisher, R. G., 1961, The effect of poliomyelitis virus Type 1 (Mahoney strain) on the phospholipid metabolism of the Hela cell, *Biochim. Biophys. Acta* **49**, 414.

Cranston, J., Malathi, V. G., and Silber, R., 1973, Further studies on RNA ligase, *Fed. Proc.* **32**, 498.

Crocker, T. T., Pfendt, E., and Spendlove, R., 1964, Poliovirus: Growth in non-nucleate cytoplasm, *Science (Wash., D.C.)* **145**, 401.

Crowell, R. L., and Philipson, L., 1971, Specific alterations of coxsackievirus B3 eluted from Hela cells, *J. Virol.* **8**, 509.

Crowther, D., and Melnick, J. L., 1961, The incorporation of neutral red and acridine orange into developing poliovirus particles making them photosensitive, *Virology* **14**, 11.

Dales, S., 1973, Early events in cell–animal virus interactions, *Bacteriol. Rev.* **37**, 103.

Dales, S., and Franklin, R. M., 1962, A comparison of the changes in fine structure of L-cells during single cycles of virus multiplication, following their infection with the viruses of Mengo and encephalomyocarditis, *J. Cell Biol.* **14**, 281.

Dales, S., Eggers, H. J., Tamm, I., and Palade, G. E., 1965, Electron microscopic study of the formation of poliovirus, *Virology* **26**, 379.

Dalgarno, L., Cox, R. A., and Martin, E. M., 1967, Polyribosomes in normal Krebs 2 ascites tumor cells and in cells infected with encephalomyocarditis virus, *Biochim. Biophys. Acta* **138**, 316.

Darnell, J. E., Jr., 1958, Adsorption and maturation of poliovirus in single and multiply infected Hela cells, *J. Exp. Med.* **107**, 633.

Darnell, J. E., Jr., 1968, Ribonucleic acids from animal cells, *Bacteriol. Rev.* **32**, 262.

Darnell, J. E., Jr., and Eagle, H., 1960, The biosynthesis of poliovirus in cell culture, *Adv. Virus Res.* **7**, 1.

Darnell, J. E., Jr., and Levintow, L., 1960, Poliovirus protein: Source of amino acids and time course of synthesis, *J. Biol. Chem.* **234**, 74.

Darnell, J. E., Jr., and Sawyer, T. K., 1960, Variation in plaque-forming ability among parental and clonal strains of Hela cells, *Virology* **8**, 223.

Darnell, J. E., Jr., Levintow, L., Thoren, M. M., and Hooper, J. L., 1961, The time course of synthesis of poliovirus RNA, *Virology* **13**, 271.

Darnell, J. E., Jr., Girard, M., Baltimore, D., Summers, D. F., and Maizel, J. V., Jr., 1967, The synthesis and translation of poliovirus RNA, *in* "The Molecular Biology of Viruses" (J. S. Colter and W. Paranchych, eds.), pp. 375–401, Academic Press, New York.

Dietzschold, B., and Ahl, R., 1970, Characterization of foot-and-mouth disease virus ribonucleic acid synthesized *in vitro, J. Gen. Virol.***8**, 73.

Dietzschold, B., Kaaden, O. R., Tokui, T., and Böhm, H. O., 1971, Polynucleotide sequence homologies among the RNAs of foot-and-mouth disease virus Types A,C, and O, *J. Gen. Virol.* **13**, 1.

Dinter, Z., and Bengtsson, S., 1964, Suppression of the inhibitory action of guanidine on virus multiplication by some amino acids, *Virology* **24**, 254.

Dixon, G. J., Rightsel, W. A., and Skipper, H. E., 1965, Indirect inhibition of protein synthesis, *Ann. N.Y. Acad. Sci.* **130**, 249.

Doyle, M., and Holland, J. J., 1972, Virus-induced interference in heterologously infected Hela cells, *J. Virol.* **9**, 22.

Dulbecco, R., and Vogt, M., 1954, Plaque formation and isolation of pure lines with poliomyelitis viruses, *J. Exp. Med.* **99**, 167.

Dulbecco, R., and Vogt, M., 1958, Studies on the induction of mutations in poliovirus by proflavin, *Virology* **5**, 236.

Duncan, J. L., and Groman, N. B., 1967, Studies of the activity of diphtheria toxin. I. Poliovirus replication in intoxicated Hela cells, *J. Exp. Med.* **125**, 489.

Dunnebacke, T. H., Levinthal, J. D., and Williams, R. C., 1969, Entry and release of poliovirus as observed by electron microscopy of cultured cells, *J. Virol.* **4**, 505.

Eagle, H., 1955, Nutrition needs of mammalian cells in tissue culture, *Science (Wash., D.C.)* **122**, 501.

Eggers, H. J., and Tamm, I., 1961, Spectrum and characteristics of the virus inhibitory action of 2-(α-hydroxybenzyl)-benzimidazole, *J. Exp. Med.* **113**, 675.

Eggers, H. J., Baltimore, D., and Tamm, I., 1963, The relation of protein synthesis to the formation of poliovirus RNA polymerase, *Virology* **21**, 281.

Ehrenfeld, E., and Hunt, T., 1971, Double-stranded poliovirus RNA inhibits initiation of protein synthesis by reticulocyte lysates, *Proc. Natl. Acad. Sci. USA* **68,** 1075.

Ehrenfeld, E., Maizel, J. V., Jr., and Summers, D. F., 1970, Soluble RNA polymerase complex from poliovirus-infected Hela cells, *Virology* **40,** 840.

Eikhom, T. S., Stockley, D. J., and Spiegelman, S., 1968, Direct participation of a host protein in the replication of viral RNA *in vitro, Proc. Natl. Acad. USA* **59,** 506.

Enders, J. F., Weller, T. H., and Robbins, F. C., 1949, Cultivation of the Lansing strain of poliomyelitis virus in cultures of various human embryonic tissues, *Science (Wash., D.C.)* **109,** 85.

Ensminger, W. D., and Tamm, I., 1970, The step in cellular DNA synthesis blocked by Newcastle disease or mengovirus infection, *Virology* **40,** 152.

Eremenko, T., Benedetto, A., and Volpe, P., 1972, Virus infection as a function of the host cell life cycle: Replication of poliovirus RNA. *J. Gen. Virol.* **16,** 61.

Falcoff, E., Falcoff, R., Lebleu, B., and Revel, M., 1972, Interferon treatment inhibits Mengo RNA and haemoglobin mRNA translation in cell-free extracts of L cells, *Nat. New Biol.* **240,** 145.

Fenwick, M. L., and Cooper, P. D., 1962, Early interactions between poliovirus and ERK cells: Some observations on the nature and significance of the rejected particles, *Virology* **18,** 212.

Fenwick, M. L., and Wall, M. J., 1972, The density of poliovirus-specific polysomes, *J. Gen. Virol.* **17,** 143.

Fenwick, M. L., Erikson, R. L., and Franklin, R. M., 1964, Replication of the RNA of bacteriophage R17, *Science (Wash., D.C.)* **146,** 527.

Fiszman, M. Y., Bucchini, D., Girard, M., and Lwoff, A., 1970, Inhibition of poliovirus RNA synthesis by supraoptimal temperatures, *J. Gen. Virol.* **6,** 293.

Fiszman, M., Reynier, M., Bucchini, D., and Girard, M., 1972, Thermosensitive block of the Sabin strain of poliovirus Type I, *J. Virol.* **10,** 1143.

Franklin, R. M., and Baltimore, D., 1962, Patterns of macromolecular synthesis in normal and virus-infected mammalian cells, *Cold Spring Harbor Symp. Quant. Biol.* **27,** 175.

Franklin, R. M., and Rosner, J., 1962, Localization of ribonucleic acid synthesis in mengovirus-infected L-cells, *Biochim. Biophys. Acta* **55,** 240.

Freda, C. E., and Buck, C. A., 1971, System of double infection between vaccinia virus and mengovirus, *J. Virol.* **8,** 293.

Garfinkle, B. D., and Tershak, D. R., 1971, Effect of temperature on the cleavage of polypeptides during growth of LSc poliovirus, *J. Mol. Biol.* **59,** 537.

Gessa, G. L., Loddo, B., Brotzu, G., Schivo, M. L., Tagliamonte, A., Spanedda, A., Bo, G., and Ferrari, W., 1966, Selective inhibition of poliovirus growth by D-penicillamine *in vitro, Virology* **30,** 618.

Ghendon, Y. A., 1966, Non-complementing rct_{40}-mutant of poliovirus, *Acta Virol.* **10,** 173.

Ghendon, Y. Z., and Yakobson, E. A., 1971, Antigenic specificity of poliovirus related particles, *J. Virol.* **8,** 589.

Ghendon, Y., Yakobson, E., and Mikhejeva, A., 1972, Study of some stages of poliovirus morphogenesis in MiO cells, *J. Virol.* **10,** 261.

Gilbert, W., and Dressler, D., 1968, DNA replication: The rolling circle model, *Cold Spring Harbor Symp. Quant. Biol.* **33,** 473.

Girard, M., 1969, *In vitro* synthesis of poliovirus ribonucleic acid: Role of the replicative intermediate, *J. Virol.* **3**, 376.

Girard, M., Baltimore, D., and Darnell, J. E., Jr., 1967, The poliovirus replication complex: Site for synthesis of poliovirus RNA, *J. Mol. Biol.* **24**, 59.

Grado, C., Fischer, S., and Contreras, G., 1965, The inhibition by actinomycin D of poliovirus multiplication in HE$_p$ 2 cells, *Virology* **27**, 623.

Grado, C., Friedlender, B., Ihl, M., and Contreras, G., 1968, Incorporation of methyl groups by viral and cellular RNA of HE$_p$ 2 cells after poliovirus infection, *Virology* **35**, 339.

Granboulan, N., and Girard, M., 1969, Molecular weight of poliovirus ribonucleic acid, *J. Virol.* **4**, 475.

Hall, L., and Rueckert, R. R., 1971, Infection of mouse fibroblasts by cardioviruses: Premature uncoating and its prevention by elevated *p*H and magnesium chloride, *Virology* **43**, 152.

Halperen, S., Eggers, H. J., and Tamm, I., 1964, Evidence for uncoupled synthesis of viral RNA and viral capsids, *Virology* **24**, 36.

Hand, R. R., and Tamm, I., 1972, Rate of DNA chain growth in mammalian cells infected with cytocidal RNA viruses, *Virology* **47**, 331.

Hand, R., Ensminger, W. D., and Tamm, I., 1971, Cellular DNA replication in infections with cytocidal RNA viruses, *Virology* **44**, 527.

Hausen, H., 1962, Cytologische Studien über die Vermehrung des ME-Virus in L-Zellen, *Z. Naturforsch.* **17b**, 158.

Hirst, G. K., 1962, Genetic recombinations with Newcastle disease virus, polioviruses, and influenza, *Cold Spring Harbor Symp. Quant. Biol.* **27**, 303.

Ho, P. P. K., and Washington, A. L., 1971, Evidence for a cellular ribonucleic acid synthesis inhibitor from poliovirus-infected Hela cells, *Biochemistry* **10**, 3646.

Hodes, H. L., Zepp, H. D., and Ainbender, E., 1960, A physical property as a virus marker. Difference of avidity of cellulose resin for virulent (Mahoney) and attenuated (LSc,2ab) strain of Type 1 poliovirus, *Virology* **11**, 306.

Holland, J. J., and Cords, C. E., 1964, Maturation of poliovirus RNA with capsid protein coded by heterologous enteroviruses, *Proc. Natl. Acad. Sci. USA* **51**, 1082.

Holland, J. J., and Kiehn, E. D., 1968, Specific cleavage of viral proteins as steps in the synthesis and maturation of enteroviruses, *Proc. Natl. Acad. Sci. USA* **60**, 1015.

Holland, J. J., and McLaren, L. C., 1959, The mammalian cell-virus relationship, II. Adsorption, reception and eclipse of poliovirus by Hela cells, *J. Exp. Med.* **109**, 487.

Holland, J. J., and Peterson, J. A., 1964, Nucleic acid and protein synthesis during poliovirus infection of human cells, *J. Mol. Biol.* **8**, 556.

Holland, J. J., McLaren, L. C., and Syverton, J. T., 1959, The mammalian cell-virus relationship, IV. Infection of naturally insusceptible cells with enterovirus nucleic acid. *J. Exp. Med.* **110**, 65.

Homma, M., and Graham, A. F., 1965, Intracellular fate of Mengo virus ribonucleic acid, *J. Bacteriol.* **89**, 64.

Horne, R. W., and Nagington, J., 1959, Electron microscope studies of the development and structure of poliomyelitis virus, *J. Mol. Biol.* **1**, 333.

Housman, D., Jacobs-Lorena, M., Rajbhandary, U. L., and Lodish, H. F., 1970, Initiation of haemoglobin synthesis by methionyl-tRNA, *Nature (Lond.)* **227**, 913.

Huang, A. S., and Baltimore, D., 1970, Initiation of polyribosome formation in poliovirus-infected Hela cells, *J. Mol. Biol.* **47**, 275.

Ikegami, N., Eggers, H. J., and Tamm, I., 1964, Rescue of drug-requiring and drug-inhibited enteroviruses, *Proc. Natl. Acad. Sci. USA* **52**, 1419.

International Enterovirus Study Group, 1963, Picornavirus group, *Virology* **19**, 114.

Jacobson, M. F., and Baltimore, D., 1968a, Morphogenesis of poliovirus. I. Association of the viral RNA with the coat protein, *J. Mol. Biol.* **33**, 369.

Jacobson, M. F., and Baltimore, D., 1968b, Polypeptide cleavages in the formation of poliovirus proteins, *Proc. Natl. Acad. Sci. USA* **61**, 77.

Jacobson, M. F., Asso, J., and Baltimore, D., 1970, Further evidence on the formation of poliovirus proteins, *J. Mol. Biol.* **49**, 657.

Johnson, T. C., and Holland, J. J., 1965, Ribonucleic acid and protein synthesis in mitotic HeLa cells, *J. Cell Biol.* **27**, 565.

Joklik, W. K., and Darnell, J. E., Jr., 1961, The adsorption and early fate of purified poliovirus in Hela cells, *Virology* **13**, 439.

Kaempfer, R., and Kaufman, J., 1973, Inhibition of cellular protein synthesis by double-stranded RNA: Inactivation of an initiation factor, *Proc. Natl. Acad. Sci.* **70**, 1222.

Katz, L., and Penman, S., 1966, The solvent denaturation of double-stranded RNA from poliovirus infected Hela cells, *Biochem. Biophys. Res. Commun.* **23**, 557.

Kerr, I. M., Martin, E. M., Hamilton, M. G., and Work, T. S., 1965, Studies on protein and nucleic acid metabolism in virus-infected mammalian cells, *Biochem. J.* **94**, 337.

Kiehn, E. D., and Holland, J. J., 1970, Synthesis and cleavage of enterovirus polypeptides in mammalian cells, *J. Virol.* **5**, 358.

King, D. W., Socolow, E. L., and Bensch, K. G., 1959, The relation between protein synthesis and lipid accumulation in L strain cells and Ehrlich ascites cells, *J. Biophys. Biochem. Cytology* **5**, 421.

Koch, G., Koening, S., and Alexander, H. E., 1960, Quantitative studies on the infectivity of ribonucleic acid from partially purified and highly purified poliovirus preparations, *Virology* **10**, 329.

Koch, G., Quintrell, N., and Bishop, J. M., 1967, Differential effect of actinomycin D on the infectivity of single- and double-stranded poliovirus RNA, *Virology* **31**, 388.

Korant, B. D., 1972, Cleavage of viral precursor proteins *in vivo* and *in vitro, J. Virol.* **10**, 751.

Korant, B. D., Lonberg-Holm, K., Noble, J., and Stasny, J. T., 1972, Naturally occurring and artificially produced components of three rhinoviruses, *Virology* **48**, 71.

Kozda, H., and Jungeblut, C. W., 1958, Effect of receptor-destroying enzyme on the growth of EMC virus in tissue culture, *J. Immunol.* **81**, 76.

LeBouvier, G., 1959, The D→C change in poliovirus particles, *Brit. J. Exp. Pathol.* **40**, 605.

Ledinko, N., 1962, Discussion, *Cold Spring Harbor Symp. Quant. Biol.* **27**, 309.

Ledinko, N., 1963a, An analysis of interference between active polioviruses Types 1 and 2 in Hela cells, *Virology* **20**, 29

Ledinko, N., 1963b, Genetic recombination with poliovirus Type I studies of crosses between a normal horse serum-resistant mutant and several guanidine-resistant mutants of the same strain, *Virology* **20**, 107.

Ledinko, N., and Hirst, G. K., 1961, Mixed infection of Hela cells with poliovirus Types 1 and 2, *Virology* **14**, 207.

Leibowitz, R., and Penman, S., 1971, Regulation of protein synthesis in Hela cells. III. Inhibition during poliovirus infection, *J. Virol.* **8**, 661.

Levintow, L., and Darnell, J. E., Jr., 1960, A simplified procedure for purification of large amounts of poliovirus: Characterization and amino acid analysis of Type 1 poliovirus, *J. Biol. Chem.* **234**, 70.

Levintow, L., Thoren, M. M., Darnell, J. E., Jr., and Hooper, J. L., 1962, Effect of *p*-fluorophenylalanine and puromycin on the replication of poliovirus, *Virology* **16**, 220.

Levy, H. B., and Carter, W. A., 1968, Molecular basis of the action of interferon, *J. Mol. Biol.* **31**, 561.

Loddo, B., Ferrari, W., Spanedda, A., and Brotzu, G., 1962, *In vitro* guanidino-resistance guanidino-dependence of poliovirus, *Experientia (Basel)* **18**, 518.

Lonberg-Holm, K., and Korant, B. D., 1972, Early interaction of rhinoviruses with host cells, *J. Virol.* **9**, 29.

Lwoff, A., 1958, L'inhibition du developpement du virus poliomyélitique à 39° et le probleme du rôle de l'hyperthermie dans l'evolution des infections virales, *C. R. Hebd. Seances Acad. Sci. Ser. D Sci. Nat.* **246**, 190.

Lwoff, A., 1965, The specific effectors of viral development, *Biochem. J.* **96**, 289.

Lwoff, A., and Lwoff, M., 1964a, Un mutant du poliovirus insensible aux effets de la deutération, *C. R. Hebd. Seances Acad. Sci. Ser. D Sci. Nat.* **258**, 2702.

Lwoff, A., and Lwoff, M., 1964b, Neutralisation par divers métabolites de l'effet inhibiteur de la guanidine sur le developpement du poliovirus, *C. R. Hedb. Seances Acad. Sci. Ser. D Sci. Nat.* **259**, 949.

Lwoff, A., and Tournier, P., 1971, Remarks on the classification of viruses, *in* "Comprehensive Virology," (K. Maramorosch and E. Kurstak, eds.), pp. 1–42, Academic Press, New York.

Lwoff, A., Dulbecco, R., Vogt, M., and Lwoff, M., 1955, Kinetics of release of poliovirus from single cells, *Virology* **1**, 128.

McCahon, D., and Cooper, P. D., 1970, Identification of poliovirus temperature-sensitive mutants having defects in virus structural protein, *J. Gen. Virol.* **6**, 51.

McCormick, W., and Penman, S., 1967, Inhibition of RNA synthesis in Hela and L cells by mengovirus, *Virology* **31**, 135.

McCormick, W., and Penman, S., 1968, Replication of mengovirus in Hela cells preinfected with nonreplicating poliovirus, *J. Virol.* **2**, 859.

McDonnell, J. P., and Levintow, L., 1970, Kinetics of appearance of the products of poliovirus-induced RNA polymerase, *Virology* **42**, 999.

McLaren, L. C., Holland, J. J., and Syverton, J. T., 1959, The mammalian cell-virus relationship. I. Attachment of poliovirus to cultivated cells of primate and non-primate origin, *J. Exp. Med.* **109**, 475.

McLean, C., and Rueckert, R. R., 1973, Picornaviral gene order: Comparison of a rhinovirus with a cardiovirus, *J. Virol.* **11**, 341.

Maizel, J. V., Jr., and Summers, D. F., 1968, Evidence for differences in size and composition of the poliovirus-specific polypeptides in infected Hela cells, *Virology* **36**, 48.

Maizel, J. V., Jr., Phillips, B. A., and Summers, D. F., 1967, Composition of artificially produced and naturally occurring empty capsids of poliovirus Type 1, *Virology* **32**, 692.

Mak, T. W., O'Callaghan, J., and Colter, J. S., 1970, Studies of the early events of the replicative cycle of three variants of Mengo encephalomyelitis virus in mouse fibroblast cells, *Virology* **42**, 1087.

Mandel, B., 1962, Early stages of virus-cell interaction as studied by using antibody, *Cold Spring Harbor Sym. Quant. Biol.* **27**, 123.

Mandel, B., 1967, The relationship between penetration and uncoating of poliovirus in Hela cells, *Virology* **31**, 702.

Marcus, P. I., and Robbins, E., 1963, Viral inhibition in the metaphase-arrest cell, *Proc. Natl. Acad. Sci. USA* **50**, 1156.

Martin, E. M., and Kerr, I. M., 1968, Virus-induced changes in host-cell macromolecular synthesis, *in* "The Molecular Biology of Viruses," Eighteenth Symposium of the Society for General Microbiology, pp. 15–46, Cambridge University Press, London.

Mikhejeva, A., Yakobson, E., and Soloviev, G. Y., 1970, Characterization of some poliovirus temperature-sensitive mutants and poliovirus-related particle formation under nonpermissive condtions, *J. Virol.* **6**, 188.

Miller, P. A., Milstrey, K. P., and Trown, P. W., 1968, Specific inhibition of viral ribonucleic acid replication by gliotoxin, *Science (Wash., D.C.)* **159**, 431.

Miller, R. L., and Plagemann, P. W. G., 1972, Purification of mengovirus and identification of an A-rich segment in its ribonucleic acid, *J. Gen. Virol.* **17**, 349.

Montagnier, L., and Sanders, F. K., 1963a, Sedimentation properties of infective ribonucleic acid extracted from encephalomyocarditis virus, *Nature (Lond.)* **197**, 1178.

Montagnier, L., and Sanders, F. K., 1963b, Replicative form of encephalomyocarditis virus ribonucleic acid, *Nature (Lond.)* **199**, 664.

Munyon, W., 1964, Inhibition of poliovirus by 2,6-diaminopurine, *Virology* **22**, 15.

Munyon, W., and Salzman, N. P., 1962, The incorporation of 5-fluorouracil into poliovirus, *Virology* **18**, 95.

Nair, C. N., and Lonberg-Holm, K. K., 1971, Infectivity and sedimentation of rhinovirus ribonucleic acid, *J. Virol.* **7**, 278.

Newman, J. F. E., Rowlands, D. J., and Brown, F., 1973, A physico-chemical sub-grouping of the mammalian picornaviruses, *J. Gen. Virol.* **18**, 171.

Noble, J., and Levintow, L., 1970, Dynamics of poliovirus-specific RNA synthesis and the effects of inhibitors of virus replication, *Virology* **40**, 634.

Noble, J., and Lonberg-Holm, K., 1973, Interactions of components of human rhinovirus 2 with Hela cells, *Virology* **51**, 270.

Noble, J., Kass, S. J., and Levintow, L., 1969, Analysis of poliovirus-specific RNA in infected Hela cells by polyacrylamide gel electrophoresis, *Virology* **37**, 535.

Öberg, B., and Philipson, L., 1969, Replication of poliovirus RNA studied by gel filtration and electrophoresis, *Eur. J. Biochem.* **11**, 305.

Öberg, B., and Philipson, L., 1971, Replicative structures of poliovirus RNA *in vivo*, *J. Mol. Biol.* **58**, 725.

Öberg, B. F., and Shatkin, A. J., 1972, Initiation of picornavirus protein synthesis in ascites cell extracts, *Proc. Natl. Acad. Sci. USA* **69**, 3589.

Öppermann, H., and Koch, G., 1973, Kinetics of poliovirus replication in Hela cells infected by isolated RNA, *Biochem. Biphys. Res. Commun.* **52**, 635.

Pearson, G. D., and Zimmerman, E. F., 1969, Inhibition of poliovirus replication by N-methylisatin-β-4′:4′-dibutylthiosemicarbazone, *Virology* **38**, 641.

Penman, S., 1965, Stimulation of the incorporation of choline in poliovirus-infected cells, *Virology* **25**, 148.

Penman, S., and Summers, D., 1965, Effects on host cell metabolism following synchronous infection with poliovirus, *Virology* **27**, 614.

Penman, S., Becker, Y., and Darnell, J. E., Jr., 1964, A cytoplasmic structure involved in the synthesis and assembly of poliovirus components, *J. Mol. Biol.* **8**, 541.

Penman, S., Rosbash, M., and Penman, M., 1970, Messenger and heterogeneous nuclear RNA in Hela cells: Differential inhibition by cordycepin, *Proc. Natl. Acad. Sci. USA* **67**, 1878.

Perlin, M., and Phillips, B. A., 1973, *In vitro* assembly of polioviruses. III. Assembly of 14 S particles into empty capsids by poliovirus-infected Hela cell membranes, *Virology* **53**, 107.

Phillips, B. A., 1969, *In vitro* assembly of polioviruses. I. Kinetics of the assembly of empty capsids and the role of extracts from infected cells, *Virology* **39**, 811.

Phillips, B. A., 1971, *In vitro* assembly of poliovirus. II. Evidence for self-assembly of 14 S particles into empty capsids, *Virology* **44**, 307.

Phillips, B. A., Summers, D. F., and Maizel, J. V., Jr., 1968, *In vitro* assembly of poliovirus-related particles, *Virology* **35**, 216.

Philipson, L., and Lind, M., 1964, Enterovirus eclipse in a cell-free system, *Virology* **23**, 322.

Plagemann, P. G. W., 1968, Reversible inhibition of induction of mengovirus RNA polymerase and of virus maturation in Novikoff rat hepatoma cells by phenethyl alcohol, *Virology* **34**, 319.

Plagemann, P. G. W., and Swim, H. E., 1968, Synthesis of RNA by mengovirus-inducted RNA polymerase *in vitro*: Nature of products and of RNase-resistant intermediate, *J. Mol. Biol.* **35**, 13.

Plagemann, P. G. W., Cleveland, P. H., and Shea, M. A., 1970, Effect of mengovirus replication on choline metabolism and membrane formation in Novikoff hepatoma cells, *J. Virol.* **6**, 800.

Pohjanpelto, P., and Cooper, P. D., 1965, Interference between polioviruses induced by strains that cannot multiply, *Virology* **25**, 350.

Pons, M., 1964, Infectious double-stranded poliovirus RNA, *Virology* **24**, 467.

Priess, H., and Eggers, H. J., 1968, Synthesis and activity of RNA polymerase of a temperature-sensitive poliovirus mutant at an elevated temperature, *Nature (Lond.)* **220**, 1047.

Pringle, C. R., 1965, Evidence of genetic recombination in foot-and-mouth disease virus, *Virology* **25**, 48.

Reich, E., Franklin, R. M., Shatkin, A. J., and Tatum, E. L., 1961, Effect of actinomycin D on cellular nucleic acid synthesis and virus production, *Science (Wash., D.C.)* **124**, 556.

Rekosh, D. M., 1972, Gene order of the poliovirus capsid proteins, *J. Virol.* **9**, 479.

Rekosh, D. M., Lodish, H. F., and Baltimore, D., 1970, Protein synthesis in *Escherichia coli* extracts programmed by poliovirus RNA, *J. Mol. Biol.* **54**, 327.

Robertson, H. D., and Mathews, M. D., 1973, Double-stranded RNA as an inhibitor of protein synthesis and as a substrate for a nuclease in extracts of Krebs II ascites cells, *Proc. Natl. Acad. Sci. USA* **70**, 225.

Roizman, B., Mayer, M. M., and Rapp, H. J., 1958, Immunochemical studies of poliovirus. III. Further studies on the immunologic and physical properties of poliovirus particles produced in tissue culture, *J. Immunol.* **81**, 419.

Rosenberg, H., Diskin, B., Oron, L., and Traub, A., 1972, Isolation and subunit structure of polycytidylate-dependent RNA polymerase of encephalomyocarditis virus, *Proc. Natl. Acad. Sci. USA* **69**, 3815.

Roumiantzeff, M., Maizel, J. V., Jr., and Summers, D. F., 1971a, Comparison of polysomal structures of uninfected and poliovirus infected Hela cells, *Virology* **44,** 239.

Roumiantzeff, M., Summers, D. F., and Maizel, J. V., Jr., 1971*b, In vitro* protein synthesis activity of membrane-bound poliovirus polyribosomes, *Virology,* 44, 249.

Roy, P., and Bishop, D. H. L., 1970, Isolation and properties of poliovirus minus strand ribonucleic acid, *J. Virol.* **6,** 604.

Rueckert, R., 1971, Picornaviral architecture *in* "Comprehensive Virology," (K. Maramorosch and E. Kurstak, eds.), pp. 225–306, Academic Press, New York.

Sabin, A. B., Henessen, W. A., and Winsser, J., 1954, Studies of variants of poliovirus. I. Experimental segregation and properties of avirulent variants of three immunologic types, *J. Exp. Med.* **99,** 551.

Salzman, N. P., 1960, The rate of formation of vaccinia deoxyribonucleic acid and vaccinia virus, *Virology* **10,** 150.

Salzman, N. P., Lockart, R. Z., and Sebring, E. P., 1959, Alterations in Hela cell metabolism resulting from poliovirus infection, *Virology* **9,** 244.

Savage, T., Granboulan, N., and Girard, M., 1971, Architecture of the poliovirus replicative intermediate RNA, *Biochimie* **53,** 533.

Saxton, R. E., and Stevens, J. G., 1972, Restriction of herpes simplex virus replication by poliovirus: A selective inhibition of viral translation, *Virology* **48,** 207.

Schaffer, F. L., 1962, Binding of proflavine and photoinactivation of poliovirus propagated in the presence of the dye, *Virology* **18,** 412.

Schaffer, F. L., and Gordon, M., 1966, Differential inhibitory effects of actinomycin D among strains of poliovirus, *J. Bacteriol.* **91,** 2309.

Schaffer, F. L., and Schwerdt, C. E., 1955, Crystallization of purified MEF-1 poliomyelitis virus particles, *Proc. Natl. Acad. Sci. USA* **41,** 1020.

Schaffer, F. L., Moore, H. F., and Schwerdt, C. E., 1960, Base composition of the ribonucleic acid of the three types of poliovirus, *Virology* **10,** 530.

Scharff, M. D., and Levintow, L., 1963, Quantitative study of the formation of poliovirus antigens in infected Hela cells, *Virology* **19,** 491.

Scharff, M. D., Shatkin, A. J., and Levintow, L., 1963*a,* Association of newly formed viral protein with specific polyribosomes, *Proc. Natl. Acad. Sci. USA* **50,** 686.

Scharff, M. D., Thoren, M. M., McElvain, N. F., and Levintow, L., 1963*b,* Interruption of poliovirus RNA synthesis by *p*-fluorophenylalanine and puromycin, *Biochem. Biphys. Res. Commun.* **10,** 127.

Scharff, M. D., Maizel, J. V., Jr., and Levintow, L., 1964, Physical and immunological properties of a soluble precursor of the poliovirus capsid, *Proc. Natl. Acad. Sci. USA* **51,** 329.

Scharff, M. D., Summers, D. F., and Levintow, L., 1965, Further studies on the effect of *p*-fluorophenylalanine and puromycin on poliovirus replication, *Ann. N.Y. Acad. Sci.* **130,** 282.

Schwerdt, C. E., and Schaffer, F. L., 1955, Some physical and chemical properties of poliomyelitis virus preparations, *Ann. N.Y. Acad. Sci.* **61,** 740.

Sedmak, G. V., Taylor, M. W., Mealey, J., and Chen, T. T., 1972, Oncolytic effect of bovine enterovirus in mouse and human tumours, *Nat. New. Biol.* **238,** 7.

Semmel, M., and Huppert, J., 1970, Encephalomyocarditis virus multiplication in the presence of pyronine, *J. Gen. Virol.* **7,** 187.

Semmel, M., Verjus, M. -A., and Huppert, J., 1973, The effect of ethidium bromide on L cells and encephalomyocarditis virus replication, *J. Gen. Virol.* **20,** 51.

Sergiescu, D., Aubert-Combiescu, A., and Crainic, R., 1969, Recombination between guanidine-resistant and dextran sulfate-resistant mutants of Type 1 poliovirus, *J. Virol.* **3**, 326.

Shea, M. A., and Plagemann, P. G. W., 1971, Effects of elevated temperatures on mengovirus ribonucleic acid synthesis and virus production in Novikoff rat Hepatoma cells, *J. Virol.* **7**, 144.

Simon, E. H., 1961, Evidence for the non-participation of DNA in viral RNA synthesis, *Virology* **13**, 105.

Smith, A. E., 1973, The initiation of protein synthesis directed by the RNA from encephalomyocarditis virus, *Eur. J. Biochem.* **33**, 301.

Smith, A. E., Marcker, K. A., and Mathews, M. B., 1970, Translation of RNA from encephalomyocarditis virus in a cell-free system, *Nature (Lond.)* **225**, 184.

Stavis, R. L., and August, J. T., 1970, The biochemistry of RNA bacteriophage replication, *Annu. Rev. Biochem.* **39**, 527.

Stoltzfus, C. M., and Rueckert, R., 1972, Capsid polypeptides of mouse Elberfeld virus. I. Amino acid compositions and molar ratios in the virion, *J. Virol.* **10**, 347.

Stoner, G. D., Williams, B., Kniazeff, A., and Shimkin, M. B., 1973, Effect of neuraminidase pretreatment on the susceptibility of normal and transformed mammalian cells to bovine enterovirus 261, *Nat. New Biol.* **245** 319.

Summers, D. F., and Levintow, L., 1965, Constitution and function of polyribosomes of poliovirus-infected Hela cells, *Virology* **27**, 44.

Summers, D. F., and Maizel, J. V., Jr., 1967, Disaggregation of Hela cell polysomes after infection with poliovirus, *Virology* **31**, 550.

Summers, D. F., and Maizel, J. V., Jr., 1968, Evidence for large precursor proteins in poliovirus synthesis, *Proc. Natl. Acad. Sci USA* **59**, 966.

Summers, D. F., and Maizel, J. V., Jr., 1971, Determination of the gene sequence of poliovirus with pactamycin, *Proc. Natl. Acad. Sci. USA* **68**, 2852.

Summers, D. F., Maizel, J. V. Jr., and Darnell, J. E. Jr., 1965, Evidence for virus-specific noncapsid proteins in poliovirus-infected Hela cells, *Proc. Natl. Acad. Sci. USA* **54**, 505.

Summers, D. F., Maizel, J. V., Jr., and Darnell, J. E., Jr., 1967, The decrease in size and synthetic activity of poliovirus polysomes late in the infectious cycle, *Virology* **31**, 427.

Summers, D. F., Shaw, E. N., Stewart, M. L., and Maizel, J. V., Jr., 1972, Inhibition of cleavage of large poliovirus specific precursor proteins in infected Hela cells by inhibitors of proteolytic enzymes, *J. Virol.* **10**, 880.

Taber, R., Rekosh, D. M., and Baltimore, D., 1971, Effect of pactamycin on synthesis of poliovirus proteins: A method for genetic mapping, *J. Virol.* **8**, 395.

Tannock, G. A., Gibbs, A. J., and Cooper, P. D., 1970, A re-examination of the molecular weight of poliovirus RNA, *Biochem. Biophys. Res. Commun.* **38**, 298.

Taylor, M. W., Cordell, B., Souhrada, M., and Prather, S., 1971, Viruses as an aid to cancer therapy: Regression of solid and ascites tumors in rodents after treatment with bovine enterovirus, *Proc. Natl. Acad. Sci. USA* **68**, 836.

Tershak, D. R., 1964, Effect of 5-fluorouracil on poliovirus growth, *Virology* **24**, 262.

Tershak, D. R., 1966, Effect of 5-fluorouracil on poliovirus-induced RNA polymerase, *J. Mol. Biol.* **21**, 43.

Tershak, D. R., 1969, Synthesis of RNA in cells infected with LSc poliovirus at elevated temperatures, *J. Virol* **3**, 297.

Tolskaya, E. A., Agol, V. I., Voroshilova, M. K. and Lipskaya, G. Y., 1966, The osmotic pressure of the maintenance medium and reproduction of poliovirus, *Virology* **29**, 613.

Vaheri, A., and Pagano, J. S., 1965, Infectious poliovirus RNA: A sensitive method of assay, *Virology* **27**, 434.

Vanden Berghe, D., and Boeyé, A., 1972, New polypeptides in poliovirus, *Virology* **48**, 604.

Vande Woude, G. F., Polatnick, J., and Ascione, R., 1970, Foot-and-mouth disease virus-induced alterations of baby hamster kidney cell macromolecular biosynthesis: Inhibition of ribonucleic acid methylation and stimulation of ribonucleic acid synthesis, *J. Virol.* **5**, 458.

Vogt, M., and Dulbecco, R., 1958, Properties of a Hela cell culture with increased resistance to poliomyelitis virus, *Virology* **5**, 425.

Wall, R., and Taylor, M. W., 1970, Mengovirus RNA synthesis in productive and restrictive cell lines, *Virology* **42**, 78.

Warner, J., Madden, M. J., and Darnell, J. E., Jr., 1963, The interaction of poliovirus RNA with *Escherichia coli* ribosomes, *Virology* **19**, 393.

Watanabe, Y., 1965, A double-stranded RNA of poliovirus-infected Hela cells: Thermal denaturation and annealing, *Biochim. Biophys. Acta* **95**, 515.

Watanabe, Y., Watanabe, K., and Hinuma, Y., 1962, Synthesis of poliovirus-specific proteins in Hela cells, *Biochim. Biophys. Acta* **61**, 976.

Watanabe, Y., Watanabe, K., Katagiri, S., and Hinuma, Y., 1965, Virus-specific proteins produced in Hela cells infected with poliovirus: Characterization of subunit-like protein, *J. Biochem.* **57**, 733.

Wecker, E., and Lederhilger, G., 1964*a,* Curtailment of the latent period by double-infection with poliovirus, *Proc. Natl. Acad. Sci. USA* **52**, 246.

Wecker, E., and Lederhilger, G., 1964*b,* Genomic masking produced by double-infection with heterotypic polioviruses, *Proc. Natl. Acad. Sci. USA* **52**, 705.

Weissmann, C., Feix, G., and Slor, H., 1968, *In vitro* synthesis of phage RNA: The nature of the intermediates, *Cold Spring Harbor Symp. Quant. Biol.* **33**, 83.

Wentworth, B. B., McCahon, D., and Cooper, P. D., 1968, Production of infectious RNA and serum-blocking antigen by poliovirus temperature-sensitive mutants, *J. Gen. Virol.* **2**, 297.

Wild, T. F., and Brown, F., 1970, Replication of foot-and-mouth disease virus ribonucleic acid, *J. Gen. Virol.* **7**, 1.

Wild, T. F., Martin, S. J., and Brown, F., 1968, A study of the heterogeneous 37 S ribonucleic acid induced by foot-and-mouth disease virus, *Biochem. J.* **107**, 395.

Willems, F. T. C., Melnick, J. L., and Rawls, W. E., 1969, Replication of poliovirus in phytohemagglutinin-stimulated human lymphocytes, *J. Virol.* **3**, 451.

Wilson, J. N., and Cooper, P. D., 1962, Photodynamic demonstration of two stages of growth of poliovirus, *Virology* **17**, 195.

Wimmer, E., 1972, Sequence studies of poliovirus RNA. I. Characterization of the 5'-terminus, *J. Mol. Biol.* **68**, 537.

Wolff, D. A., and Bubel, H. C., 1964, The disposition of lysosomal enzymes as related to specific viral cytopathic effects, *Virology* **24**, 502.

Yin, F. H., Lonberg-Holm, K., and Chan, S. P., 1973, Lack of a close relationship between three strains of human rhinoviruses as determined by their RNA sequences, *J. Virol.* **12**, 108.

Yogo, Y., and Wimmer, E., 1972, Polyadenylic acid at the 3'-terminus of poliovirus RNA, *Proc. Natl. Acad. Sci. USA* **69**, 1877.

Yogo, Y., and Wimmer, E., 1973, Poly(A) and poly(U) in poliovirus double-stranded RNA, *Nat. New Biol.* **242**, 171.

Young, N. A., 1973a, Polioviruses, coxsackieviruses, and echoviruses: Comparison of their genomes by RNA hybridization, *J. Virol.* **11**, 832.

Young, N. A., 1973b, Size of gene sequences shared by polioviruses types 1, 2, and 3, *Virology* **56**, 400.

Young, N. A., Hoyer, B. H., and Martin, M. A., 1968, Polynucleotide sequence homologies among polioviruses, *Proc. Natl. Acad. Sci. USA* **61**, 548.

Zajac, I., and Crowell, R. L., 1965, Effect of enzymes on the interaction of enteroviruses with living Hela cells, *J. Bacteriol.* **89**, 574.

CHAPTER 4

Reproduction of Togaviruses

Elmer R. Pfefferkorn

Microbiology Department
Dartmouth Medical School
Hanover, New Hampshire 03755

and

Daniel Shapiro

Department of Microbiology
Colorado State University
Fort Collins, Colorado 80521

1. INTRODUCTION

The togaviruses may be more familiar to some readers under the old term "arboviruses." Arboviruses (*ar*thropod-*bo*rne), as originally defined, generally are transmitted to their vertebrate hosts by the bite of an infected arthropod, usually a mosquito or a tick. In this natural cycle, the arthropod does not play a passive role; instead, active multiplication of virus in the arthropod host is essential. As Casals (1971) has pointed out, this essentially ecological classification no longer suffices to define a morphologically and biochemically related group of viruses and hence should be abandoned.

Although the first "arboviruses" isolated seemed to form a relatively homogeneous group, as more recent isolates have been examined by modern electron microscopic and biochemical techniques, it has become apparent that a wide variety of viruses can multiply in and be transmitted by arthropods. Among the viruses found to fit this definition have been pox-, picorna-, rhabdo-, diplorna-, and arenaviruses (Casals, 1971). No doubt additional viral groups will be added to this list when as yet uncharacterized "arboviruses" are further studied. Clearly these various viral groups have nothing in common but the potential role of an arthropod in their transmission.

Many of the viruses classified as "arboviruses" can be assigned to the recently defined togaviruses (Wildy, 1971), i.e., enveloped single-stranded RNA viruses in which the nucleocapsid probably has icosahedral symmetry. Omission of arthropod transmission from this definition serves to emphasize that viruses with no known arthropod vector may also be classed as togaviruses. Among these are rubella virus and lactic dehydrogenase virus. This chapter, however, will be confined to those viruses previously classified as group A and group B arboviruses. We propose to continue part of this traditional nomenclature by terming these viruses group A and group B togaviruses.* These groupings were originally based on antigenic cross-reaction, as detected by neutralization, complement fixation, and hemagglutination inhibition (reviewed by Casals and Clarke, 1965; Clarke and Casals, 1965). Antigenic cross reaction among viruses generally implies both evolution from a common ancestor and substantial biochemical and morphological similarity. As Schlesinger (1971) has indicated, the complex natural cycle of arthropod transmission provides a strong selective pressure for the rapid emergence of viruses of new antigenic types. This probably accounts for the large number of group A (about 20 types) and group B (about 40 types) togaviruses now known. Although notable differences exist between group A and group B togaviruses, we are impressed by the similarity that exists within each group. Thus, discrepancies in data concerning the general morphology or the biochemistry of replication of, for example, two group A togaviruses are likely to represent subtle effects of experimental technique rather than fundamental differences between related viruses. In preparing our chapter, we have, in fact, presumed homogeneity within each of these two antigenically defined groups and pooled the data on the viruses listed in Table 1. Indeed, without pooling data from related viruses, we could not prepare as coherent an account of the replication of togaviruses. In constructing our composite pictures of viral replication, we have not always indicated the identity of the virus used in a particular experiment, although assignment to group A or B should be apparent at those places in which we consider it important. When a

---

* Editor's note: The names alphaviruses and flavoviruses have been approved by the International Committee on Nomenclature of Viruses (ICNV) for groups A and B of the togaviruses, respectively [H. F.-C.].

TABLE 1

Togaviruses Widely Used in the Study of Viral Replication

Group A	Group B
Chikungunya	Dengue
Eastern equine encephalitis	Japanese encephalitis
Semliki Forest	Kunjin
Sindbis	St. Louis encephalitis
Venezuelan equine encephalitis	
Western equine encephalitis	

virus is not named in the text, its identity can be determined by inspection of the reference list, which includes titles.

2. STRUCTURE AND COMPOSITION

2.1. Morphology and Stability

2.1.1. Electron Microscopy

A wide variety of togaviruses have been examined by electron microscopy using thin sectioning, negative staining, and freeze etching. Representative electron micrographs are presented in Figs. 1 and 2. The sum of the evidence from these studies is that togaviruses are nonrigid membrane-coated spheres with an electron-dense core or nucleocapsid. Not surprisingly, there is some discrepancy in the diameters assigned to the virions since this measurement can vary with the method of preparation. Furthermore, an heritable difference in size has been noted in individual clones of a group A virus (Tsilinsky et al., 1971). Inspection of a large number of reports suggests that the group A viruses have a somewhat greater diameter, 45–75 nm, than the group B viruses, 37–50 nm (e.g., earlier results, tabulated by Mussgay, 1964; Nishimura and Kitaoka, 1964; Yasuzumi et al., 1964; Ota, 1965; Murphy et al., 1968; Simpson and Hauser, 1968; Smith et al., 1970; Tsilinsky et al., 1971; Brown et al., 1972; Cardiff et al., 1973a). We wish to reemphasize that the true sizes of group A and group B virions probably do not vary over as great a range as those noted above. Indeed, the measurements of a given investigator using a single technique on one virus vary less than 10%.

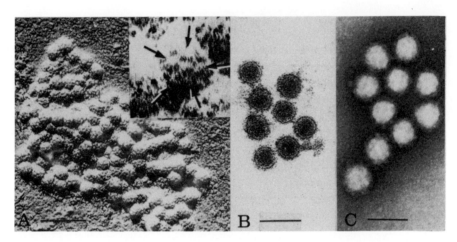

Fig. 1. The morphology of Sindbis, a group A togavirus. (A) Surface replica of freeze-dried nucleocapsids prepared by treating Sindbis virus with deoxycholate. The insert shows one nucleocapsid that displays a fivefold axis of symmetry. The magnification bar is 100 nm for the figure and 20 nm for the insert. From Brown *et al.* (1972). Reproduced by permission of the American Society for Microbiology. (B and C) Sindbis virions prepared for electron microscopy by ultrathin sectioning and negative staining, respectively. The magnification bars are 100 nm. Photographs kindly supplied by Dr. Dennis Brown.

Negatively stained group A virions have irregular surface projections (Simpson and Hauser, 1968), but these are not as prominent as the "spikes" that project from the surface of myxoviruses. Freeze-etching studies show that these projections in Sindbis virus are in the form of 4-nm subunits packed with a center-to-center spacing of 6 nm (Brown *et al.*, 1972). They may be equivalent to the surface subunits of a group B virion seen by negative staining to be about 7 nm in diameter (Smith *et al.*, 1970). These surface projections are probably composed of the viral glycoproteins (see section 2.2.3).

2.1.2. Properties of Virions and Nucleocapsids

Densities of togavirions have been measured by centrifugation to equilibrium in cesium chloride, potassium tartrate, or sucrose. We mistrust values obtained in cesium chloride because of the marked loss of infectivity (Pfefferkorn and Hunter, 1963a; Stevens and Schlesinger, 1965). Recorded densities for both group A and B virions vary from 1.18 to 1.24 g/ml (Pfefferkorn and Hunter, 1963a; Mussgay and Horzinek, 1966; Smith *et al.*, 1970; Fuscaldo *et al.*, 1971; Shapiro *et al.*, 1971a; Stinski and Gruber, 1971; Weiss and Schlesinger, 1973).

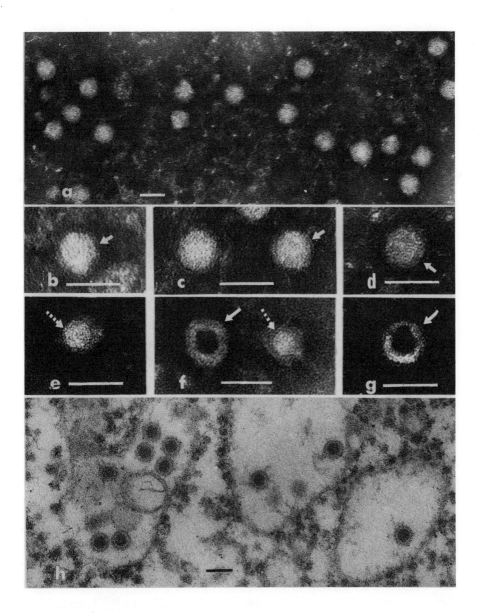

Fig. 2.   Morphology of dengue 2 virions. Negatively stained preparations of virions (a–d) reveal their average size to be 50 mn. The solid arrows indicate the viral envelope. The virion surface is composed of ill-defined subunits. Osmotic shock reveals a nucleocapsid (e, f–broken arrow) and a hollow envelope (f, g–solid arrow). Thin sections (h) clearly reveal the virion envelope and nucleocapsid. The magnification bars are 50 nm. From Matsumura *et al.* (1971). Reproduced by permission of Academic Press.

Again this is probably a greater variation than truly exists. The density of togavirions, measured in sucrose solutions, is probably about 1.20 g/ml. In keeping with their larger diameter, group A virions appear to have greater sedimentation coefficients, about 280 S, than group B virions, about 208 S (Strauss *et al.*, 1968; Boulton and Westaway, 1972).

Like most enveloped viruses, togavirions are labile. Thermal inactivation of group A viruses occurs at a significant rate, even under the relatively mild conditions of incubation in tissue culture medium, a fact which can lead to the misinterpretation of growth curves (Purifoy *et al.*, 1968). The thermal inactivation of group A togaviruses proceeds through two different and independent reactions, one predominating at temperatures below 40°C and the other at higher temperatures (Barnes *et al.*, 1969; Fleming, 1971*a*). Thus, the HR mutant of Sindbis virus, selected for increased resistance to thermal inactivation at 60°C, is inactivated at 40°C at a rate indistinguishable from that of the wild type (Burge and Pfefferkorn, 1966*a*). Although virions of group B are even more thermolabile than those of group A, a thermostable mutant of Japanese encephalitis virus has been isolated (Iwasaki and Inoue, 1961).

All togaviruses are sensitive to detergents and ether by virtue of the lipid in their envelopes. The effects of a battery of different organic solvents on the infectivity and antigenicity of Western equine encephalitis virus has been reported (Ventura and Scherer, 1970).

Exposure to various enzymes reduces the infectivity of group A togaviruses. As noted above, the proteolytic enzyme bromalein removes the envelope proteins of Sindbis virus and yields a bald, noninfectious particle (Compans, 1971). Contrary to an earlier report (Cheng, 1958) that trypsin sensitivity distinguishes between group A and group B togaviruses, Gorman and Goss (1972) noted that both group A and B viruses are inactivated by proteases. Lipases also inactivate virions, but, surprisingly, some 45% of the phospholipid of Semliki Forest virus can be removed by treatment with phospholipase C without reducing the infectivity of the virions; these virions, however, then become more labile (Friedman and Pastan, 1969). Japanese encephalitis virus is also inactivated by lipase, but no detailed kinetics are available (Takehara and Hotta, 1961).

Agents which reduce disulfide bonds, particularly dithiothreitol, rapidly inactivate representative group A and B togaviruses under conditions that fail to affect picornaviruses (Carver and Seto, 1968). In the case of Sindbis virus, this inactivation is partially reversed by treatment with oxidized glutathione. A similar reversibility of Semliki

Forest virus inactivation by the denaturing agents urea and guanidine–HCl has been observed by Fleming (1971b). Although Sindbis
virus is uniformly stable over the pH range 6.8–9.0 (Pfefferkorn,
unpublished observation), group B togaviruses are maximally stable at
pH 8–9 (Igarashi et al., 1963).

Treatment with nonionic detergents or mild ionic detergents such
as deoxycholate will remove the envelope of togavirions. Since the 40-
nm nucleocapsids survive this treatment, they can be freed from the
resulting envelope fragments by velocity gradient or isopycnic centrifugation (Strauss et al., 1968; Stollar, 1969; Shapiro et al., 1971a).
Greater yields of group A nucleocapsids can be prepared from infected
cells (Acheson and Tamm, 1970a), but here purification is more difficult and the best products still contain some adsorbed cellular protein.

Reported sedimentation coefficients of nucleocapsids isolated
from group A or group B virions range from 140 to 150 S (Strauss et
al., 1968; Stollar, 1969; Acheson and Tamm, 1970a; Kääriäinen and
Söderlund, 1971). The only comparative study (Boulton and Westaway, 1972) notes that the nucleocapsids of group A and B virions
have identical sedimentation coefficients. The density of the
nucleocapsid of Semliki Forest virus is 1.30 g/ml in potassium tartrate
and 1.47 g/ml in cesium chloride (Acheson and Tamm, 1970a). The
density of group B nucleocapsids is about 1.30 g/ml in both sucrose–deuterium oxide and potassium tartrate gradients (Shapiro et al.,
1971a; Trent and Qureshi, 1971).

Nucleocapsids of togaviruses contain the viral RNA and a single
species of protein (see Sect. 2.2.3). The general principles of construction lead us to expect that these nucleocapsids should exhibit helical or
icosahedral symmetry. Although this symmetry has never been
unequivocally revealed by electron microscopy, most observers favor
an icosahedral structure. Horzinek and Mussgay (1969) isolated
nucleocapsids from Sindbis virions and studied them by negative
staining. Their pictures are consistent with an icosahedron having 32
hexamer–pentamer morphological units and a triangulation number of
three. Hints of icosahedral symmetry were also reported by Simpson
and Hauser (1968) who examined negatively stained virions and by
Brown et al. (1972) who used isolated nucleocapsids (see Fig. 1).
Further evidence for icosahedral symmetry comes from the observation
of regular arrays of intracellular nucleocapsids (Morgan et al., 1961).
The sole report of helical symmetry comes from electron microscopy
of Venezuelan equine encephalitis virus preparations in which a small
number of virions was apparently disrupted, and released an obviously

helical structure (Klimenko *et al.*, 1965). We suspect that this observation is invalid because of contaminating virions of a different species.

In contrast to those virions that are simply naked icosahedrons (e.g., poliovirus), togaviral nucleocapsids are susceptible to RNase which, at low concentrations, degrades the virion RNA to small fragments (Acheson and Tamm, 1970c; Kääriäinen and Söderlund, 1971; Boulton and Westaway, 1972). Since the infectivity of intact virions is not reduced by RNase, the envelope presumably serves to protect the viral RNA from enzymatic attack. Although nucleocapsids contain infectious RNA, they are not infectious because they fail to adsorb to susceptible cells (Bose and Sagik, 1970b). Thus, adsorption to cells is presumably another function of the viral envelope.

2.2. Chemical Composition

2.2.1. Purification and Overall Composition

Togaviruses are relatively easily purified because they are released into tissue culture fluid without overt lysis of the infected cell. In purification, the first step is usually concentration of virus from tissue culture medium by ultracentrifugation or, preferentially, by precipitation with ammonium sulfate (Strauss *et al.*, 1969) or polyethylene glycol (Qureshi and Trent, 1973). Virus in the resulting small volume can then be purified by sequential velocity and equilibrium ultracentrifugation in sucrose gradients (Strauss *et al.*, 1969; Stollar *et al.*, 1966).

Chemical analyses of virions purified in this manner show the presence of RNA, protein, lipid, and carbohydrate. The overall analyses of group A viruses that are available are in general agreement (Wachter and Johnson, 1962; Pfefferkorn and Hunter, 1963a). Correcting the earlier determinations with recent values for the carbohydrate content of viral glycoproteins (Strauss *et al.*, 1970) yields the following composition: RNA, 5.5%; protein, 61%; lipid, 27%; carbohydrate (in glycoprotein), 6.5%. Other partial analyses, e.g., protein: lipid ratios, are in accord with this overall composition (Renkonen *et al.*, 1971).

In contrast to the relatively consistent data reported for group A viruses, overall analyses of group B togaviruses show widely disparate results. This lack of agreement probably reflects the fact that group B viruses do not produce such high titers in tissue culture, and thus contamination with cellular debris is more serious. Purification of virus from tissues of infected animals is even more difficult. In general, the RNA content reported for group B viruses is about 7%, slightly higher than that of the group A viruses. This difference is perhaps to be expected, for both groups have an RNA molecule of about the same size, but the group B virions are smaller. Reports of the protein: lipid ratios for group B virions vary from 7:1 (Ada *et al.*, 1962), to 1:4 (Trent, 1973), to 1:1.7 (Nozima *et al.*, 1964). It is unlikely that the growth of these closely related viruses in different cells can so profoundly affect viral composition. Thus, for the present, these values only suggest the range in which the true composition of group B togaviruses is likely to lie.

2.2.2. Viral RNA

The phenolic or detergent extraction of infectious RNA from a variety of togaviruses (e.g., Wecker, 1959; Igarashi *et al.*, 1963) is the best proof for an RNA genome. Analyses of the extracted viral RNAs by velocity gradient centrifugation yield sedimentation coefficients ranging from 40 to 49 S (Sonnabend *et al.*, 1967; Friedman *et al.*, 1966; Marcus and Salb, 1966; Simmons and Strauss, 1972a; Stollar *et al.*, 1967; Boulton and Westaway, 1972; Igarashi *et al.*, 1964; Trent *et al.*, 1969). We assume that these various values reflect differences in experimental technique rather than true heterogeneity in the sedimentation behavior of togaviral RNA, particularly since both the largest and smallest values are reported for RNA from the same virus, Sindbis. We know of no experiments in which differentially labeled togaviral RNAs have been directly compared by cosedimentation or coelectrophoresis. Comparison by parallel electrophoresis of RNAs from representative group A and B virions showed them to be indistinguishable (Boulton and Westaway, 1972), although a slight difference in sedimentation was noted.

The calculation of molecular weights of single-stranded RNA from sedimentation coefficients in aqueous medium is unreliable because the secondary structure of these molecules makes prediction of their hydrodynamic behavior difficult. Thus we prefer molecular weight determinations based upon polyacrylamide gel electrophoresis, which yield an average value of about 4.2×10^6 daltons for the molecular weights of both group A and group B togaviral RNA (Dobos and Faulkner, 1970; Boulton and Westaway, 1972).

The structure of group A togaviral RNA was long a matter of

some dispute. Treatment with mild denaturing conditions (heat, dimethyl sulfoxide, or urea) that were unlikely to break phosphodiester bonds appeared to convert group A viral RNA into a more slowly sedimenting (26 S) form (e.g., Dobos and Faulkner, 1969; Sreevalsan and Lockart, 1966). Boulton and Westaway (1972) have recently reported exactly parallel results with the RNA of a group B virus, Kunjin, suggesting that this *seeming* susceptibility to denaturing agents may be a property of both groups. Two models were proposed to explain these observations: the virion RNA was assumed either to be segmented and held together by short base-paired regions or to have an alternate, more slowly sedimenting, physical form.

Both of these models can now be discarded because the original observations were almost certainly artifacts. Careful studies by Arif and Faulkner (1972) have demonstrated conclusively that the RNA of Sindbis virus is indeed a single, continuous polynucleotide chain that is unaltered by exposure to denaturing conditions which were even more drastic than those noted above. This critical result has been confirmed by Simmons and Strauss (1972a). The key to this success was careful extraction of RNA from highly purified virus. In the absence of such precautions, contaminating ribonuclease presumably nicks the viral RNA at a limited number of defined sites; the extensive secondary structure (Sreevalsan *et al.*, 1968) of the viral RNA then masks these nicks until the nucleic acid is exposed to denaturing conditions.

Although no one has yet reported that the RNA of group B togaviruses retains its integrity after exposure to denaturing conditions, we suspect that it is also a continuous polynucleotide chain that is highly susceptible to the same "nicking" artifact that misled investigators of group A viral RNA.

Sensitivity to ribonuclease (e.g., Pfefferkorn *et al.*, 1967; Stollar *et al.*, 1966) indicates that togaviral RNA is single-stranded, a conclusion confirmed by the base ratios recorded in Table 2. These ratios are clearly inconsistent with a base-paired structure. Indirect, but on the whole convincing, evidence suggests that togaviral RNA is "plus" stranded. We are here using the convention suggested by Baltimore (1971) in which the "plus" strand has the base sequence of messenger RNA and the "minus" strand is complementary to it. The direct demonstration of messenger activity, synthesis of identifiable viral polypeptides in a cell-free system directed by virion RNA, is lacking. However, as noted above, togaviral RNAs are intrinsically infectious, a property shared with the "plus-stranded" polio RNA and lacking in the "minus-stranded" virion RNA of myxoviruses, paramyxoviruses, and rhabdoviruses. Furthermore, the RNAs of Sindbis virus (group A)

TABLE 2

Base Ratios of the Virion RNA of Various Togaviruses

Virus	Group	Ade-nine	Ura-cil	Gua-nine	Cyto-sine	Reference
		\multicolumn{4}{c}{Moles per 100 moles of base}		
Sindbis	A	29.6	19.7	25.8	24.9	Pfefferkorn and Hunter (1963a)
Semliki Forest	A	27.4	22.2	26.1	24.4	Sonnabend et al. (1967)
Semliki Forest	A	29.1	19.5	25.5	25.9	Kääriäinen and Gomatos (1969)
Western equine encephalitis	A	29.6	22.7	22.3	25.3	Sreevalsan et al. (1968)
Chikungunya	A	32.9	23.5	21.3	22.2	Nagatomo (1972)
Dengue	B	30.6	21.6	26.4	21.3	Stollar et al. (1966)
Murray Valley encephalitis	B	25.5	25.5	27.5	21.5	Ada et al. (1962)
St. Louis encephalitis	B	30.7	21.4	26.2	21.7	Trent et al. (1969)

and of St. Louis encephalitis virus (group B) have both been shown to contain polyadenylic acid (Johnston and Bose, 1972a,b; Brawner et al., 1973), a hallmark of most mammalian messenger RNA. The observations on Sindbis viral RNA have been extended and confirmed by Eaton and Faulkner (1972) who report substantial heterogeneity in the length of the polyadenylic acid segment. The bulk of the RNA extracted from Sindbis virus fails to bind to millipore filters under conditions generally used to bind mammalian mRNA by virtue of its polyadenylic acid content. This RNA passes through the filter because its polyadenylic acid sequence of 60–80 nucleotides is too short to be bound. The small fraction of virion RNA found bound to millipore filter has a polyadenylic acid sequence 150–250 nucleotides long. Surprisingly, both species of viral RNA are equally infectious. At present, it is not known if these differences in length of the polyadenylic acid sequence are genetically determined.

2.2.3. Viral Proteins and Glycoproteins

2.2.3(a). Group A Viruses

The first polyacrylamide gel electrophoretic analysis of amino acid-labeled Sindbis virus detected but two virus-specific proteins, one associated with the nucleocapsid and the other with the envelope (Strauss *et al.*, 1968). Subsequent analyses of other group A togaviruses have either confirmed this observation (Kennedy and Burke, 1972; Dorsett and Acton 1970; Hay *et al.*, 1968) or suggested the presence of an additional capsid protein (Horzinek and Mussgay, 1969; Friedman, 1968*b*). This second capsid protein, however, is almost certainly an artifact resulting from dimerization of the capsid protein (Acheson and Tamm, 1970*b*).

More recent investigations (M. J. Schlesinger *et al.*, 1972; Simons *et al.*, 1973) have disclosed an additional envelope protein in group A togaviruses. Continuous polyacrylamide gel electrophoresis in the presence of sodium dodecyl sulfate fails to resolve the two envelope

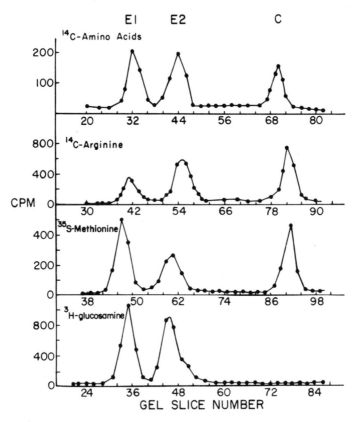

Fig. 3. Structural proteins of purified Sindbis virions resolved by discontinuous SDS polyacrylamide gel electrophoresis. Radioactive labeling is indicated in the figure. E1 and E2 are envelope proteins and C is the capsid protein. From M. J. Schlesinger *et al.* (1972). Reproduced by permission of Academic Press.

TABLE 3

Nomenclature and Properties of Togavirion Proteins

Virus	Protein	Location	Glyco-sylation	Approximate mol. wt. daltons $\times 10^3$
Group A	C	Nucleocapsid	0	30–32
	E1	Envelope	+	50–53
	E2	Envelope	+	50–53
Group B	V-1	Envelope	0	8–9
	V-2	Nucleocapsid	0	13–14
	V-3	Envelope	+	50–60

proteins; thus, they probably have about the same molecular weight. However, as shown in Fig. 3, application of a discontinuous electrophoretic technique, which affords greater resolution, readily demonstrates these two proteins. These proteins are undoubtedly distinct for they differ in amino acid composition and tryptic peptide maps (M. J. Schlesinger et al., 1972; Simons et al., 1973). The properties and the standard nomenclature for the virion proteins of group A togaviruses are summarized in Table 3.

Electrophoretic analysis of purified amino acid-labeled nucleocapsids shows only the C (capsid) protein of molecular weight 30,000–32,000 daltons (Strauss et al., 1968; Acheson and Tamm, 1970a). Amino acid analyses of the C protein show that it has an N-terminal lysine and is relatively hydrophilic, a property consistent with its extensive interaction with viral RNA. The mixture of both envelope proteins (E1 and E2) contains only one N-terminal amino acid, valine, and it is more hydrophobic in its amino acid content, as befits proteins that interact primarily with lipids (Kennedy and Burke, 1972).

As shown in Fig. 3, both proteins E1 and E2 of Sindbis virus are glycoproteins (Burge and Strauss, 1970; M. J. Schlesinger et al., 1972). Most analyses of the carbohydrate moiety of these proteins have been performed on the unresolved mixture of E1 and E2, which contains about 14% carbohydrate by weight (Strauss et al., 1970). Pronase digestion yields three prominent glycopeptides of different molecular weights and carbohydrate compositions (Burge and Strauss, 1970). If the two envelope proteins are equally glycosylated, as indicated by the preliminary results of M. J. Schlesinger et al. (1972), each envelope protein contains 3–4 glycopeptides. A carbohydrate analysis of the envelope glycoproteins of a group A togavirus is recorded in Table 4.

Both envelope proteins appear to occupy a superficial position in group A togavirions for they can be completely stripped away by treatment with a protease (Compans, 1971). Further evidence for the superficial location of proteins E1 and E2 comes from enzymatic iodination specific for proteins exposed to the external medium (Sefton *et al.*, 1973). Only the envelope proteins of intact Sindbis virions are labeled with ^{125}I. Prior disruption with detergent is required to allow labeling of the C protein. Similar results were obtained by Gahmberg *et al.* (1972) using a membrane-impermeable alkylating agent. An exclusively superficial location of Sindbis virus envelope proteins has been suggested by the X-ray diffraction studies of Harrison *et al.* (1971). These authors conclude that neither the external glycoproteins nor the internal capsid protein penetrate into the lipid layer although both are closely opposed to it. However, their data do not exclude penetration through the lipid bilayer by a limited segment of a glycoprotein. Such an internal representation of the virus-modified membrane would allow easy recognition by a nucleocapsid about to mature by budding (see Sect. 3.8.1).

The group A togaviral proteins can also be distinguished by serological methods. Treatment with detergent yields envelope fragments which contain lipid and the envelope proteins. These envelope fragments can agglutinate red cells under the conditions used for viral

TABLE 4

Carbohydrate Residues in the Envelope Proteins of Sindbis Virus[a]

Carbohydrate	Monosaccharide residues per mole of envelope protein[b]
Mannose plus galactose	17 ± 2
Glucosamine	19 ± 6
Sialic acid (virus grown in chick cells)	1.2 ± 0.1
(virus grown in BHK cells)	2.3 ± 0.2
Fucose	1.8 ± 0.5
Total	39 ± 7

[a] From Strauss *et al.* (1970). Reproduced by permission of Academic Press.
[b] Assuming equal glycosylation of proteins E1 and E2.

hemagglutination and also adsorb neutralizing antibodies (Appleyard et al., 1970). Thus, the envelope proteins represent both the hemagglutinin and the neutralization antigen. At present, it is not known which of these properties reside in proteins E1 and E2 or, indeed, if a complex of both is required for one or both activities. In contrast, the capsid antigen can only readily be detected by complement fixation (Bose and Sagik, 1970a); it is antigenically distinct from the envelope proteins. Preliminary evidence (Dalrymple et al., 1973) obtained by radioimmunoprecipitation suggests that several representatives of the group A togaviruses have a similar or identical capsid antigen and that they differ primarily in their envelope antigen(s).

2.2.3(b).   Group B Viruses

Group B togavirions also contain three polypeptides, but they are markedly different from those of group A virions. As shown in Fig. 4, these three proteins are readily resolved by continuous polyacrylamide gel electrophoresis (Stollar, 1969; Westaway and Reedman, 1969; Shapiro et al., 1971a, 1972a; Trent and Qureshi, 1971; Westaway, 1973); discontinuous gel electrophoresis fails to reveal any additional components. Occasionally, however, electropherograms of purified virus contain a polypeptide that migrates more slowly than V-3 and has an apparent molecular weight of about 93,000 daltons. We suspect that this polypeptide is a dimer of V-3 because both are glycosylated (Shapiro et al., 1973a); it is not likely to represent contamination with the intracellular nonstructural virus-specified protein of similar molecular weight because that nonstructural protein is not glycosylated. The standard terminology and properties of group B togavirion proteins are reviewed in Table 3. The estimated molecular weight of protein V-1 may be inaccurate because it is so small.

Nucleocapsids released from group B togavirions by treatment with nonionic detergents contain only the structural polypeptide V-2, while V-3 and V-1 remain in the envelope fraction (Stollar, 1969; Shapiro et al., 1971a; Trent and Qureshi, 1971; Boulton and Westaway, 1972). However, the assignment of protein V-1 to the envelope is somewhat ambiguous, for when virions are disrupted with deoxycholate, the nucleocapsid fraction contains both V-2 and V-1 (Trent and Qureshi, 1971). It would be of interest to study group B virions by enzymatic iodination of surface proteins to determine whether protein V-1 is exposed at the surface of viral envelope or is

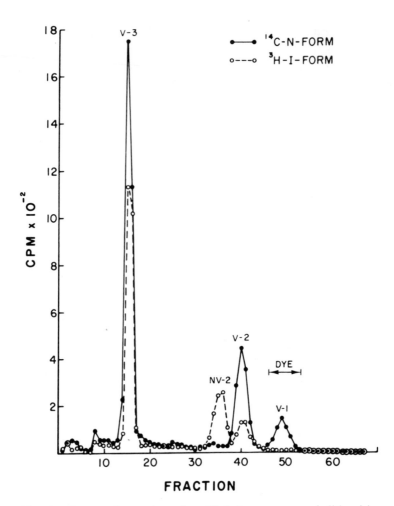

Fig. 4. Structural proteins of purified Japanese encephalitis virions resolved by continuous SDS polyacrylamide gel electrophoresis. The extracellular (N-form) virions are labeled with ^{14}C-amino acids. The intracellular (I-form, see Sect. 3.7) virions are labeled with ^{3}H-amino acids. V-1, V-3, and NV-2 are envelope proteins and V-2 is the capsid protein. From Shapiro *et al.* (1972c). Reproduced by permission of Academic Press.

inaccessible because it is buried within the lipid bilayer or at its inner surface.

The smaller envelope protein, V-1, also differs from the envelope proteins of group A virions in that it is not glycosylated. The sole glycoprotein in group B virions is the large envelope protein, V-3 (Stollar, 1969; Shapiro *et al.*, 1972c; Qureshi and Trent, 1973). Although no detailed carbohydrate analyses are available, the glycoprotein V-3 can be labeled with and presumably contains glucosamine, galactose, and mannose (Shapiro *et al.*, 1973*a*).

None of the antigens of group B viruses can be assigned to an individual structural protein. However, by analogy with other enveloped viruses, we predict that the principal antigen involved in neutralization of infectivity will be associated with the envelope glycoprotein V-3.

Qureshi and Trent (1973) have reported a surprising antigenic cross-reaction between the large viral envelope protein, V-3, and the capsid protein, V-2. We suspect that this cross-reaction is an artifact due to impurities or aggregation of viral polypeptides which would not be detected under their conditions of electrophoresis.

2.2.4. Viral Lipids

Togaviruses contain a large amount of lipid, presumably as a part of their envelope. The lipid/protein ratio of group A togaviruses has been reported to range from 0.44 in Sindbis virus (Pfefferkorn and Hunter, 1963*a*) to 0.44–0.39 in Semliki Forest virus, depending on the clone of BHK cells in which the virus was grown (Renkonen *et al.*, 1971). Extensive analyses of these viral lipids show significant variations from laboratory to laboratory and virus to virus, probably reflecting (1) systematic errors in lipid determinations on small samples, (2) the possibility that virions are contaminated with adventitious lipid despite rigorous attempts at purification, and (3) the effect of the host cell on the lipid composition of virions (Heydrick *et al.*, 1971). Despite these difficulties, the lipid analyses of group A viruses falls into a general pattern. Some 25% (Pfefferkorn and Hunter, 1963*a*) to 31% (Renkonen *et al.*, 1971) of the total lipid, by weight, is neutral lipid, in each case almost entirely unesterified cholesterol. Most of the remaining lipids are represented by four phospholipids: phosphatidylcholine, phosphatidylethanolamine, phosphatidylserine, and sphingomyelin. Phosphatidylcholine is generally found to be the principal phospatide (Pfefferkorn and Hunter, 1963*a*; Friedman and Pastan, 1969; Heydrick *et al.*, 1971; Renkonen *et al.*, 1971). However, David (1971) found phosphatidylethanolamine to be the most prominent phosphatide of Sindbis virus. It should be noted that David found more phosphatidylethanolamine than phosphatidylcholine in the plasma membrane of BHK cells, a result which also fails to agree with the report of Renkonen *et al.* (1971). The available analyses of viral fatty acids agree that oleic, palmitic, and stearic acids predominate

TABLE 5

Lipid Composition of Semliki Forest Virus and the Plasma
Membrane of the BHK Cells Used to Grow the Virus[a]

| | Molar ratio of individual lipid classes to phospholipid[b] | |
Lipid	Plasma membrane of BHK cells	Semliki Forest virus
Cholesterol	0.56	0.97
Sphingoglycolipids	0.08	0.09
Phosphatidylethanolamine	0.21	0.26
Phosphatidylcholine	0.40	0.34
Phosphatidylserine	0.07	0.12
Phosphatidylinositol	0.03	0.01
Sphingomyelin	0.17	0.21

[a] From Renkonen et al. (1971). Reproduced by permission of Academic Press.
[b] The total phospholipids consist of several minor components in addition to the major ones listed in the table.

(David, 1971; Renkonen et al., 1971; Laine et al., 1972). A typical lipid analysis for a group A togavirus is recorded in Table 5. On the basis of these data and other analyses, Renkonen et al. (1971) calculate that there are about 10,000 cholesterol–phospholipid pairs in each Semliki Forest virion, more than enough to form a complete bilayer surrounding the nucleocapsid.

The most striking illustration of the effect of the host cell on the lipid composition of togaviruses comes from a comparison of Semliki Forest virions grown in BHK cells and in *Aedes albopictus* cells. Renkonen et al. (1974) found that the virus grown in the insect cells resembles its host in lipid composition, but is so different from mammalian cell virus that they have only 36% of their lipids in common.

3. REPLICATION

3.1. Growth Curves

3.1.1. In Cultured Vertebrate Cells

The growth of group A togaviruses is rapid. After only two hours, vertebrate cells infected at temperatures close to 37°C begin to release infectious virus into the extracellular medium. After a relatively brief exponential phase, viral production continues at a more or less constant rate up to 10–12 hours after infection. During this linear phase, the rate of virus production may approach 1000 PFU/cell/hr, and the total yield may approach 10^{10} PFU/ml (Pfefferkorn and Hunter, 1963b). Group A viruses grow to some extent in most cultured vertebrate cells, but the highest titers are achieved in primary chick embryo cells and in BHK cells. As a viral cytopathic effect becomes apparent by light microscopy, the rate of virus production falls markedly. In most vertebrate cultures, the cells are ultimately destroyed, although chronically infected BHK (Schwöbel and Ahl, 1972) and mouse cell cultures (Inglot et al., 1973) have been described. In the latter case, interferon is instrumental in maintaining the persistent infection.

In contrast to the group A viruses, group B togavirus grow slowly in cultured vertebrate cells. When cells are infected at a high multiplicity, the latent period is about 12 hours (Stollar et al., 1967; Trent et al., 1969; Shapiro et al., 1971a); a further 10–20 hours are required to achieve maximal titers of extracellular virus. These titers are often low; a yield of 10^6–10^7 PFU/ml is not uncommon. Such titers may indicate extensive inactivation of virions that are unstable at the temperature and pH generally used in cell cultures (see Sect. 2.1.2). Growth at a lower temperature and at an alkaline pH increases the yield of Japanese encephalitis virus, but this result was at least partly ascribed to decreased synthesis of interferon (Chiang-Shem et al., 1966). Careful attention to certain empirical details can improve the yield of group B viruses (Singh et al., 1973). Specific factors shown to be effective include increased magnesium concentration (Matsumura et al., 1970) and the presence of polyions in the medium (Ozaki and Kumagi, 1972).

In some cultured cells, particularly hamster kidney (Karabatsos and Buckley, 1967) and pig kidney (Lee et al., 1958; Diercks and Hammon, 1958; Inoue and Ogura, 1962; Stim and Henderson, 1969), group B viral infection produces an obvious cytopathic effect. In many instances, however, infection is without any cytopathic effect that can be seen by light microscopy (Scherer and Syverton, 1954; McCollum and Foley, 1956). In fact, the first reported plaque assay of a group B virus was performed with cells that showed no cytopathic effect (Porterfield, 1959). Cultures of vertebrate cells chronically infected with various group B viruses can be established (Wiebenga, 1961; Furusawa et al., 1969); these cultures are refractory to superinfection with certain unrelated viruses, a state that may be mediated by intrinsic interference (cf. Marcus and Carver, 1967) or by interferon.

3.1.2. In Cultured Arthropod Cells

Although the ability to grow in arthropod cells is no longer part of the definition of togaviruses, it remains a pivotal feature of both group A and B viruses. At present, a thorough understanding of the replication of these viruses in arthropod cells is lacking. The ability of group A and B viruses to grow in these cells cannot be explained simply by the trivial capacity for adsorption and penetration. Peleg (1969*a*) has made the intriguing observation that infectious RNA from a picornavirus fails to replicate in mosquito cultures that can be infected by togaviral RNA.

In contrast to their generally destructive effect in cultures of vertebrate cells, the group A and B togaviruses produce chronic infections in arthropod cultures. It is of interest to note that this behavior resembles *in vivo* infections of mosquitoes and ticks in which togaviruses characteristically produce asymptomatic life-long infections. Their natural species tropism is also reflected in tissue culture: tick-borne viruses grow best in tick cell cultures while mosquito-borne viruses grow best in mosquito cultures (Singh, 1971).

The initial response of *Aedes albopictus* cultures to togaviral infection is the production of virus at rates and titers which are roughly comparable to those achieved in vertebrate cells at equivalent low temperatures (Singh and Paul, 1968*a,b*; Stevens, 1970; Yunker, 1971). This high yield of virus is accompanied by a cytopathic effect that includes cytolysis, the development of syncytia, and phagocytosis. There is, in fact, sufficient cell damage to allow the use of *A. albopictus* in a plaque assay (Suitor, 1969; Cory and Yunker, 1972). Most cultures in liquid medium recover from this initial cytopathic response and become chronically infected, yielding much less virus (Banerjee and Singh, 1968; Paul *et al.*, 1969; Stevens, 1970; Peleg, 1969*a,b*, 1972). It is not certain what percentage of the cells are infected at this stage. In *Aedes aegypti* cultures, only a small fraction of the cells appears to be infected by group B virus, and a chronic infection can be established with or without an initial cytopathic effect (Filshie and Rehacek, 1968; Rehacek, 1968).

The mechanism by which chronically infected arthropod cultures maintain their viability is unknown. An important clue may be the observation that the mosquito cultures chronically infected with a group A virus contain 12 S double-stranded virus-specific RNA; this evidence suggests that defective-interfering particles (see Sect. 3.8) may play a role in this mechanism (Stollar and Shenk, 1973). Other possible mechanisms are interferon, which has been detected in *A. al-*

bopictus cultures persistently infected with a group A virus (Enzmann, 1973), and intrinsic interference of the sort described by Marcus and Carver (1967).

Mosquito cultures chronically infected with one group A or B virus can be superinfected with another group A or B virus (Rehacek, 1968; Stollar and Shenk, 1973). However, at least in the case of group A viruses, superinfection with the homologous virus is blocked (Stollar and Shenk, 1973). The basis for this homologous interference is unknown but, as noted above, defective-interfering particles may well play a role.

3.2. Cytopathology

Although light microscopy fails to reveal marked cytopathic changes during the most rapid release of group A togaviruses, electron microscopy readily discloses extensive changes in the cytoplasm of infected cells. Virions are produced by budding of nucleocapsids through areas of cell membranes which are modified by the presence of virus-specified envelope proteins (see Sect. 3.6). Various investigators have reported two principal sites of viral budding: (1) the plasma membrane (Acheson and Tamm, 1967; Brown *et al.*, 1972), as illustrated in Fig. 5, and (2) intracellular vacuoles that apparently do not communicate with the extracellular fluid (Morgan *et al.*, 1961; Grimley *et al.*, 1968). Grimley *et al.*, (1968) have termed these vacuoles "type 2 cytopathic vacuoles." They are illustrated in Fig. 6. In any given preparation, one site of maturation or another predominates, presumably depending on some unidentified variable. At both of these sites, examination of thin sections by electron microscopy reveals nucleocapsids closely apposed to the cytoplasmic side of the membrane, and occasionally in the process of budding through it.

Those virions that bud into the intracellular vacuoles are presumed to be released by subsequent fusion of the vacuole with the plasma membrane of the infected cell. In those cells in which maturation takes place at the plasma membrane, the entire surface of the cell is not involved, at any one time at least, in the production of the virus. Localized regions, in which the budding of the virions is concentrated, have been detected by electron microscopy using both freeze etching, as shown in Fig. 5, and ferritin-labeled antiviral antibody (Pederson and Sagik, 1973).

In addition to the obvious sites of viral budding, other ultrastructural changes occur within the cytoplasm of infected cells.

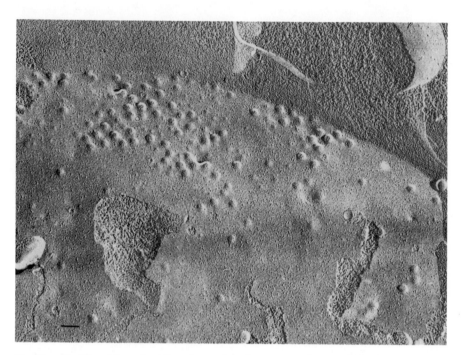

Fig. 5. Sindbis virions budding from the plasma membrane of an infected chick embryo fibroblast as demonstrated by freeze etching. The magnification bar is 100 nm. From Brown *et al.* (1972). Reproduced by permission of the American Society for Microbiology.

Grimley *et al.*, (1968) have described another type of cytopathic vacuole (CPV-1) that occurs early in the exponential phase of Semliki Forest virus growth. These 0.6–2-μm vacuoles bear regularly spaced, 50-nm, membranous spherules that project from their interior surfaces (Fig. 6). The spherules are clearly neither virions nor nucleocapsids. Their appearance is independent of cellular RNA synthesis as shown by actinomycin D studies. However, antimetabolites that block viral RNA or protein synthesis also limit formation of CPV-1s. Thus, they are likely to represent a virus-specific structure (Grimley *et al.*, 1972). Autoradiographic experiments performed in the presence of actinomycin D show that the CPV-1 is a site of viral RNA synthesis (Grimley *et al.*, 1968).

Cells infected by group B togaviruses also show characteristic ultrastructural changes during the early period of active virus release, but they are significantly different from those described above (Ota, 1965; Matsumura *et al.*, 1971; Murphy *et al.*, 1968). Initially, there is a proliferation of cytoplasmic vacuoles, of smooth and rough endoplasmic

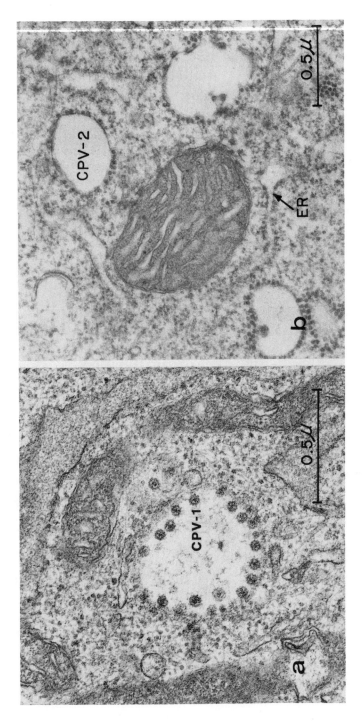

Fig. 6. Intracellular vacuoles characteristic of group A togavirus infection. (a) Type 1 cytopathic vacuoles (CPV-1) in an L cell infected with Semliki Forest virus. The spherules lining the vacuole are not nucleocapsids. Vacuoles of this type may be the site of viral RNA synthesis. Photograph kindly supplied by Dr. Philip Grimley. (b) Type 2 cytopathic vacuoles (CPV-2) in a mouse brain cell infected with Semliki Forest virus. The vacuoles are surrounded by nucleocapsids. ER, endoplasmic reticulum. From Grimley *et al.* (1968). Reproduced by permission of the American Society for Microbiology.

reticulum, and of Golgi membranes, particularly within the perinuclear region (see Fig. 7). Lining the cytoplasmic side of many of the vacuoles and cisternae are ill-defined, electron-dense, ragged but generally round structures, about 26–28 nm in diameter, which may be nucleocapsids. Ota (1965) has suggested that viral morphogenesis occurs by budding of these particles through cytoplasmic membranes. Support for this mechanism at present is weak. The "precursor" particles have not been unequivocally identified as nucleocapsids and, in contrast to studies with other enveloped viruses, no virions have ever been definitely observed in the process of budding. Cell-associated virus is sometimes seen in contact with vacuolar membranes, but only through amorphous, electron-dense material (Cardiff et al., 1973a). Thus, there is little concrete morphological evidence as to the mechanism of the envelopment of group B virions. It may resemble the budding of group A virions or it may be quite different. Regardless of the mechanism, many of the intracellular vacuoles and vesicles are found later in infection to contain virions that are morphologically indistinguishable from extracellular virions. [As we shall see (Sect. 3.4.2), these intracellular virions differ in their polypeptide composition from normal virions.]

As infection with group B virions proceeds, the membrane-enclosed virions apparently migrate from the perinuclear region of the cell and approach the plasma membrane. The virions are released through exocytosis of individual particles through narrow caniculi or through fusion of virus-containing vacuoles with the plasma membrane, as previously described in cells infected by group A viruses. Degenerating cells release virus by lysis.

Yasuzumi et al. (Yasuzumi et al., 1964; Yasuzumi and Tsuba, 1965a,b) have suggested the possibility of nuclear involvement in the morphogenesis of group B virions. They find that pleomorphic precursor particles and virions appear first in the nucleus. However, the interpretation of some of their electron micrographs seems equivocal because of degenerative nuclear changes. At least one other report (Murphy et al., 1968) indicates the presence of intranuclear virions and possibly nucleocapsids while the nuclei remain apparently undamaged. Some biochemical and autoradiographic evidence has also been put forth to support a primary role for the nucleus in early viral development (see Sect. 3.5.1), but, on the whole, more evidence is needed before a nuclear role can be accepted.

Immunofluorescence studies show that group B antigens are present in the cytoplasm of infected cells (Bhamarapravati et al., 1964;

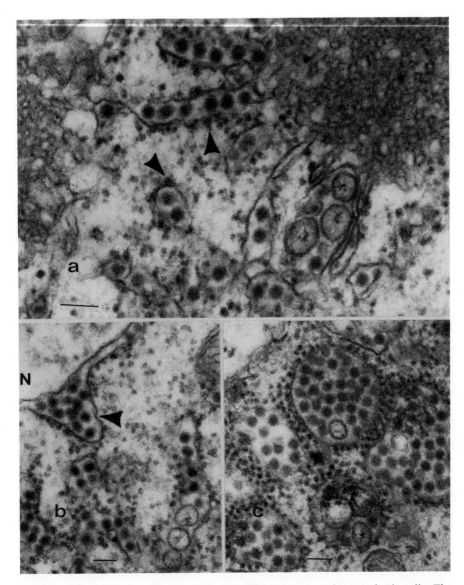

Fig. 7.   Ultrastructure of St. Louis encephalitis virus-infected mouse brain cells. The cells contain proliferated membranes of the endoplasmic reticulum and Golgi complex that are most prominent in the perinuclear region early in infection. The nucleus (N) appears normal. Intracellular virions are found within the cisternae of the endoplasmic reticulum (a), within the inner and outer nuclear membranes (arrow, b), and within vacuoles (a, b, c). Many of the vacuoles bear on their surface possible nucleocapsid precursor particles (arrows, a) that are difficult to distinguish from ribosomes. Continuity of the envelope of intracellular virus with the vacuolar membrane is not apparent. The bars represent 100 nm. From Murphy *et al.* (1968). Reproduced by permission of the Williams and Wilkins Company.

El Dadah and Nathanson, 1967). By using specific antisera and fixation procedures which allow the differentiation of structural and nonstructural antigens, Cardiff *et al.,* (1973*a*) have found that both virion and nonvirion antigens first appear late in latency in a confined perinuclear zone. As virus is released, virion antigens appear in the cytoplasm as a granular fluorescence. These results are quite different from those obtained with group A togavirus-infected cells. Here the immunofluorescence is seen both diffusely in the cytoplasm and at the plasma membrane. The absence of immunofluorescence at the plasma membrane of cells infected with group B viruses is a reflection of the fact that viral maturation does not take place at the cell surface.

3.3. Genetics

Our discussion of togavirus genetics is not intended to be exhaustive, but is merely to serve as an introduction to several mutants used in experiments to be discussed in subsequent sections. Mutations affecting the virulence, plaque morphology, and thermostability of togaviruses have been described. Since, by and large, these mutants have not contributed to our understanding of viral replication, they will not be considered here. In contrast, temperature-sensitive mutants have proven to be a useful tool in the dissection of various stages in viral growth.

Togaviruses are ideal for the selection of temperature-sensitive mutants since their alternate growth in vertebrate and arthropod hosts provides a natural selection for replication over a broad range of temperature. Two extensive catalogues of temperature-sensitive mutants of group A togaviruses are available. Although isolated from two different viruses, Sindbis (Burge and Pfefferkorn, 1966*a*) and Semliki Forest virus (Tan *et al.,* 1969), these mutants exhibit a similar spectrum of physiological defects. Many are incapable of virus-specific RNA synthesis (RNA⁻) at the restrictive temperature and probably have a temperature-sensitive lesion in some virus-determined component of the RNA polymerase. In some of these RNA⁻ mutants, viral nucleic acid synthesis, once begun at the permissive temperature, continues unabated in cultures shifted to the restrictive temperature; this evidence suggests that the polymerase, once made in a functional conformation, remains stable (Pfefferkorn and Burge, 1967). In other mutants, such a temperature shift promptly suppresses virus-specific RNA synthesis, indicating a heat-labile polymerase (Waite and Pfefferkorn, 1970b). These latter RNA⁻ mutants are particularly useful because they allow the study of infected cells in which viral RNA synthesis has been curtailed by a shift in the temperature (see Sect. 3.4.4).

Mutants with no apparent lesion in viral RNA synthesis (RNA⁺) fall into three physiological classes (Burge and Pfefferkorn, 1968) whose properties are summarized in Table 6. These RNA⁺ mutants have been most useful in the isolation of viral polyribosomes and in the discovery of precursor proteins (see Sect. 3.6).

At present, it is difficult to assign these late temperature-sensitive defects to individual structural proteins of the virion because of the probability that these proteins are derived by post-translational cleavage of a high-molecular-weight precursor (see Sect. 3.6.). An amino acid substitution anywhere in a precursor protein may affect its conformation and subsequent cleavage and thus interfere with the formation of specific structural proteins. One temperature-sensitive defect can probably be assigned unequivocally. Mutant *ts* 23 of Sindbis virus fails to induce hemadsorption in cells infected at the restrictive temperature. More specifically, however, virions of this mutant produced at the permissive temperature show a reversibly thermolabile hemagglutinin (Yin, 1969; Scheele and Pfefferkorn, 1970). Hence, mutant *ts* 23 is likely to have a defect in the polypeptide (E1 or E2) responsible for hemagglutination.

TABLE 6

Properties of Temperature-Sensitive Mutants of Sindbis Virus

Comple-mentation group	Repre-sentative mutant	Phenotype in infection at the restrictive temperature
A	*ts* 4	RNA⁻; parental RNA fails to enter the replicative form
B	*ts* 6	RNA⁻; parental RNA fails to enter replicative form
C	*ts* 2	RNA⁺; nucleocapsids are not assembled
D	*ts* 10	RNA⁺; hemadsorption is absent
E	*ts* 20	RNA⁺; both hemadsorption and nucleocapsid assembly are normal but infectious virions are not produced

Genetic characterization of Sindbis virus mutants has proceeded in parallel with physiological studies of this virus. Complementation tests measuring the yield from mixed infections at the restrictive temperature were sufficient to define five nonoverlapping groups (Table 6) which are concordant with those defined by the physiological defects described above (Burge and Pfefferkorn, 1966b). With the exception of tests using the RNA$^-$ mutant *ts* 6, the complementation is quite inefficient, although the patterns are reproducible (Pfefferkorn and Burge, 1967). Curiously, attempts to secure comparable patterns of complementation with the catalogue of Semliki Forest virus mutants failed to yield consistent results. The reason for this failure is unknown.

Most attempts to demonstrate genetic recombination between mutants of group A togaviruses have met with failure (Burge and Pfefferkorn, 1966b). A preliminary report suggests that prior clumping of infecting virions may promote recombination (Brawner and Sagik, 1971). This observation may open the way for the construction of a genetic map based on frequency of recombination.

3.4.   Effect of Infection on Cellular Biosynthetic Activities

Studies on the synthesis of macromolecules in infected cells generally depend on the incorporation of labeled precursors. Comparisons between infected and uninfected cells are made with the tacit assumptions that infection does not alter the size of precursor pools or kinetics with which they are labeled. Given these assumptions, infection with group A viruses profoundly alters cellular biosynthesis. During the first three hours of infection, amino acid incorporation into cellular protein falls to a low level, allowing ready detection of virus-specific proteins (Strauss *et al.*, 1969). The mechanism of this inhibition is unknown. The reduction of cellular protein synthesis, however, may not be uniform since the first four hours of Semliki Forest virus infection are marked by significant increases in four cytoplasmic enzymes, the dehydrogenases for glucose-6-phosphate, isocitrate, malate, and lactate (Cassells and Burke, 1973). The possibility that these increases simply represent enzyme activations should be borne in mind. However, since actinomycin D, which has no effect on viral replication, blocks these increases, new cellular messenger RNA may well be involved.

Group A virus infection gradually suppresses cellular RNA synthesis during the first three hours of infection (Taylor, 1965). Again, the mechanism is unknown but the components of the infecting virion are apparently insufficient for the inhibition. Infection with an RNA⁻ temperature-sensitive mutant of Semliki Forest virus at the restrictive temperature fails to halt cellular RNA synthesis. However, incubation of the infected cells at the permissive temperature for only one hour before shifting to the restrictive temperature was sufficient to cause a marked suppression of cellular RNA synthesis while allowing only minimal production of virus (Tan *et al.,* 1969). Thus, only slight viral RNA synthesis is required to suppress the production of cellular RNA.

Infection of chick embryo fibroblasts with Sindbis virus causes a progressive reduction of phospholipid synthesis that affects all the principal phosphatides to about the same extent (Pfefferkorn and Hunter, 1963*b*; Waite and Pfefferkorn, 1970*b*). In temperature-shift experiments similar to those described above, it was shown that limited replication of viral RNA is required to affect phospholipid synthesis. Indeed, the effect on phospholipid synthesis may well be secondary to the viral inhibition of cellular protein and/or RNA synthesis, for in uninfected chick cells treatment with actinomycin D or inhibitors of protein synthesis suppresses phospholipid synthesis (Waite and Pfefferkorn, 1970*b*). These antimetabolites have no immediate effect on phospholipid synthesis in BHK cells. Similarly, Sindbis virus infection of BHK cells does not suppress phospholipid synthesis even though the production of cellular RNA and protein are sharply curtailed.

We know less of the effect of group B viral infection on cellular biosynthetic activities. In general, it would appear that group B viruses, in keeping with their milder cytopathic effect, have a less drastic biochemical effect on the cells they infect. In particular, a substantial fraction of total protein synthesized during the period of maximal viral production is cellular. This continued production of cellular protein makes identification of minor viral polypeptides difficult. Treatment of infected cells with actinomycin D is generally used to suppress cellular protein synthesis in infected cells, but even in its presence as much as 40% of the newly synthesized protein may be cellular (Westaway, 1973).

Again in contrast to infections by group A viruses, the synthesis of phospholipids is stimulated by infection with group B viruses. This response may reflect the proliferation of perinuclear membranous structures (see Sect. 3.2) since short pulses of ³H-choline label perinuclear membranes to a greater extent than cytoplasmic membranes (Zebovitz *et al.,* 1974).

3.5. Synthesis of Viral RNA

3.5.1. Intracellular Virus-Specific RNAs

3.5.1(a). Group A Viruses

Togaviral RNA synthesis is easily observed in infected cells treated with actinomycin D and labeled with a radioactive nucleic acid precursor such as ^{3}H-uridine. Under these conditions, cellular RNA synthesis is suppressed without affecting viral replication. Group A viral RNA synthesis reaches levels detectable by incorporation of precursors about two hours after infection (Kääriäinen and Gomatos, 1969), rises to nearly maximal rates within the next hour, and then continues throughout the period of viral release.

The two principal forms of single-stranded RNA found in group A togavirus-infected cells are the virion RNA (approximately 42 S) and a lower-molecular-weight, single-stranded RNA which sediments at 26 S and is most conveniently termed "interjacent RNA" (Sreevalsan and Lockart, 1966; Friedman *et al.*, 1966). In crude cytoplasmic extracts of infected cells these two species of viral RNA are found associated with proteins (Friedman and Berezesky, 1967; Sreevalsan and Allen, 1968). The virion RNA is contained in nucleocapsids that sediment at 140 S (see Sect. 3.1.2). Interjacent RNA sediments at 65 S because of association with an as yet unidentified component that is probably derived from breakdown of polyribosomes (Mowshowitz, 1973). Interjacent RNA has about the same base ratios as virion RNA (Sonnabend *et al.*, 1967; Sreevalsan *et al.*, 1968). However, the suggestion that interjacent RNA is simply a different physical form of virion RNA now has no experimental support. Reports that the interjacent RNA is intrinsically infectious (Sreevalsan and Lockart, 1966) are suspect because in these experiments the 26 S region of their sucrose gradient was undoubtedly contaminated with viral replicative intermediate, which is now known to be infectious (Yoshinaka and Hotta, 1971). However, the interjacent RNA is not simply an artifact resulting from the degradation of virion RNA before or after extraction. Convincing hybridization experiments in which interjacent and virion RNA competed for the "minus strand" of denatured, labeled, virus-specific, double-stranded RNA show that interjacent RNA contains only about one-third of the sequences of virion RNA (Simmons and Strauss, 1972*a*). Thus interjacent RNA represents a very specific segment of the viral genome.

Several minor viral single-stranded RNAs have also been noted by some investigators in cells infected with group A arboviruses. Two of these migrate between virion and interjacent RNA, 38 S and 33 S (Levin and Friedman, 1971), and one is smaller, 20–22 S (Kääriäinen and Gomatos, 1969). Nothing more is known about these RNAs, but the smallest species may indicate the presence of defective-interfering particles (see Sect. 3.8).

Although direct evidence is scant, replication of the RNA of togaviruses undoubtedly proceeds through a multiple-stranded replicative intermediate similar to that described in the well-studied picornavirus and RNA bacteriophage systems. Short pulses with ^{3}H-uridine given to cells infected with a group A virus disclose a rapidly sedimenting polydisperse (up to 30 S) structure with properties consistent with those of a replicative intermediate (Friedman, 1968a). This structure is partially resistant to RNase, and infectious single-stranded RNA can be derived from it by denaturation. RNase treatment of RNA extracted from cells infected with a group A virus yields double-stranded replicative forms that are derived from replicative intermediates or exist before digestion. These double-stranded forms are generally reported to sediment at about 20 S (Friedman and Berezesky, 1967; Cartwright and Burke, 1970; Eaton and Faulkner, 1973; Shenk and Stollar, 1972).

Pulse-chase experiments using crude virus-specific RNA polymerase (see Sect. 3.5.2) also support the role of multiple-stranded RNA as an intermediate in the synthesis of single-stranded RNA (Michel and Gomatos, 1973). Similar experiments are, in general, difficult to perform in intact cells because the nucleotide pool is large and slow to equilibrate during the chase. However, glucosamine treatment allows pulse-chase studies to be performed with labeled uridine. Under these conditions, Scholtissek et al., (1972) were able to trace the flow of radioactivity through RNase-resistant RNA into the single-stranded RNA species. Significantly, they could not chase the radioactivity from interjacent to virion RNA, thus showing that interjacent RNA is unlikely to be a precursor.

The origin of interjacent RNA remains a puzzle. The most coherent explanation has been provided by Simmons and Strauss (1972a,b). Since their findings with respect to replicative forms differ somewhat from those described above, we shall present a fuller account of their data. Simmons and Strauss have found three replicative forms of viral RNA in infected cells and have assigned them the following sedimentation coefficients and molecular weights: 23.5 S (8.8×10^6 daltons), 20 S (5.6×10^6 daltons), 16 S (2.9×10^6 daltons). Funda-

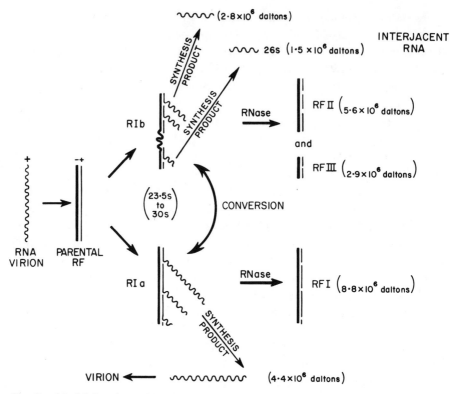

Fig. 8.   Model for the replication of group A viral RNA. The wavy lines represent single-stranded RNA and single-stranded regions of replicative intermediates. Double-stranded RNAs are shown as straight lines with the "minus" strand heavy and the "plus" strand light. Placement of RF-III at the 5′ end of RIb is arbitrary. Modified from Simmons and Strauss (1972*b*). Reproduced by permission of Academic Press.

mental to their model (see Fig. 8) are the following observations: (1) Molecular hybridization shows that the largest replicative form (23.5 S) is the double-stranded homologue of virion RNA. Note that the sedimentation coefficient for this double-stranded RNA is somewhat greater than the 20 S value mentioned earlier. This discrepancy may well represent some minor technical difference. We assume that the 20 S replicative form reported by others corresponds to the 23.5 S form of Simmons and Strauss. (2) Interjacent RNA, with due allowance for minor contamination with virion RNA, is homologous to the smallest (16 S) replicative form. (3) Simmons and Strauss argue that if independent replicative intermediates gave rise to each of the three replicative forms, the small replicative forms should be derived from more slowly sedimenting replicative intermediates. However, when the replicative intermediate(s) from infected cells are resolved on a velocity gradient and various fractions are treated with RNase to produce replicative forms, both the rapidly and slowly sedimenting replicative intermediates yield the same distribution of the three replicative forms. Simmons and Strauss thus hypothesize that the RNase treatment not only converts replicative intermediates into replicative forms by removing nascent RNA strands, but that it also cleaves the "minus strands" of some replicative intermediates at a specific site to yield the two smaller replicative forms. The RNase attack on the "minus strand" is assumed to occur within a short single-stranded region that results from termination of transcription. Reinitiation of RNA synthesis upon the remainder of the template is presumed to occur distal to the termination site. Consistent with the Simmons and Strauss model is their observation that the two smaller replicative forms are found in a molar ratio of 1:1 throughout the infection. They conclude that transcription of the smallest segment of the replicative intermediate yields interjacent RNA. Transciption of the longer segment is much less frequent and presumably yields a minor species of viral messenger RNA. Indeed, an RNA of the appropriate molecular weight (sedimenting at 33 S) has recently been found independently by two groups examining the polysomal RNAs of Sindbis virus-infected cells (see Sect. 3.6.1).

An obvious concern in relying too heavily on the hypothesis presented above is that the multiple replicative forms might have been the result of mixed infections with inadvertently admixed defective-interfering particles (see Sect. 3.8). Other workers have indicated that the presence of multiple replicative forms is characteristic of coinfection with defective particles, while infection with standard virus yields but a single replicative form. Against this interpretation is the absence in Simmons and Strauss's data of the 12 S replicative form and the 20 S single-stranded RNA that seem to be the hallmarks of infection with defective interfering particles of Sindbis virus.

The foregoing model is attractive in that it explains the synthesis of the principal virus-specific single-stranded RNAs. However, alternative hypotheses, e.g., those involving independent production of segments of the genome followed by ligation to make virion RNA (Michel and Gomatos, 1973), cannot be excluded.

Transcription of group A viral RNA is apparently regulated during the course of infection. The synthesis of virion RNA becomes maximal only during the phase of rapid release of virions, while interjacent RNA is made at a more or less constant rate beginning near the end of the latent period (Mécs *et al.*, 1967; Sonnabend *et al.*, 1967; Kääriäinen and Gomatos, 1969). Manipulation of experimental conditions can also distort the ratio of newly synthesized virion to interjacent RNA. If an RNA⁻ mutant of Sindbis virus is allowed to infect cells at the permissive temperature and these infected cells are later shifted to the nonpermissive temperature, synthesis of interjacent RNA is preferentially inhibited (Scheele and Pfefferkorn, 1969*b*). A similar effect is seen in cells infected by wild-type virus when *de novo* protein synthesis is inhibited early in the course of infection (Scheele and Pfefferkorn, 1969*b*). Finally, Mécs *et al.*, (1967) noted that interferon selectively inhibits the production of virion RNA.

There is general agreement that group A viral RNA synthesis is associated with some cytoplasmic membranous structure. A membrane-associated replication complex containing viral RNA polymerase and replicative intermediate was identified by pulse labeling infected cells with ³H-uridine. Partial purification of this structure resulted in a concentration of the type 1 cytopathic vacuoles (Fig. 6). Grimley *et al.* (1968) suggest that these vacuoles may actually represent the membranous site of viral RNA synthesis, and they have presented autoradiographic evidence to support their contention. This question cannot be settled until the membrane-associated replication complex can be purified from other contaminating structures. Further evidence for replication of group A viral RNA in association with cytoplasmic membranes comes from experiments in which radioactive RNA of infecting virions is traced. It should be remembered that this type of experiment has an intrinsic defect in that the majority of the added virions do not cause infection, and thus most of the input radioactivity is irrelevant to the course of infection. Fortunately, the particle: PFU ratio is relatively low for group A arboviruses (Pfefferkorn and Hunter, 1963*a*). Friedman and Sreevalsan (1970) traced the labeled RNA of Semliki Forest virus into a structure that is similar in its sedimentation properties to a membrane-bound replication complex. Only about one-third of the cell-associated viral RNA is found in these structures, but this is consistent with estimated particle:PFU ratios. Cycloheximide inhibits the membrane association of input viral RNA suggesting that protein synthesis, presumably virus-specified, is required. Sreevalsan (1970) used the "M-band" technique (Tremblay *et al.*, 1969) to isolate membrane-associated replicating viral RNA and were able to follow the attachment of labeled input viral RNA to membranes and its subsequent detachment later in infection. Use of an RNA⁻ mutant in infection at the restrictive temperature showed that viral RNA replication is not required for attachment but is needed for subsequent release.

3.5.1(b).   Group B Viruses

In most studies with group B togaviruses, viral RNA synthesis cannot be detected by actinomycin D-resistant incorporation of ^{3}H-uridine until the end of the latent period, about 10–12 hours after infection (Stollar *et al.*, 1967; Nishimura and Tsukeda, 1971; Takehara, 1971; Zebovitz *et al.*, 1972). However, viral RNA synthesis clearly begins earlier, as Stollar *et al.* (1966) found that virus production was curtailed when nucleoside analogues were present during the latter half of the latent period and then removed. The only direct evidence for this early viral RNA synthesis comes from the experiments of Trent *et al.* (1969). They found a biphasic synthesis of viral RNA with an early burst at about 6 hours after infection and a later rise at the end of latency. The appearance of infectious RNA seemed to parallel this biphasic pattern. Other investigators have not noted this early burst of viral RNA synthesis, but their experimental points may not have been spaced closely enough. All observers agree that the incorporation of precursors into group B viral RNA is greatest as the rate of viral release is reaching its maximal value.

Various intracellular species of group B virus-specific RNA have been detected by sucrose gradient centrifugation or polyacrylamide gel electrophoresis. Nearly all reports record the presence of 42–45 S RNA that is infectious (virion RNA) and 20 S RNase-resistant RNA, presumably the replicative form. This latter RNA can be denatured in dimethyl sulfoxide to yield single-stranded RNA which sediments at 45 S (Stollar *et al.*, 1967). An additional RNA species which sediments at about 26 S has been reported to be RNase-resistant (Trent *et al.*, 1969), RNase-sensitive (Zebovitz *et al.*, 1972), a mixture of sensitive and resistant molecules (Nishimura and Tsukeda, 1971), or absent from infected cells (Stollar *et al.*, 1966). Some of this disagreement may result from differing experimental conditions or variable degradation of virion RNA. It would be useful to know if the group B viruses resemble the group A viruses in the formation of an interjacent RNA that serves as messenger. Other partially RNase-resistant RNA molecules that sediment at 8 S (Zebovitz *et al.*, 1972) or 10–20 S (Nishimura and Tsukeda, 1971) remain to be characterized. The possibility that these latter RNAs are associated with the presence of defective-interfering particles should be considered.

Studies of the kinetics with which these various species of group B virus-specific RNA are labeled have yielded results that cannot easily be reconciled (Trent *et al.*, 1969; Nishimura and Tsukeda, 1971). It would appear that virion RNA is slowest to be labeled. Virion RNA could be synthesized on a single replicative intermediate, or segments of it could be produced by smaller·replicative intermediates and then joined to make a single molecule. RNA synthesis is probably regulated, for Stollar *et al.* (1967) found that both strands of 20 S RNA are synthesized early in dengue virus infection but only the "plus" strand is synthesized late. Similar regulation was not detected, however, in St. Louis encephalitis virus-infected cells (Trent *et al.*, 1969).

The intracellular site of group B viral RNA synthesis has not been unequivocally determined. On the basis of autoradiographic data, Takeda *et al.* (1965) reported that viral RNA synthesis is confined to the nucleus, is maximal prior to viral release, and declines thereafter. However, they did not present their autoradiograms, their grain counts were greater over the cytoplasm than over the nucleus, and their kinetic results differ from those in all other studies. We therefore cannot accept their evidence. Takehara (1971, 1972) reported the presence of a substantial fraction of putative virus-specified RNA polymerase in a nuclear and a "large-particle" cytoplasmic fraction. However, their nuclear preparation was crude and probably contaminated with perinuclear cytoplasm. Brawner *et al.* (1973) reported the presence of viral RNA in detergent-washed nuclei; in contrast, Zebovitz *et al.* (1974) reported that detergent treatment removed essentially all virus-specified RNA from isolated nuclei. We have already summarized immunofluorescent and electron microscopic evidence indicating that the perinuclear region, but not the nucleus, is an important site of virus-directed activity (see Sect. 3.2). We suspect that the nucleus *per se* is not primarily involved in the replication of group B togaviruses. Definitive proof could come from an analysis of virus replication in cells enucleated by cytochalasin B (Pollack and Goldman, 1973).

3.5.2. Viral RNA Polymerase

When present at the time of infection, inhibitors of protein synthesis such as puromycin, totally block the synthesis of togaviral RNA (Wecker and Richter, 1962; Sreevalsan and Lockart, 1964). This requirement for newly synthesized protein undoubtedly represents, at least in part, the virus-specific RNA polymerase. Such an enzyme has been demonstrated in extracts of group A and B virus-infected cells

(Martin and Sonnabend, 1967; Sreevalsan and Yin, 1969; Nishimura and Tsukeda, 1971; Takehara, 1971; Qureshi and Trent, 1972; Cardiff *et al.*, 1973*b*). Conditions necessary to demonstrate this enzymatic activity are similar to those reported for other viral RNA polymerases. The polymerase is membrane-associated, and it sediments with the particulate matter of cell homogenates, probably in the form of a membrane-bound replication complex. This replicative complex can be pulse labeled *in vivo* with RNA precursors, and contains both RNA polymerase and virus-specific RNA as replication forms and intermediates as well as some single-stranded molecules (Friedman *et al.*, 1972; Qureshi and Trent, 1972). Friedman *et al.* (1972) examined the ultrastructure of partially purified replication complex from cells infected by Semliki Forest virus and noted numerous type 1 cytopathic vacuoles (CPV-1, Fig. 6) that contained newly synthesized viral RNA. These vacuoles may bear the replication complex, but definitive proof is lacking.

In crude cytoplasmic extracts of group A virus-infected cells the principal product of *in vitro* RNA synthesis is double-stranded (Martin and Sonnabend, 1967). Resolution of the cytoplasmic extract on sucrose gradients yields a preparation that catalyses the synthesis of both 20 S double-stranded and virion-length single-stranded RNA (Sreevalsan and Yin, 1969). Michel and Gomatos (1973) have also noted the *in vitro* synthesis of virion-length RNA as well as interjacent RNA and a small species of single-stranded RNA which sediments at 22 S. Once synthesized, the three single-stranded RNAs apparently become associated with particles sufficiently different in size that they can be resolved by centrifugation. Michel and Gomatos (1973) comment that the replicative forms present in their extracts were at best only half the molecular weight required for a template corresponding to virion RNA. RNA synthesized in a cell-free system by a group B viral polymerase is heterogeneous with peaks corresponding to 20 S and 26 S. Surprisingly, both of these species of RNA are sensitive to ribonuclease, but the digestion was carried out at rather low ionic strength with high enzyme concentration (Cardiff *et al.*, 1973*b*).

The information for at least some of the polypeptides that make up the virus-specific RNA polymerase is likely to be encoded in the viral genome; this has been shown by isolation from group A viruses of temperature-sensitive mutants with a specific defect in viral RNA synthesis (Burge and Pfefferkorn 1966*a*; Tan *et al.*, 1969). However, examination of the virus-induced RNA polymerase of a number of temperature-sensitive mutants of Semliki Forest virus has failed to disclose any marked increase in thermolability (Martin, 1969). In these mutants, the polymerase once formed at the permissive temperature may simply be relatively stable. A similar effect has been noted in temperature-shift experiments with cultures infected by most RNA⁻ mutants of Sindbis virus: once viral RNA synthesis is proceeding at the maximal rate at the permissive temperature, shift to the restrictive temperature has little effect on the subsequent production of virus (Pfefferkorn and Burge, 1967).

At present, no preparation of togaviral polymerase has been significantly purified or made dependent upon exogenous template. Neither the possible role of cellular proteins nor the number of virus-specific polypeptides has been determined. However, it is likely that more than one viral component is involved since at least two well-defined complementation groups of mutants defective in RNA synthesis have been detected (Pfefferkorn and Burge, 1967).

3.6. Synthesis of Virus-Specific Proteins

3.6.1. Messenger RNA

The nature of the viral RNA species that serve as messenger in togavirus-infected cells has yet to be determined unequivocally. The principal difficulties standing in the way of isolation of virus-specific RNA from polyribosomes of cells infected by a group A virus are twofold. The first difficulty is that the nucleocapsid, which accumulates within infected cells, sediments in velocity gradients into the region in which polyribosomes might be expected; this problem has been circumvented by using temperature-sensitive mutants with a specific defect in the assembly of nucleocapsids. The second and greater difficulty is the simple inability to isolate polyribosomes from most cells infected with group A togaviruses, even with techniques that yield apparently undegraded polysomes from uninfected cells.

Despite these difficulties, three recent reports describe the isolation of polyribosomal messenger RNA from group A togavirus-infected cells. Kennedy (1972) and Mowshowitz (1973) agree that the principal virus-specific messenger is interjacent RNA. The main messenger found by Rosemond and Sreevalsan (1973) sediments slightly more rapidly than interjacent RNA, perhaps, as they suggest, because of increased content of polyadenylic acid. The general agreement among these three reports is gratifying because recent studies on viral protein synthesis reviewed below (Sect. 3.6.2) suggest that the main polypeptide produced in infected cells should have a minimal molecular weight of 129,000 daltons. The interjacent RNA, with its molecular weight of about 1.6×10^6 daltons, is an appropriate messenger for such a high-molecular-weight protein. In addition to this principal species of messenger RNA, Mowshowitz (1973) and Kennedy (1972) also note that a 33 S RNA is represented among virus-specific polysomal RNAs. In contrast, Rosemond and Sreevalsan (1973) find an additional, more slowly sedimenting, 15–18 S messenger RNA. The role of these minor species of RNA, assuming they are not artifacts, remains to be determined.

Nothing is known of the messenger RNAs of group B togaviruses.

3.6.2. Intracellular Virus-Specific Proteins

3.6.2(a). Group A Viruses

The rapid suppression of host protein synthesis by group A togaviral infection simplifies the task of identifying intracellular virus-specific proteins. All virus-specified proteins appear to be associated with cellular membranes, at least during the early stages of infection (Bose and Brundige, 1972). Analysis by polyacrylamide gel electrophoresis of extracts of infected cells labeled with amino acid precursors shows a pattern markedly different from that of uninfected cells (e.g., Friedman, 1968b; Strauss et al., 1968). The number of intracellular virus-specific polypeptides reported varies from 6 to 20 depending, to some extent, upon the confidence of individual observers. The one outstanding feature of these various studies is that the production of virus-specified proteins is efficiently regulated (Fig. 9). Only those polypeptides destined for incorporation into the virion are made in substantial quantities. The mechanism by which this control of virus-specific protein synthesis is exercised remains unclear, although preferential translation of messenger RNA(s) corresponding to viral structural proteins is a reasonable hypothesis. Baltimore (reviewed, 1971) has suggested that the protein-synthetic machinery of mammalian cells is incapable of directly producing the individual polypeptide specified by a polycistronic messenger RNA. Instead, translation of polycistronic messenger RNA yields a high-molecular-weight precursor protein which is then cleaved by a proteolytic mechanism to yield functional molecules. The evidence for such a mechanism in cells infected by picornaviruses is quite convincing. However, the demonstration of high-molecular-weight precursor proteins has proven to be more difficult in cells infected with group A to-

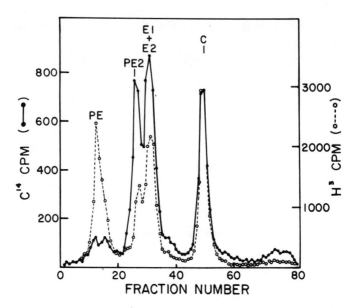

Fig. 9. Comparison of Sindbis virus proteins synthesized in chick cells with those synthesized in BHK cells. Chick embryo fibroblasts were labeled with ¹⁴C-amino acids 9–9.5 hours after infection (●). BHK cells were labeled with ³H-amino acids 9–12 hours after infection (○). The mixed extracts were analyzed by continuous polyacrylamide gel electrophoresis, which does not resolve envelope proteins E1 and E2. Modified from Strauss *et al.* (1969). Reproduced by permission of Academic Press.

gaviruses. Neither very short pulses of labeled amino acids nor treatment with a battery of amino acid analogues gave more than a hint of high-molecular-weight, virus-specific proteins in cells infected with Sindbis virus (Friedman, 1969; Scheele and Pfefferkorn, 1970). However, several independent lines of evidence now indicate that precursor proteins can be found in cells infected by group A togaviruses. Several temperature-sensitive mutants of Sindbis virus have been shown to accumulate a protein of molecular weight $1–1.6 \times 10^5$ daltons during incubation of infected cells at the nonpermissive temperature (Strauss *et al.*, 1969; Scheele and Pfefferkorn, 1970; Waite, 1973). A protein of similar molecular weight was observed in Semliki Forest virus-infected cells (Burrell *et al.*, 1970). Finally, a somewhat smaller protein, presumably also a precursor, was detected in infected cells treated with the chloromethylketone derivative of tosylphenylalanine, an inhibitor of enzymes with the specificity of chymotrypsin (Pfefferkorn and Boyle, 1972), and in wild-type infected cells pulse-labeled at 28°C (Waite, 1973).

M. J. Schlesinger and Schlesinger (1973) have presented tryptic peptide maps of the high-molecular-weight protein accumulated by cells infected at the restrictive temperature by the RNA$^+$ Sindbis virus mutant ts-2. These maps show convincingly that this presumed precursor encompasses all three of the principal polypeptides of Sindbis virus, C, E1, and E2 (see Sect. 2.2.3). Since there is no established nomenclature for the precursor proteins, we propose to call the polypeptide accumulated by mutant ts-2-infected cells PEC (precursor of envelope and capsid proteins). S. Schlesinger and Schlesinger (1972) have presented preliminary data suggesting that the C protein lies at the amino terminus of PEC. Pulse labeling with amino acids in the presence of sufficient pactamycin to inhibit initiation preferentially showed an initial reduction of incorporation into the C protein.

As shown in Fig. 9, the use of BHK cells instead of chick cells for wild-type Sindbis virus infection allows the detection of a smaller precursor protein (Strauss et al., 1968; Igarashi, 1970). Radioactive amino acids incorporated into this protein during a pulse are lost, at least in part, during the subsequent chase (M. J. Schlesinger and Schlesinger, 1973). Tryptic peptide maps of this presumed precursor display the pattern of both envelope proteins of the virion (M. J. Schlesinger and Schlesinger, 1973). We propose to call this precursor PE. The smallest intracellular precursor protein is readily identified in all types of infected cells. It has a molecular weight of about 60,000 daltons and migrates only slightly more slowly than the envelope proteins in SDS polyacrylamide gel electrophoresis. Both S. Schlesinger and Schlesinger (1972) and Simons et al., (1973) have shown through pulse-chase experiments and peptide maps that this polypeptide (PE2) is a precursor of the envelope protein E2. This suggestion is further strengthened by the description of a temperature-sensitive mutant that is defective in the conversion of PE2 to E2 in infections carried out at the restrictive temperatures (Simons et al., 1973). Since the difference in electrophoretic mobility between PE2 and E2 is slight, the conversion may involve glycosylation rather than proteolysis, although the latter is more likely. Simons et al. (1973) have detected a small intracellular glycopeptide that may result from the cleavage of PE2 to E2. A working model for the processing of group A viral proteins is shown in Fig. 10.

In summary, it is likely that the synthesis of structural proteins of group A togaviruses is directed by a polycistronic messenger RNA (probably interjacent RNA) that is first translated into a high-molecular-weight precursor. It should be noted that no precursor pro-

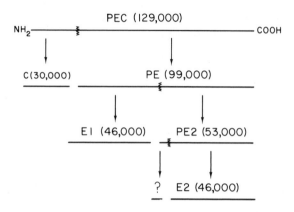

Fig. 10. Hypothetical model for the cleavage of precursors to yield the three structural proteins of group A togaviruses. C, E1, and E2. The parenthetical molecular weights are estimates for the polypeptide moiety only. The contribution of the glycoprotein carbohydrate has been subtracted. Although the C protein is thought to be at the amino terminal end of PEC, nothing is known of the relative locations of PE2 and E1. Their placement is arbitrary. Based on the data of Schlesinger and Schlesinger (1972, 1973).

tein corresponding to translation of the entire viral genome has as yet been detected. It is reasonable to suppose that virion RNA should function as polycistronic messenger early in infection. Unfortunately, detection of virus-specific proteins is most difficult in the interval immediately after infection.

Glycosylation may be an important factor in the processing of viral precursor proteins and in their ultimate appearance at the virus-modified membrane in the form of the glycoproteins E1 and E2. The precursor PE2 is known to be glycosylated (Ranki *et al.*, 1972). Incubation of infected cells in the presence of 2-deoxy-D-glucose distorts the glycosylation of PE2 and inhibits its cleavage (Kaluza *et al.*, 1973).

Little is known about the control of the glycosylation of proteins in togavirus-infected cells. In the uninfected cell, carbohydrate residues are transferred to acceptor proteins by a battery of specific transferases. The possibility that new virus-determined transferases are synthesized after infection cannot be excluded, but current evidence points to at least partial utilization of cellular enzymes. Two of these transferases have been assayed in infected and control cells and have been found to have the same specificities and specific activities (Grimes and Burge, 1971).

The specificity of cellular enzymes seems to control incorporation of sialic acid into the virions, as there is less of this residue in Sindbis virus grown in chick cells than in virus grown in hamster cells. The glycoprotein(s) of Sindbis virus grown in chick cells can be further glycosylated by sialyl transferase from hamster cells (Grimes and Burge, 1971). Furthermore, after removal of terminal sialic acid residues, the glycopeptides of two totally unrelated enveloped viruses, Sindbis and vesicular stomatitis virus, grown in the same cell contained an array of glycopeptides indistinguishable on the basis of molecular weight (Burge and Huang, 1970), again pointing to a dominant influence of cellular enzymes on the glycosylation of viral proteins. The ability of togaviruses to grow in phylogenetically distant arthropod cells offers an excellent opportunity to test this theory, but no data are available at present.

3.6.2(b). Group B Viruses

Radioactively labeled virus-specific proteins in group B virus-infected cells have been detected only during the phase of virus release. Actinomycin D treatment is generally sufficient to suppress host protein synthesis in infected cells and allow detection of newly synthesized viral proteins (Westaway, 1973; Shapiro et al., 1973b). Six prominent polypeptides with molecular weights ranging from about 93,000 to about 8,000 daltons are always present; they include two virion polypeptides (V-3 and V-2) and four nonvirion polypeptides (NV-5, NV-4, NV-2, and NV-1) (Fig. 11). Polypeptides V-3 and NV-2 are glycosylated (Shapiro et al., 1973a). Several investigators have noted additional, poorly resolved, somewhat variable, radioactive peaks called NV-3 (a glycosylated shoulder on the leading edge of V-3), NV-X (between NV-3 and NV-2), and NV-2½ (a shoulder on the trailing edge of NV-2) (Westaway, 1973; Shapiro et al., 1971a). All virus-specified proteins are membrane bound and probably none are freely soluble in the cytoplasm to any significant degree (Shapiro et al., 1972b).

Pulse-chase and amino acid-analogue-incorporation experiments have not revealed the presence of high-molecular-weight precursors (Trent and Qureshi, 1971; Westaway, 1973). It should be remembered that this approach has also failed to disclose most of the precursors of group A viral proteins. Perhaps additional attacks, such as the use of temperature-sensitive mutants, will also be required in the study of group B togaviruses. Pulse-chase experiments do reveal some apparent

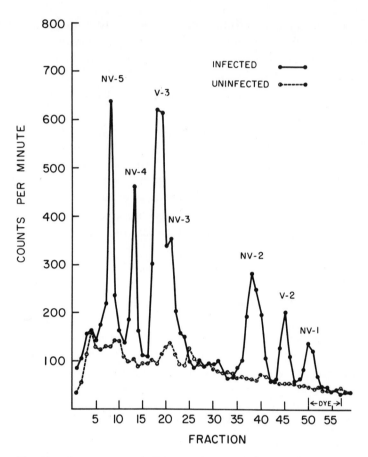

Fig. 11.   Japanese encephalitis virus-specified intracellular proteins.
Virus-infected chick embryo cells treated with inhibitors synthesize
at least six proteins, as demonstrated by polyacrylamide gel electrophoresis, that are apparently absent from uninfected cells. Two of
these (V-3 and V-2) are virion structural proteins. Most notable is
the absence of V-1 (the small virion envelope protein) from infected
cells (see Sect. 3.7.2). From Shapiro *et al.* (1971*a*). Reproduced by
permission of Academic Press.

instability in viral proteins. The core protein V-2 loses its radioactivity
more rapidly than other proteins (Westaway, 1973). More dramatic
changes in the protein-labeling pattern, particularly with respect to
NV-5, were noted when actinomycin D-treated cells were briefly pulse-
inhibited with cycloheximide and then labeled at various times after removal of the cycloheximide (Trent and Qureshi, 1971). Because the
combined drug treatment interferes with normal virus replication, and

because cells appear to require a prolonged "recovery" period, the significance of these changes is not clear.

When electropherograms of intracellular virus-specific proteins and virion proteins are compared, the single most striking observation is the absence of the smaller virion envelope protein V-1 in infected cells (Shapiro *et al.*, 1971a; Westaway, 1973). The significance of this absence will be considered later (Sect. 3.7.2).

3.7. Morphogenesis

3.7.1. Group A Viruses

There are three general steps in the morphogenesis of group A togaviruses: (1) assembly of nucleocapsids from the C protein and the virion RNA, (2) modification of a cellular membrane by the addition of the polypeptides E1 and E2, and (3) budding of the nucleocapsid through the modified cellular membrane to release complete virions into the extracellular fluid. None of these steps is well understood, nor has any of them been reproduced in a cell-free system.

The entire process of viral morphogenesis is comparatively rapid; only 20 minutes after labeled amino acids are supplied to infected cells, virions containing labeled protein are released into the extracellular medium (Scheele and Pfefferkorn, 1969a). Assembly of the nucleocapsid appears to be slightly more rapid than modification of cellular membranes because the first labeled virions released after a pulse of amino acids are preferentially labeled in C protein (Scheele and Pfefferkorn, 1969a; S. Schlesinger and Schlesinger 1972). The supply of C protein is apparently the limiting factor in the assembly of nucleocapsids. There is no intracellular pool of free capsid protein; it is incorporated into nucleocapsids immediately after synthesis (Friedman and Grimley, 1969). It is likely that the formation of nucleocapsids is a self-assembly process similar to that observed with RNA bacteriophages.

The appearance of virus-specific proteins on the plasma membrane of infected cells can be monitored by several methods. Historically, the first to be used was hemadsorption; this method depends upon the appearance in the plasma membrane of the viral envelope protein responsible for hemagglutination. In general, the kinetics of this process are what would be expected from the growth curve of the group A togaviruses. Hemadsorption begins approximately 2½ hours after infection and rises to a maximal level over the next 90 minutes

(Burge and Pfefferkorn, 1967). No doubt, modification of the cellular membrane continues after hemadsorption becomes maximal. Steric considerations simply limit the number of red cells that can adsorb to an infected cell.

An alternative method for detecting virus-specific proteins at the surface of infected cells is enzymatic iodination of their tyrosine residues with the aid of the enzyme lactoperoxidase. This method is quite specific for superficial proteins of the plasma membrane since the enzyme required for the reaction does not penetrate into the cells. However, it is not specific for viral proteins; therefore, these must be defined by a careful comparison of infected and uninfected cells. Sefton *et al.* (1973) have used this method to study the plasma membrane of cells infected with Sindbis virus. Enzymatic iodination of the virion shows that the envelope protein E2 is preferentially iodinated, as compared with the protein E1. This difference in iodination is apparently a steric effect, since both proteins have comparable amounts of tyrosine. Quite similar results were obtained by enzymatic iodination of infected cells. Again, the envelope protein E2 is more heavily iodinated than E1. Interestingly, PE2, the precursor of E2, is not iodinated in intact infected cells. Sefton *et al.* (1973) suggest that PE2 migrates to the inner surface of the plasma membrane where cleavage allows E2 to assume an external position.

Another reflection of an altered plasma membrane in cells infected by a group A virus is the increased agglutinability by the lectin concanavalin A (Birdwell and Strauss, 1973). This change is observed during the interval in which hemadsorption increases, but the relationship between these two phenomena is unknown.

Any explanation of how the viral envelope proteins make their way onto cellular membranes must take into account two facts. First, the virion, and consequently the viral envelope, contains no detectable cellular proteins. Cells which are labeled only before infection do not contribute preformed labeled proteins to Sindbis virus (Pfefferkorn and Clifford, 1964). Analysis of purified Semliki Forest virus by staining polyacrylamide gels showed only the same structural proteins previously detected by radioactive methods (Hay *et al.*, 1968). A morphological representation of the loss of cellular protein during the viral modification of the plasma membrane is the absence in the viral envelope of 6–10-nm structures found between the lipid bilayer leaflets of the normal plasma membrane (Brown *et al.*, 1972).

The second important consideration in explaining viral modification of cellular membranes is the fact that the viral-envelope lipids are derived from preexisting cellular material. This was proven by labeling cells with $^{32}PO_4$ before infection and tracing the incorporation of preformed phosphatides into virions (Pfefferkorn and Hunter, 1963*b*). Furthermore, the lipid composition of Sindbis virus most closely resembles that of the plasma membrane, the presumed site of viral budding (David, 1971; Renkonen *et al.*, 1971).

Pederson and Sagik (1973), using ferritin-labeled antibody, noted that viral nucleocapsids are only found at the inner surface of the plasma membrane at sites that contain viral envelope antigen. The mechanism by which the nucleocapsid finds a modified patch of cellular membrane suitable for budding is unknown. Extension of an envelope protein through the lipid bilayer would provide a convenient signal. Alternatively, if these proteins are entirely external, the internal surface of a virus-modified membrane may be uniquely denuded since cellular proteins are absent from virions. Finally, the presence of the precursor PE2 at the inner surface of a cellular membrane may mark a site undergoing viral modification.

Although viral budding is easily detected by electron microscopy using thin sections or freeze-etch methods (see Sect. 3.2), it is not readily open to direct experimental manipulation. Waite and Pfefferkorn (1970*a*) have suggested one approach that may be of use in the study of viral budding. They observed that reducing the ionic strength of the tissue culture medium markedly inhibits the appearance of Sindbis virus in the extracellular fluid. This reduction in virus yield could not be accounted for by any deficiency in the synthesis of viral nucleic acid or virus-specific proteins, the modification of cellular membranes as demonstrated by hemadsorption, or the assembly of nucleocapsids. Clearly a late step in the production of virus was affected. The nature of this late block was suggested by electron microscopic studies (Waite *et al.*, 1972) that used the freeze-etch method to examine the surface of infected cells. Cells infected in medium of normal ionic strength show occasional clusters of budding virions, in numbers that would be expected for a virus released from the cell in less than two minutes (Rubin *et al.*, 1955). Budding virions are extremely rare in cells exposed to medium of low ionic strength, suggesting that budding is inhibited. When cells infected in low-ionic-strength mediums are shifted to normal mediums, infectious virus is released for a few minutes at a much greater than normal rate (Waite and Pfefferkorn, 1968). Electron microscopic examination of cells during such a shift reveals numerous buds over large areas of the cell surface. These observations indicate that a medium of reduced ionic strength provides a readily reversible inhibition of viral budding. Thus it was of interest to examine the metabolic requirements for virus release during the shift to normal medium. Waite and Pfefferkorn (1970*a*) used inhibitors of protein synthesis and of both glycolysis and of oxidative phosphorylation to demonstrate that neither new protein nor a supply of energy is required for the release of virus. It may well be that the final stage of budding is akin to a self-assembly process. We envision that the nucleocapsid makes contact with a patch of membrane already modified through the addition of E1 and E2 to its outer surface. Interactions between the capsid protein and the internal face of the modified membrane may then proceed to allow the nucleocapsid to become progressively wrapped in the modified membrane which finally fuses and allows the release of the completed virion into the extracellular fluid.

3.7.2. Group B Viruses

We have already commented on the absence of a virion protein, V-1, in extracts of infected cells [see Sect. 3.6.2.(b)]. To provide the background for our explanation of this absence and its relationship to morphogenesis, we must first describe two additional forms of Japanese encephalitis virus. Normal (N) virions released into the extracellular medium contain two envelope proteins, the large glycoprotein V-3 and the small, nonglycosylated protein V-1 (see Sect. 2.2.3). However, intracellular (I) virions purified from artificial lysates of infected cells, lack V-1 and contain instead the glycoprotein NV-2 (Fig. 4). Furthermore, on a molar basis, these I virions contain a higher ratio of envelope proteins to capsid protein than do the N virions. The I virions are notably less infectious than the N virions. Shapiro *et al.* (1972*c*) have suggested that the intravacuolar, cell-associated I virions are initially assembled with an excess of envelope that contains glycoproteins V-3 and NV-2. Viral maturation proceeds within the vacuole. Probably near the time of virus release, the glycosylated moiety of NV-2 is cleaved, leaving only the nonglycosylated segment V-1 in the virion. Excess envelope may also be removed at this time to form the subviral particle described below. This cleavage can be inhibited by medium that contains Tris (Shapiro *et al.*, 1973*c*). Cells infected in this medium release T-form virions, which resemble I-form virions in their protein composition.

The medium of cultures infected by group B togaviruses contains both virions and a more slowly sedimenting (70 S) subviral particle which, since it is not infectious, can be most readily detected by its hemagglutinin. (Stollar, 1969; Smith *et al.*, 1970; Cardiff *et al.*, 1971;

Shapiro *et al.*, 1971*a*). Electron microscopy of this subviral particle (also called slowly sedimenting hemagglutinin) shows that it is composed of 13–14-nm "doughnut" structures containing a 5–7-nm central "hole." Although such particles are not part of the surface substructure of the virion, they are sometimes found adhering to virions (Kitaoka *et al.*, 1971). The 70 S hemagglutinating particles produced by treating virions with Tween-80 and ether (Brandt *et al.*, 1970) differ from naturally occurring subviral particles in both morphology and density; thus, naturally occurring subviral particles are probably not a result of viral degradation.

Polypeptide analysis of subviral particles shows that they lack the capsid protein V-2, while they contain three envelope proteins, V-3, NV-2, and V-1. The apparent proportions of the latter two varies with the labeling conditions. After a short exposure of infected cells to labeled amino acids, NV-2 is prominent with respect to V-1, while the opposite holds true with longer labeling periods (Shapiro *et al.*, 1971*b*). This subviral particle may be produced during the maturation of intracellular virions to the normal extracellular forms.

3.8. Defective-Interfering Particles

Serial passage of many animal viruses at a high multiplicity of infection has been shown to yield defective-interfering particles; these lack intrinsic infectivity and both depend upon and interfere with the multiplication of standard virus. In those instances that have been carefully analyzed, the defective-interfering particles appear to be deletion mutants. Defective-interfering particles of Sindbis virus have been described independently by three laboratories. It is not surprising that their observations differ in some respects, for subtle differences in selection pressure or pure chance may give rise to defective-interfering particles with different properties. For example, Shenk and Stollar (1973) find that most isolates of defective-interfering particles are slightly more dense than standard virions and contain only virion-length RNA. Weiss and Schlesinger (1973), on the other hand, note no difference in density, but report heterogeneous RNA in the virion.

A common feature of the reports of Shenk and Stollar (1973) and Eaton and Faulkner (1973) is that the only replicative form observed when defective-interfering particles are rigorously excluded from the inoculum sediments at 20 S and is presumably a double-stranded homologue of virion RNA. In contrast, coinfection with standard and defective interfering particles yields a new, lower-molecular-weight, replicative form which sediments at about 12 S. In addition, several new single-stranded RNA species smaller than virion RNA and a new virus-specified protein are found in these mixedly infected cells.

Defective-interfering particles are themselves of substantial interest for they may be useful in unraveling certain problems in both the biochemistry and the genetics of togaviruses. They also stand as a warning to unwary investigators whose results may be confounded by the presence of undetected defective-interfering particles.

ACKNOWLEDGMENTS

We are indebted to the following persons for preprints, illustrations, and helpful comments: D. Brown, B. Burge, J. Dalrymple, P. Grimley, F. Murphy, O. Renkonen, M. Schlesinger, S. Schlesinger, R. W. Schlesinger, D. Simmons, D. Stollar, and E. Zebovitz.

The personal research reported in this chapter was supported by NIH grant AI 08238. Daniel Shapiro received support from Special NIH Research Fellowship GM 53687 during the preparation of this chapter.

4. REFERENCES

Acheson, N. H., and Tamm, I., 1967, Replication of Semliki Forest virus: an electron microscopic study, *Virology* **32**, 128.

Acheson, N. H., and Tamm, I., 1970*a*, Purification and properties of Semliki Forest virus nucleocapsids, *Virology* **41**, 306.

Acheson, N. H., and Tamm, I., 1970*b*, Structural proteins of Semliki Forest virus and its nucleocapsid, *Virology* **41**, 321.

Acheson, N. H., and Tamm, I., 1970*c*, Ribonuclease sensitivity of Semliki Forest virus nucleocapsids, *J. Virol.* **5**, 714.

Ada, G. L., Abbott, A., Anderson, S. G., and Collins, F. D., 1962, Particle count and some chemical properties of Murray Valley encephalitis virus, *J. Gen. Microbiol.* **29**, 165.

Appleyard, G., Oram, J. D., and Stanley, J. L., 1970, Dissociation of Semliki Forest virus into biologically active components, *J. Gen. Virol.* **9**, 179.

Arif, B. M., and Faulkner, P., 1972, Genome of Sindbis virus, *J. Virol.* **9**, 102.

Baltimore, D., 1971, Expression of animal virus genomes, *Bacteriol. Rev.* **35**, 235.

Banerjee, K., and Singh, K. R. P., 1968, Establishment of carrier cultures of *Aedes albopictus* cell line infected with arboviruses. *Ind. J. Med. Res.* **56**, 812.

Barnes, R., Vogel, H., and Gordon, I., 1969, Temperature of compensation: significance for virus inactivation, *Proc. Natl. Acad. Sci. USA* **69**, 263.

Bhamarapravati, N., Halstead, S. B., Sookavachana, P., and Boonyapaknavik, V.,

1964, Studies on dengue virus infection. 1. Immunofluorescent localization of virus in mouse tissue, *Arch. Pathol.* **77**, 538.

Birdwell, C. R., and Strauss, J. H., Jr., 1973, Agglutination of Sindbis virus and of cells infected with Sindbis virus by plant lectins, *J. Virol.* **11**, 502.

Bose, H. R., and Brundige, M. A., 1972, Selective association of Sindbis virion proteins with different membrane fractions of infected cells, *J. Virol.* **9**, 785.

Bose, H. R., and Sagik, B. P., 1970a, Immunological activity associated with the nucelocapsid and envelope components of an arbovirus, *J. Virol.* **5**, 410.

Bose, H. R., and Sagik, B. P., 1970b, The virus envelope in cell attachment, *J. Gen. Virol.* **9**, 159.

Boulton, R. W., and Westaway, E. G., 1972, Comparisons of togaviruses: Sindbis virus (group A) and Kunjun virus (group B), *Virology* **49**, 283.

Brandt, W. E., Cardiff, R. D., and Russell, P. K., 1970, Dengue virions and antigens in brain and serum of infected mice, *J. Virol.* **6**, 500.

Brawner, T. A., and Sagik, B. P., 1971, Rescue of ultraviolet-inactivated Sindbis virus, *Abstr. Annu. Meet. Am. Soc. Microbiol.* 218.

Brawner, T. A., Lee, J. C., and Trent, D. W., 1973, Nuclear and cytoplasmic localization of polyadenylate-rich St. Louis encephalitis virus-induced RNA, *Abstr. Annu. Meet. Am. Soc. Microbiol.* 202.

Brown, D. T., Waite, M. R. F., and Pfefferkorn, E. R., 1972, Morphology and morphogenesis of Sindbis virus as seen with freeze-etching techniques, *J. Virol.* **10**, 524.

Burge, B. W., and Huang, A. S., 1970, Comparison of membrane protein glycopeptides of Sindbis virus and vesicular stomatitis virus, *J. Virol.* **6**, 176.

Burge, B. W., and Pfefferkorn, E. R., 1966a, Isolation and characteristics of temperature-sensitive mutants of Sindbis virus, *Virology* **30**, 204.

Burge, B. W., and Pfefferkorn, E. R., 1966b, Complementation between temperature-sensitive mutants of Sindbis virus, *Virology* **30**, 214.

Burge, B. W., and Pfefferkorn, E. R., 1967, Temperature-sensitive mutants of Sindbis virus: biochemical correlates of complementation, *J. Virol.* **1**, 956.

Burge, B. W., and Pfefferkorn, E. R., 1968, Functional defects of temperature-sensitive mutants of Sindbis virus, *J. Mol. Biol.* **35**, 193.

Burge, B. W., and Strauss, J. H., Jr., 1970, Glycopeptides of the membrane glycoprotein of Sindbis virus, *J. Mol. Biol.* **47**, 449.

Burrell, C. J., Martin, E. M., and Cooper, P. D., 1970, Posttranslational cleavage of virus polypeptides in arbovirus-infected cells, *J. Gen. Virol.* **6**, 319.

Cardiff, R. D., Brandt, W. E., McCloud, T. O., Shapiro, D., and Russell, P. K., 1971, Immunological and biophysical separation of dengue-2 antigens, *J. Virol.* **7**, 15.

Cardiff, R. D., Russ, S. B., Brandt, W. E., and Russell, P. K., 1973a, Cytological localization of dengue-2 antigens: an immunological study with ultrastrucutral correlation, *Infect. Immun.* **7**, 809.

Cardiff, R. D., Dalrymple, J. M., and Russell, P. K., 1973b, RNA polymerase in group B arbovirus (dengue-2) infected cells, *Arch. Ges. Virus* **40**, 392.

Cartwright, K. L., and Burke, D. C., 1970, Virus nucleic acids formed in chick embryo cells infected with Semliki Forest virus, *J. Gen. Virol.* **6**, 231.

Carver, D. H., and Seto, D. S. Y., 1968, Viral inactivation by disulfide bond reducing agents, *J. Virol.* **2**, 1482.

Casals, J., 1971, Arboviruses: incorporation into a general system of virus classification, *in* "Comparative Virology," (K. Maramorosch and E. Kurstak, eds.), pp. 307–333, Academic Press, New York.

Casals, J., and Clarke, D. H., 1965, Arbovirus; group A, *in* "Viral and Rickettsial Infections of Man" (F. L. Horsfall and I. Tamm, eds.) pp. 583–605, Lippincott, Philadelphia.

Cassells, A. C., and Burke, D. C., 1973, Changes in the constitutve enzymes of chick cells following infection with Semliki Forest virus, *J. Gen. Virol.* **18,** 135.

Cheng, P.-Y., 1958, The inactivation of group B arthropod-borne animal viruses by proteases, *Virology* **6,** 129.

Chiang-Shem, M., Chen-Hsiang, H., and Chiang-Show, H., 1966, The effect of temperature and *p*H on the production of Japanese B encephalitis virus and interferon in embryo cell cultures, *Acta Microbiol. Sin.* **12,** 152.

Clarke, D. H., and Casals, J., 1965, Arboviruses; group B *in* "Viral and Rickettsial Infections of Man" (F. L. Horsfall and I. Tamm, eds.), pp. 606–658, Lippincott, Philadelphia.

Compans, R. W., 1971, Location of the glycoprotein in the membrane of Sindbis virus, *Nat. New Biol.* **229,** 114.

Cory, J., and Yunker, C. E., 1972, Arbovirus plaques in mosquito cell monolayers, *Acta Virol.* **16,** 90.

Dalrymple, J. M., Vogel, S. N., Teramoto, A. Y., and Russell, P. K., 1973, Antigenic components of group A arbovirus virions, *J. Virology* **12,** 1034.

David, A. E., 1971, Lipid composition of Sindbis virus, *Virology* **46,** 711.

Diercks, F. D., and Hammon, W. McD., 1958, Hamster kidney cell tissue cultures for propagation of Japanese B encephalitis. *Proc. Soc. Exp. Biol. Med.* **97,** 627.

Dobos, P., and Faulkner, P., 1969, Properties of 42 S and 26 S Sindbis viral ribonucleic acid species, *J. Virol.* **5,** 429.

Dobos, P., and Faulkner, P., 1970, Molecular weight of Sindbis virus ribonucleic acid as measured by polyacrylamide gel electrophoresis, *J. Virol.* **6,** 145.

Dorsett, P. H., and Acton, J. D., 1970, Synthesis of virus macromolecules in L-929 cells infected with Mayaro virus, *J. Gen. Virol.* **9,** 133.

Eaton, B. T., and Faulkner, P., 1972, Heterogeneity in the poly(A) content of the genome of Sindbis virus, *Virology* **50,** 865.

Eaton, B. T., and Faulkner, P., 1973, Altered pattern of viral RNA synthesis in cells infected with standard and defective Sindbis virus, *Virology* **51,** 85.

El Dadah, N., and Nathanson, N., 1967, Pathogenesis of West Nile virus encephalitis in mice and rats. II. Virus multiplication, evolution, of immunofluorescence, and development of histological lesions in the brain, *Am. J. Epidemiol.* **86,** 776.

Enzmann, P. J., 1973, Induction of an interferon-like substance in persistently infected *Aedes albopictus* cells, *Arch. Ges. Virus.* 40:382.

Filshie, B. K., and Rehacek, J., 1968, Studies of the morphology of Murray Valley encephalitis and Japanese encephalitis viruses growing in cultured mosquito cells, *Virology* **34,** 435.

Fleming, P., 1971*a*, Thermal inactivation of Semliki Forest virus, *J. Gen. Virol.* **13,** 385.

Fleming, P., 1971*b*, Inactivation and reactivation of Semliki Forest virus by urea and guanidine hydrochloride, *J. Gen. Virol.* **13,** 393.

Friedman, R. M., 1968*a*, Replicative intermediate of an arbovirus, *J. Virol.* **2,** 547.

Friedman, R. M., 1968*b*, Structural and nonstructural proteins of an arbovirus, *J. Virol.* **2,** 1076.

Friedman, R. M., 1969, Primary gene products of an arbovirus, *Biochem. Biophys. Res. Commun.* **37,** 369.

Friedman, R. M., and Berezesky, I. K., 1967, Cytoplasmic fractions associated with Semliki Forest virus ribonucleic acid replication, *J. Virol.* **1,** 374.

Friedman, R. M., and Grimley, P. M., 1969, Inhibition of arbovirus assembly by cycloheximide, *J. Virol.* **4,** 292.

Friedman, R. M., and Pastan, I., 1969, Nature and function of the structural phospholipids of an arbovirus, *J. Mol. Biol.* **40,** 107.

Friedman, R. M., and Sreevalsan, T., 1970, Membrane binding of input arbovirus ribonucleic acid: Effect of interferon or cycloheximide, *J. Virol.* **6,** 169.

Friedman, R. M., Levy, H. R., and Carter, W. B., 1966, Replication of Semliki Forest virus: three forms of viral RNA produced during infection, *Proc. Natl. Acad. Sci. USA* **56,** 440.

Friedman, R. M., Levin, J. G., Grimley, P. M., and Berezesky, I. K., 1972, Membrane-associated replication complex in arbovirus infection, *J. Virol.* **10,** 504.

Furusawa, E., Furusawa, S., and Cutting, W., 1969, Refractoriness of KB cell cultures carrying Japanese B encephalitis virus to encephalomyocarditis virus infection. *Proc. Soc. Exp. Biol. Med.* **131,** 951.

Fuscaldo, A. A., Aaslestad, H. G., and Hoffman, E. J., 1971, Biological, physical and chemical properties of eastern equine encephalitis virus, *J. Virol.* **7,** 233.

Gahmberg, C. G., Simons, K., Renkonen, O., and Kääriäinen, L., 1972, Exposure of proteins and lipids in the Semliki Forest virus membrane, *Virology* **50,** 259.

Gorman, B., and Goss, P., 1972, Sensitivity of arboviruses to proteases, *J. Gen. Virol.* **16,** 83.

Grimes, W. J., and Burge, B. W., 1971, Modification of Sindbis virus glycoprotein by host-specified glycosyl transferases, *J. Virol.* **7,** 309.

Grimley, P. M., Berezesky, I. K., and Friedman, R. M., 1968, Cytoplasmic structures associated with an arbovirus infection: loci of viral ribonucleic acid synthesis, *J. Virol.* **2,** 1326.

Grimley, P. M., Levin, J. G., Berezesky, I. K., and Friedman, R. M., 1972, Specific membranous structures associated with the replication of group A arboviruses, *J. Virol.* **10,** 492.

Harrison, S. C., David, A. E., Jumblatt, J., and Darnell, J. E., Jr., 1971, Lipid and protein organization in Sindbis virus, *J. Mol. Biol.* **60,** 523.

Hay, A. J., Skehel, J. J., and Burke, D. C., 1968, Proteins synthesized in chick cells following infection with Semliki Forest virus, *J. Gen. Virol.* **3,** 175.

Heydrick, F. P., Comer, J. F., and Wachter, R. F., 1971, Phospholipid composition of Venezuelan equine encephalitis virus, *J. Virol.* **7,** 642.

Horzinek, M., and Mussgay, M., 1969, Studies on the nucleocapsid structure of a group A arbovirus, *J. Virology* **4,** 514.

Igarashi, A., 1970, Protein synthesis and formation of Chikungungya virus in infected BHK21 cells, *Biken J.* **13,** 289.

Igarashi, A., Kitano, H., Fukunaga, T., and Fukai, K., 1963, Infectivity of the ribonucleic acid fraction from mouse brain infected with Japanese encephalitis virus, *Biken J.* **6,** 165.

Igarashi, A., Fukunaga, T., and Fukai, K., 1964, Sedimentation characteristics of Japanese encephalitis virus ribonucleic acid, *Biken J.* **7,** 111.

Inglot, A. D., Albin, M., and Chudzio, T., 1973, Persistent infection of mouse cells with Sindbis virus: role of virulence of strains, auto-interfering particles and interferon, *J. Gen. Virol.* **20,** 105.

Inoue, Y. K., and Ogura, R., 1962, Studies on Japanese B encephalitis virus. III.

Propagation and assay of Japanese B encephalitis virus in a stable line of porcine kidney cells, *Virology* **16**, 205.

Iwasaki, T., and Inoue, Y. K., 1961, Studies on Japanese B encephalitis virus. II. Isolation of a heat-resistant mutant of Japanese B encephalitis virus, *Virology* **51**, 81.

Johnston, R. E., and Bose, H. R., 1972a, An adenylate-rich segment in the virion RNA of Sindbis virus, *Biochem. Biophys. Res. Commun.* **46**, 712.

Johnston, R. E., and Bose, H. R., 1972b, Correlation of messenger RNA function with adenylate-rich segments in the genomes of single-stranded RNA viruses, *Proc. Natl. Acad. Sci. USA* **69**, 1514.

Kääriäinen, L., and Gomatos, P. J., 1969, A kinetic analysis of the synthesis in BHK 21 cells of RNAs specific for Semliki Forest virus, *J. Gen. Virol.* **5**, 251.

Kääriäinen, L., and Söderlund, H., 1971, Properties of Semliki Forest virus nucleocapsid. I. Sensitivity to pancreatic ribonuclease, *Virology* **43**, 291.

Kaluza, G., Scholtissek, C., and Rott, R., 1972, Inhibition of the multiplication of enveloped RNA-viruses by glucosamine and 2-deoxy-D-glucose, *J. Gen. Virol.* **14**, 251.

Kaluza, G., Schmidt, M. F. G., and Scholtissek, C., 1973, Effect of 2-deoxy-D-glucose on the multiplication of Semliki Forest virus and the reversal of the block by mannose, *Virology* **54**, 179.

Karabatsos, N., and Buckley, S. M., 1967, Susceptibility of the baby-hamster kidney-cell line (BHK-21) to infection with arboviruses, *Am. J. Trop. Med. Hyg.* **16**, 99.

Kennedy, S. I. T., 1972, Isolation and identification of the virus-specified RNA species found on membrane-bound polyribosomes of chick embryo cells infected with Semliki Forest virus, *Biochem. Biophys. Res. Commun.* **48**, 1254.

Kennedy, S. I. T., and Burke, D. C., 1972, Studies on the structural proteins of Semliki Forest virus, *J. Gen. Virol.* **14**, 87.

Kitaoka, M., Shimizu, A., Tuchinda, P., and Chandana, K. A., 1971, Electron microscopic observations on dengue type 2 virus, *Biken J.* **14**, 361.

Klimenko, S. M., Yershov, F. I., Gofman, Y. P., Nabatnikov, A. P., and Zhdanov, V. M., 1965, Architecture of Venezuelan equine encephalitis virus, *Virology* **27**, 125.

Laine, R., Kettunen, M.-L., Gahmberg, C. G., Kääriäinen, L., Renkonen, O., 1972, Fatty acids of different lipid classes of Semliki Forest virus and host cell membranes, *J. Virol.* **10**, 433.

Lee, H. W., Hinz, R. W., and Scherer, W. F., 1958, Porcine kidney cell cultures for propagation and assay of Japanese encephalitis virus, *Proc. Soc. Exp. Biol. Med.* **99**, 579.

Levin, J. G., and Friedman, R. M., 1971, Analysis of arbovirus ribonucleic acid forms by polyacrylamide gel electrophoresis, *J. Virol.* **7**, 504.

McCollum, R. W., and Foley, J. F., 1956, Japanese B encephalitis virus in tissue culture. *Proc. Soc. Exp. Biol. Med.* **94**, 556.

Marcus, P. I., and Carver, D. H., 1967, Intrinsic interference: a new type of viral interference, *J. Virol.* **1**, 334.

Marcus, P. I., and Salb, J. M., 1966, Molecular basis of interferon action: inhibition of viral RNA translation, *Virology* **30**, 502.

Martin, E. M., 1969, Studies on the RNA polymerase of some temperature-sensitive mutants of Semliki Forest virus, *Virology* **39**, 107.

Martin, E. M., and Sonnabend, J. A., 1967, Ribonucleic acid polymerase catalyzing synthesis of double-stranded arbovirus ribonucleic acid, *J. Virol.* **1**, 97.

Matsumura, T., Stollar, V., and Schlesinger, R. W., 1970, Effect of magnesium chloride on yield of dengue virus from Vero cells, *Abstr. Annu. Meet. Am. Soc. Microbiol.* 190.

Matsumura, T., Stollar, V., and Schlesinger, R. W., 1971, Studies on the nature of dengue viruses. V. Structure and development of dengue virus in Vero cells, *Virology* **46**, 344.

Mécs, E., Sonnabend, J. A., and Martin, E. M., 1967, The effect of interferon on the synthesis of RNA in chick cells infected with Semliki Forest virus, *J. Gen. Virol.* **1**, 25.

Michel, M. R., and Gomatos, P. J., 1973, Semliki Forest virus-specific RNAs synthesized in vitro by enzyme from infected BHK cells, *J. Virol.* **11**, 900.

Morgan, C., Howe, C., and Rose. H. M., 1961, Structure and development of viruses as observed in the electronmicroscope. V. Western equine encaphalomyelitis virus, *J. Exptl. Med.* **113**, 219.

Mowshowitz, D., 1973, Identification of polysomal RNA in BHK cells infected by Sindbis virus, *J. Virol.* **11**, 535.

Murphy, F. A., Harrison, A. K., Gary, G. W., Whitfield, S. G., and Forrester, F. T., 1968, St. Louis encephalitis virus infection of mice. Electron microscopic studies of central nervous system, *Lab. Invest.* **19**, 652.

Mussgay, M., 1964, Growth cycle of arboviruses in vertebrate and arthropod cells, *Prog. Med. Virol.* **6**, 193.

Mussgay, M., and Horzinek, M., 1966, Investigations on complement-fixing subunits of a group A arbovirus (Sindbis), *Virology* **29**, 199.

Nagatomo, Y., 1972, The characterization of Chikungunya virus RNA, *Archiv. Ges. Virus* **39**, 63.

Nishimura, C., and Kitaoka, M., 1964, Purification of Japanese encephalitis virus and its antigenic particles from infected suckling mouse brains, *Jap. J. Med. Sci. Biol.* **17**, 295.

Nishimura, C., and Tsukeda, H., 1971, Replication and synthesis of Japanese encephalitis virus ribonucleic acids in Vero cells, *Jap. Microbiol.* **15**, 309.

Nozima, T., Mori, Hl, Minobe, Y., and Yamamoto, S., 1964, Some properties of Japanese encephalitis virus, *Acta Virol.* **8**, 97.

Ota, Z., 1965, Electron microscopic study of the development of Japanese B encephalitis virus in porcine kidney stable (PS) cells, *Virology* **25**, 372.

Ozaki, Y., and Kumagi, K., 1972, Effect of polyions on Japanese encephalitis virus, *Arch. Ges. Virus* **39**, 83.

Paul, S. D., Singh, K. R. P., and Bhat, U. K. M., 1969, A study on the cytopathic effect of arboviruses on cultures from *Aedes albopictus* cell line, *Ind. J. Med. Res.* **57**, 339.

Pederson, C. E., Jr., and Sagik, B. P., 1973, Sindbis virus maturation, *J. Gen. Virol.* **18**, 375.

Peleg, J., 1969a, Behaviour of infectious RNA from four different viruses in continuously subcultured *Aedes aegypti* mosquito embryo cells, *Nature (Lond.)* **221**, 193.

Peleg, J., 1969b, Inapparent persistent virus infection in continuously grown *Aedes aegypti* mosquito cells, *J. Gen. Virol.* **5**, 463.

Peleg, J., 1972, Studies on the behavior of arboviruses in an *Aedes aegypti* mosquito cell line, *Arch. Ges. Virus* **37**, 54.

Pfefferkorn, E. R., and Boyle, M. K., 1972, Selective inhibition of the synthesis of Sindbis virion proteins by an inhibitor of chymotrypsin, *J. Virol.* **9**, 187.

Pfefferkorn, E. R., and Burge, B. W., 1967, Genetics and biochemistry of arbovirus temperature-sensitive mutants, *in* "The Molecular Biology of Viruses" (J. Colter, ed.), pp. 403–426, Academic Press, New York.

Pfefferkorn, E. R., and Clifford, R. L., 1964, The origin of the protein of Sindbis virus, *Virology* **23**, 217.

Pfefferkorn, E. R., and Hunter, H. S., 1963a, Purification and partial chemical analysis of Sindbis virus, *Virology* **20**, 433.

Pfefferkorn, E. R., and Hunter, H. S., 1963b, The source of the ribonucleic acid and phospholipid of Sindbis virus, *Virology* **20**, 446.

Pfefferkorn, E. R., Burge, B. W., and Coady, H. M., 1967, Intracellular conversion of the RNA of Sindbis virus to a double-stranded form, *Virology* **33**, 239.

Pollack, R., and Goldman, R, 1973, Synthesis of infective poliovirus in BSC-1 monkey cells enucleated with cytochalasin B, *Science* (*Wash., D.C.*) **179**, 915.

Porterfield, J. S., 1959, Plaque production with yellow fever and related arthropod-borne virus, *Nature* (*Lond.*) **183**, 1069.

Purifoy, D. J. M., Purifoy, J. A., and Sagik, B. P., 1968, A mathematical analysis of concomitant virus replication and heat inactivation, *J. Virol.* **2**, 275.

Qureshi, A. A., and Trent, D. W., 1972, Saint Louis encephalitis viral ribonucleic acid replication complex, *J. Virol.* **9**, 565.

Qureshi, A. A., and Trent, D. W., 1973, Group B arbovirus structural and nonstructural antigens I. Serological identification of Saint Louis encephalitis virus soluble antigens. *Infect. Immun.* **7**, 242.

Ranki, M., Kääriäinen, L., and Renkonen, O., 1972, Semliki Forest virus glycoproteins and canavanine, *Acta Pathol. Microbiol. Scand.* (*B*) **80**, 760.

Rehacek, J., 1968, Persistent infection of mosquito cells grown *in vitro* with Murray Valley encephalitis and Japanese encephalitis viruses, *Acta Virol.* **12**, 340.

Renkonen, O., Kääriäinen, L., Simons, K., and Gahmberg, C. G., 1971, The lipid class composition of Semliki Forest virus and of plasma membranes of the host cells, *Virology* **46**, 318.

Renkonen, O., Luukkonen, A., Brotherus, J., and Kääriäinen, L., 1974, Composition and turnover of membrane lipids in Semliki Forest virus and in host cells, *in* "Control of Proliferation in Animal Cells" (B. Clarkson and R. Baserga, eds.), Cold Spring Harbor Monograph, Cold Spring Harbor, New York.

Rosemond, H., and Sreevalsan, T., 1973, Viral RNAs associated with ribosomes in Sindbis virus-infected HeLa cells, *J. Virol.* **11**, 399.

Rubin, H., Baluda, M., and Hotchkin, J. E., 1955, The maturation of Western equine encephalomyelitis virus and its release from chick embryo cells in suspension, *J. Exp. Med.* **101**, 205.

Scheele, C. M., and Pfefferkorn, E. R., 1969a, The kinetics of incorporation of structural proteins into Sindbis virions, *J. Virol.* **3**, 369.

Scheele, C. M., and Pfefferkorn, E. R., 1969b, Inhibition of interjacent RNA (26 S) synthesis in cells infected by Sindbis virus, *J. Virol.* **4**, 117.

Scheele, C. M., and Pfefferkorn, E. R., 1970, Virus-specific proteins synthesized in cells infected with RNA⁺ temperature-sensitive mutants of Sindbis virus, *J. Virol.* **5**, 329.

Scherer, W. F., and Syverton, J. T., 1954, The viral range *in vitro* of a malignant human epithelial cell (strain HeLa, Gey). II. Studies with encephalitis viruses of the eastern, western, West Nile, St. Louis, and Japanese B types, *Am. J. Pathol.* **30**, 1075.

Schlesinger, M. J., and Schlesinger, S., 1973, Large-molecular-weight precursors of Sindbis virus proteins, *J. Virol.* **11**, 1013.

Schlesinger, M. J., Schlesinger, S., and Burge, B. W., 1972, Identification of a second glycoprotein in Sindbis virus, *Virology* **47**, 539.

Schlesinger, S., and Schlesinger, M. J., 1972, Formation of Sindbis virus proteins: identification of a precursor for one of the envelope proteins, *J. Virol.* **10**, 925.

Schlesinger, S., Schlesinger, M. J., and Burge, B. W., 1972, Defective virus particles from Sindbis virus, *Virology* **48**, 615.

Schlesinger, R. W., 1971, Some speculations on the possible role of arthropods in the evolution of arboviruses, *Curr. Top. Microbiol. Immun.* **55**, 241.

Scholtissek, C., Kaluza, G., and Rott, R., 1972, Stability and precursor relationships of virus RNA, *J. Gen. Virol.* **17**, 213.

Schwöbel, W., and Ahl, R., 1972, Persistence of Sindbis virus in BHK-21 cell structures, *Archiv. Ges. Virus* 38:1.

Sefton, B. M., Wickus, G. G., and Burge, B. W., 1973, Enzymatic iodination of Sindbis virus proteins, *J. Virol.* **11**, 730.

Shapiro, D., Brandt, W. E., Cardiff, R. D., and Russell, P. K., 1971*a*, The proteins of Japanese encephalitis virus, *Virology* **44**, 108.

Shapiro, D., Cardiff, R. D., Brandt, W. E., and Russell, P. K., 1971*b*, Properties of dengue-2 and Japanese encephalitis virus slowly sedimenting hemagglutinins, *Abstr. Annu. Meet. Am. Soc. Microbiol.* 182.

Shapiro, D., Trent, D., Brandt, W. E., and Russell, P. K., 1972*a*, Comparison of the virion polypeptides of group B arboviruses, *Infect. Immun.* **6**, 206.

Shapiro, D., Kos, K. A., Brandt, W. E., and Russell, P. K., 1972*b*, Membrane-bound proteins of Japanese encephalitis virus-infected, chick embryo cells, *Virology* **48**, 360.

Shapiro, D., Brandt, W. E., and Russell, P. K., 1972*c*, Change involving a viral membrane glycoprotein during morphogenesis of group B arboviruses, *Virology* **50**, 906.

Shapiro, D., Kos, K. A., and Russell, P. K., 1973*a*, Japanese encephalitis virus glycoproteins, *Virology* **56**, 88.

Shapiro, D., Kos, K. A., and Russell, P. K., 1973*b*, Protein synthesis in Japanese encephalitis virus infected chick embryo cells, *Virology* **56**, 95.

Shenk, T. E., and Stollar, V., 1972, Viral RNA species in BHK-21 cells infected with Sindbis virus serially passaged at high multiplicity of infection, *Biochem. Biophys. Res. Commun.* **49**, 60.

Shenk, T. E., and Stollar, V., 1973, Defective-interfering particles of Sindbis virus. I. Isolation and some chemical and biological properties, *Virology* **53**, 162.

Simmons, D. T., and Strauss, J. H., Jr., 1972*a*, Replication of Sindbis virus. I. Relative size and genetic content of 26 S and 49 S RNA, *J. Mol. Biol.* **71**, 599.

Simmons, D. T., and Strauss, J. H., Jr., 1972*b*, Replication of Sindbis virus. II. Multiple forms of double-stranded RNA isolated from infected cells, *J. Mol. Biol.* **71**, 615.

Simons, K., Keränen, S., and Kääriäinen, L., 1973, Identification of a precursor for one of the Semliki Forest virus membrane proteins, *FEBS (Fed. Eur. Biochem. Soc.) Lett.* 29:87.

Simpson, R. W., and Hauser, R. E., 1968, Basic structure of group A arbovirus strains

Middelburg, Sindbis and Semliki Forest examined by negative staining, *Virology* **34,** 358.

Singh, B., Chang, I. C., and Hammon, W. McD., 1973, Semi-commercial-scale production of Japanese B encephalitis virus vaccines from tissue culture, *Appl. Microbiol.* **25,** 945.

Singh, K. R. P., 1971, Propagation of arboviruses in Singh's *Aedes* cell lines. I. Growth of arboviruses in *Aedes albopictus* and *A. aegypti* cell lines, *Curr. Top. Microbiol. Immunol.* **55,** 127.

Singh, K. R. P., and Paul, S. D., 1968a, Susceptibility of *Aedes albopictus* and *Aedes aegypti* cell lines to infection by arbo- and other viruses, *Ind. J. Med. Res.* **56,** 815.

Singh, K. R. P., and Paul, S. D., 1968b, Multiplication of arboviruses in cell lines from *Aedes albopictus* and *Aedes aegypti, Curr. Sci. (Banglore)* **37,** 65.

Smith, T. J., Brandt, W. E. Swanson, J. L., McCown, J. M., and Buescher, E. L., 1970, Physical and biological properties of dengue-2 virus and associated antigens, *J. Virol.* **5,** 524.

Sonnabend, J. A., Martin, E. M., and Mécs, E., 1967, Viral specific RNAs in infected cells, *Nature (Lond.)* **213,** 365.

Sreevalsan, T., 1970, Association of viral ribonucleic acid with cellular membranes in chick embryo cells infected with Sindbis virus, *J. Virol.* **6,** 438.

Sreevalsan, T., and Allen, P. T., 1968, Replication of Western equine encephalomyelitis virus. II. Cytoplasmic structure involved in the synthesis and development of the virions, *J. Virol.* **2,** 1038.

Sreevalsan, T., and Lockart, R. Z., Jr., 1964, Inhibition by puromycin of the initiation of synthesis of infectious RNA and virus by chicken embryo cells infected with Western equine encephalomyelitis virus, *Virology* **24,** 91.

Sreevalsan, T., and Lockart, R. Z., Jr., 1966, Heterogeneous RNA's occurring during the replication of western equine encephalomyelitis virus, *Proc. Natl. Acad. Sci. USA* **55,** 974.

Sreevalsan, T., and Yin, F. H., 1969, Sindbis virus-induced viral ribonucleic acid polymerase, *J. Virol.* **3,** 599.

Sreevalsan, T., Lockart, R. Z., Jr., Dodson, M. L., Jr., and Hartman, K. A., 1968, Replication of western equine encephalomyelitis virus. I. Some chemical and physical characteristics of viral ribonucleic acid, *J. Virol.* **2,** 558.

Stevens, T. M., 1970, Arbovirus replication in mosquito cell lines (Singh) grown in monolayer or suspension culture (34793), *Proc. Soc. Exp. Biol. Med.* **134,** 356.

Stevens, T. M., and Schlesinger, R. W., 1965, Studies on the nature of dengue viruses. I. Correlation of particle density, infectivity, and RNA content of type 2 virus, *Virology* **27,** 103.

Stim, T. B., and Henderson, J. R., 1969, Arbovirus plaquing in a clonal line (PS Y-15) of porcine kidney, *Appl. Microbiol.* **17,** 246.

Stinski, M. F., and Gruber, J., 1971, Distribution of arbovirus antigens in density gradients, *Proc. Soc. Exp. Biol. Med.* **136,** 1347.

Stollar, V., 1969, Studies on the nature of dengue viruses. IV. The structural proteins of type 2 dengue virus, *Virology* **39,** 426.

Stollar, V., and Shenk, T. E., 1973, Homologous viral interference in *Aedes albopictus* cultures chronically infected with Sindbis virus, *J. Virol.* **11,** 592.

Stollar, V., Stevens, T. M., and Schlesinger, R. W., 1966, Studies on the nature of dengue viruses. II. Characterization of viral RNA and effects of inhibitors of RNA synthesis, *Virology* **30,** 303.

Stollar, V., Schlesinger, R. W., and Stevens, T. M., 1967, Studies on the nature of dengue viruses. III. RNA synthesis in cells infected with type 2 dengue virus, *Virology* **33**, 650.

Strauss, J. H., Jr., Burge, B. W., Pfefferkorn, E. R., and Darnell, J. E., Jr., 1968, Identification of the membrane protein and "core" protein of Sindbis virus, *Proc. Natl. Acad. Sci. USA* **59**, 533.

Strauss, J. H., Jr., Burge, B. W., and Darnell, J. E., Jr., 1969, Sindbis virus infection of chick and hamster cells: synthesis of virus-specific proteins, *Virology* **37**, 367.

Strauss, J. H., Jr., Burge, B. W., and Darnell, J. E., Jr., 1970, Carbohydrate content of the membrane protein of Sindbis virus, *J. Mol. Biol.* **47**, 437.

Suitor, E. C., 1969, Plaque formation by an arbovirus in a mosquito cell line, *J. Gen. Virol.* **5**, 545.

Takeda, H., Yamada, M., and Aoyama, Y., 1965, Demonstration of RNA synthesis caused by Japanese encephalitis virus infection in PS (Y-15) cells with the aid of chromomycin A_3, *Jap. J. Med. Sci. Biol.* **18**, 111.

Takehara, M., 1971, Comparative studies on nucleic acid synthesis and virus-induced RNA polymerase activity in mammalian cells infected with certain arboviruses, *Arch. Ges. Virus* **34**, 266.

Takehara, M., 1972, Inhibition of nuclear protein synthesis in BHK-21 cells infected with arboviruses, *Arch. Ges. Virus* **39**, 163.

Takehara, M., and Hotta, S., 1961, Effect of enzymes on partially purified Japanese B encephalitis and related arboviruses, *Science (Wash., D.C.)* **134**, 1878.

Tan, K. B., Sambrook, J. F., and Bellett, A. J. D., 1969, Semliki Forest virus temperature-sensitive mutants: isolation and characterization, *Virology* **38**, 427.

Taylor, J., 1965, Studies on the mechanism of action of interferon. I. Interferon action and RNA synthesis in chick embryo fibroblasts infected with Semliki Forest virus, *Virology* **25**, 340.

Tremblay, G. Y., Daniels, M. J., and Schaechter, M., 1969, Isolation of a cell membrane-DNA nascent RNA complex from bacteria, *J. Mol. Biol.* **40**, 65.

Trent, D. W., 1973, Phospholipid composition of Saint Louis encephalitis (SLE) virus and host cell membranes, *Abstr. Annu. Meet. Am. Soc. Microbiol.*, 240.

Trent, D. W., and Qureshi, A. A., 1971, Structural and nonstructural proteins of Saint Louis encephalitis virus, *J. Virol.* **7**, 379.

Trent, D. W., Swenson, C. C., and Qureshi, A. A., 1969, Synthesis of Saint Louis encephalitis virus ribonucleic acid in BHK-21/13 cells, *J. Virol.* **3**, 385.

Tsilinsky, Y. Y., Butshin, B. V., Klimenko, S. M., and Lvov, D. K., 1971, Variations of virion sizes in different clones of Venezuelan equine encephalomyelitis virus, *Archiv. Ges. Virus* **34**, 301.

Ventura, A. K., and Scherer, W. F., 1970, Different effects of deoxycholate, ether, chloroform, hydrocarbons, acid alcohols on Venezuelan encephalitis viral infection, hemagglutination and complement fixation, *Proc. Soc. Exp. Biol. Med.* **133**, 711.

Wachter, R. F., and Johnson, E. W., 1962, Lipid content of the equine encephalitis viruses, *Fed. Proc.* **21**, 461.

Waite, M. R. F., 1973, Protein synthesis directed by an RNA^- temperature-sensitive mutant of Sindbis virus, *J. Virol.* **11**, 198.

Waite, M. R. F., and Pfefferkorn, E. R., 1968, Effect of altered osmotic pressure on the growth of Sindbis virus, *J. Virol.* **2**, 759.

Waite, M. R. F., and Pfefferkorn, E. R., 1970a, Inhibition of Sindbis virus production by media of low ionic strength: intracellular events and requirements for reversal, *J. Virol.* **5**, 60.

Waite, M. R. F., and Pfefferkorn, E. R., 1970*b*, Phospholipid synthesis in Sindbis virus-infected cells, *J. Virol.* **6**, 637.

Waite, M. R. F., Brown, D. T., and Pfefferkorn, E. R., 1972, Inhibition of Sindbis virus release by media of low ionic strength: an electron microscope study, *J. Virol.* **10**, 537.

Wecker, E., 1959, The extraction of infectious virus nucleic acid with hot phenol, *Virology* **7**, 241.

Wecker, E., and Richter, A., 1962, Conditions for the replication of infectious viral RNA, *Cold Spring Harbor Symp. Quant. Biol.* **27**, 137.

Weiss, B., and Schlesinger, S., 1973, Defective interfering passages of Sindbis virus: chemical composition, biological activity and mode of interference, *J. Virology* **12**, 862.

Westaway, E. G., 1973, Proteins specified by group B togaviruses in mammalian cells during productive infections, *Virology* **51**, 454.

Westaway, E. G., and Reedman, B. M., 1969, Proteins of the group B arbovirus Kunjin, *J. Virol.* **4**, 688.

Wiebenga, N. H., 1961, The cultivation of dengue-1 (Hawaiian) virus in tissue culture. I. Carrier culture of human skin cells infected with dengue-1 virus, *Am. J. Hyg.* **73**, 350.

Wildy, P., ed., 1971, International Committee on Nomenclature of Viruses, Classification and nomenclature of viruses: First report 1966–1970, *in* "Monographs in Virology," Vol. 5, pp. 52–54, Karger, Basel.

Yasuzumi, G., and Tsubo, I., 1965*a*, Analysis of the development of Japanese B encephalitis (JBE) virus. II. Electron microscopic studies of neurons infected with JBE virus, *J. Ultrastruct. Res.* **12**, 304.

Yasuzumi, G., and Tsubo, I., 1965*b*, Analysis of the development of Japanese B encephalitis virus. III. Electron microscopic studies on inclusion bodies appearing in neurons and microglial cells infected with JBE virus, *J. Ultrastruct. Res.* **12**, 217.

Yasuzumi, G., Tsubo, I., Sugihara, R., and Nakai, Y., 1964, Analysis of the development of Japanese B encephalitis virus. I. Electron microscope studies of microglia infected with JBE virus, *J. Ultrastruct. Res.* **11**, 213.

Yin, F. H., 1969, Temperature-sensitive behavior of the hemagglutinin in a temperature-sensitive mutant virion of Sindbis, *J. Virol.* **4**, 547.

Yoshinaka, Y., and Hotta, S., 1971, Infectivity of virus-specific RNA's of a group A arbovirus, Chikungunya, *Virology* **45**, 524.

Yunker, C. E., 1971, Arthropod tissue culture in the study of arboviruses and rickettsiae: a review, *in* "Arthropod cell cultures and their application to the study of viruses" (E. Weiss, ed.), pp. 113–126, Springer-Verlag, Berlin.

Zebovitz, E., Leong, J. K., and Doughty, S. C., 1972, Japanese encephalitis virus replication: a procedure for the selective isolation and characterization of viral RNA species, *Arch. Ges. Virus* **38**, 319.

Zebovitz, E., Doughty, S. C., and Scott, R. E., 1974, Involvement of the host cell nuclear envelope in the replication of Japanese encephalitis virus, *Infect. Immun.* in press.

CHAPTER 5

Reproduction of Reoviridae

Wolfgang K. Joklik

Department of Microbiology and Immunology
Duke University Medical Center
Durham, North Carolina 27710

1. INTRODUCTION

The discovery by Gomatos and Tamm (1963a) that reovirus RNA is double-stranded caused great interest since, although double-stranded RNA was at that time under active investigation as the replicative form of viral genomes consisting of single-stranded RNA, it provided the first source of stable double-stranded RNA. Equally significant was the subsequent demonstration that the reovirus genome consists of a unique set of several distinct molecules; this upset the previously held notion that the genomes of all viruses consist of a single nucleic acid molecule.

Reovirus was but the first of several viruses that proved to contain double-stranded RNA. The majority resemble each other sufficiently in morphology as well as in genome size and structure for the suggestion to be made that they should all be grouped together within a single family, the diplornaviruses (Verwoerd, 1970). Recently, fungal viruses have been discovered which also contain genomes of double-stranded RNA, but which differ from the above at least as much as, say, adenoviruses differ from papovaviruses. It has therefore been proposed by a subcommittee of the International Committee for the Nomenclature of Viruses that all "reovirus-like" viruses be placed into a family to be known as the *Reoviridae*, and that the other double-stranded-RNA-containing viruses be constituted into other appropriate families, just as double-stranded-DNA-containing viruses are grouped into several families.

The criteria for classification as a member of the Reoviridae are based primarily on morphology and genome size and structure: viruses must possess quasispherical capsids 60–80 nm in diameter that exhibit icosahedral symmetry elements, and their genomes must consist of about 10–12 molecules of double-stranded RNA with a combined molecular weight of about 15×10^6. The four groups of viruses which meet these criteria are: (1) The genus *Orthoreovirus* (abbreviated to reovirus below); host range, vertebrates. It includes primarily the three morphologically identical serotypes of reovirus. (2) The genus *Orbivirus*; host range, insects and vertebrates. Until recently these viruses were classified as arboviruses since, with few exceptions, they have been isolated only from insects. The most intensively studied *Orbivirus* is bluetongue virus (BTV). (3) A genus comprising the cytoplasmic polyhedrosis viruses (CPV); host range, insects. (4) A genus comprising primarily wound tumor virus (WTV), rice dwarf virus (RDV), Fiji disease virus (FDV), and maize rough dwarf virus (MRDV); host range, plants and insects.

There is no evidence of any serologic relationship between the members of these four genera (Gamez *et al.*, 1967), nor are they genetically related, as judged by the fact that their nucleic acids do not hybridize with each other (Shatkin and Rada, 1967*a*; Verwoerd and Huismans, 1969; Black and Knight, 1970).

The viruses which are currently classified as members of the Reoviridae are listed in Table 1.

The dual novelty of RNA double-strandedness and genome segmentation, coupled with the fact that it multiplies to high titers in established cell lines, has caused reovirus to become one of the most intensively studied animal viruses, and it is now a useful model system for the study of transcription and translation in mammalian cells. Studies of bluetongue virus have also recently begun along similar lines, but work on the molecular virology of the cytoplasmic polyhedrosis viruses and the plant virus members of this family has so far been limited almost entirely to investigations of their structure and components. The bulk of this review will of necessity be devoted to an examination of the structure and replication of reovirus. Wherever possible, however, current knowledge concerning the viruses belonging to the other three genera will also be discussed so as to permit comparison and perception of relationships.

TABLE 1

Members of the Family Reoviridae

Genus	Virus	Vector
Orthoreovirus		
	(i) Mammalian (human)reovirus (3 serotypes)	—
	(ii) Avian (chicken) reovirus (5 serotypes)	—
	(iii) Nelson Bay virus	?
	(iv) Nebraska calf diarrhea virus	—
	(v) Epizootic diarrhea of infant mice	—
	(probable member)	
Orbivirus		
	(i) Bluetongue subgroup	
	Bluetongue virus (16 serotypes)	Culicoides
	Epizootic hemorrhagic disease of deer	?
	Ib Ar 22619	Culicoides
	Ib Ar 33853	Culicoides
	Eubenangee	Mosquitoes
	B 1327	Mosquitoes
	(ii) Corriparta subgroup	
	Corriparta	Mosquitoes
	Acado	Mosquitoes
	(iii) Changuinola subgroup	
	Changuinola	Phlebotomines
	Irituia	?
	Be Ar 35646	Phlebotomines
	Be Ar 41067	Phlebotomines
	BT 2164	Phlebotomines
	BT 104	Phlebotomines
	Co Ar 2837	Phlebotomines
	(iv) Colorado tick fever	Ticks
	(v) Kemerovo subgroup	
	Kemerovo	Ticks
	Tribec	Ticks
	Chenuda	Ticks
	Mono Lake	Ticks
	Huacho	Ticks
	Wad Medani	Ticks
	Bakan	Ticks
	Bauline	Ticks
	Yaquina Head	Ticks
	Great Island	Ticks
	(vi) Palyam subgroup	
	Palyam	Mosquitoes
	Vellore	Mosquitoes
	Kasba	Mosquitoes
	D'Aguilar	Mosquitoes

Table 1—Continued

Genus	Virus	Vector
Orbivirus (*Continued*)		
	(vii) Abadina subgroup	
	Abadina	?
	MP 359	Mosquitoes
	Ib H 11306	—
	Ib H 13019	—
	(viii) Lebombo	Mosquitoes
	(ix) Warrego (Ch 9935)	Culicoides
	Mitchell River (MRM 10434)	Culicoides
	Wallal (Ch 12048)	—
	(x) African horsesickness (9 serotypes)	—
	(xi) Simian virus SA-11	—
	(xii) Equine encephalosis	—
	(xiii) XBM/67 (from bovine serum)	—
	(xiv) Aus MK 6357	Mosquitoes
	(xv) USA T5-0616	—
	(xvi) USA 69V2161	—
	Probable members	
	Ibaraki virus	—
	Rabbit syncytium virus	—
	Equine viral arteritis	—
Cytoplasmic poly-hedrosis virus		
	Numerous serologically distinct viruses	—
Plant virus		
	(i) Wound tumor virus	Leafhoppers
	(ii) Rice dwarf virus	Leafhoppers
	(iii) Fiji disease virus	Leafhoppers
	(iv) Maize rough dwarf virus	Leafhoppers
	Rice black-streaked dwarf virus	Leafhoppers

The following recent reviews of reovirus and related viruses will be found invaluable in conjunction with this chapter: diplornaviruses (Verwoerd, 1970; Wood, 1973), reovirus (Rosen, 1968; Shatkin, 1968, 1969, 1972; Gauntt and Graham, 1969; Joklik, 1970, 1973*a,b*), blue-tongue virus (Howell and Verwoerd, 1971), cytoplasmic polyhedrosis virus (Aruga and Tanada, 1971), wound tumor virus (Black, 1965, 1972), and maize rough dwarf virus (Harpaz, 1972).

2. THE NATURE OF THE VIRION

2.1. Occurrence in Nature

2.1.1. Reovirus

Reoviruses have been recovered from man and lower animals in all parts of the world (Rosen, 1968). Human reoviruses, isolated both from individuals with mild febrile respiratory disease and diarrhea and from healthy individuals, were first classified with the echo (*enteric cytophathic human orphan*) viruses as type 10 because like them they could be isolated from stools, multiplied in monkey kidney cells, lacked pathogenicity for newborn mice, and agglutinated erythrocytes. However it was soon recognized that they differed from echo viruses in several important respects: they caused cytoplasmic inclusions not produced by other echo viruses, they agglutinated human type O erythrocytes, the cellular receptors for them could be inactivated with periodate, and they were larger than echo viruses. They were therefore reclassified as a new virus group and named reoviruses (*respiratory enteric orphan*) (Sabin, 1959). Shortly thereafter it was found that two viruses previously isolated from *Macaca* monkeys, SV12 and SV59, were identical with two human reovirus serotypes (types 1 and 2, respectively), and that a virus originally isolated from suckling mice and designated hepatoencephalomyelitis virus (Stanley *et al.*, 1953) was identical with human reovirus type 3 (Stanley, 1961). Reoviruses have also been isolated from a wide variety of other mammals, as well as birds and reptiles. All these viruses, no matter what their origin, with the exception of these isolated from chickens, can be classified by hemagglutination-inhibition and neutralization tests into three serotypes which share a common complement-fixing antigen (Sabin, 1959); the chicken reoviruses can be classified into a similar group of five serotypes which is not related to the other group (Kawamura and Tsubahara, 1966). Reoviruses have also been recovered from mosquitoes, but there is no evidence that they can multiply in these or any other insects (Simpson *et al.*, 1965).

Reoviruses do not cause overt disease in any adult animals. However, in newborn rodents type 1 and type 3 can cause a great variety of diseases (e.g., Walters *et al.*, 1963, 1965; Stanley and Walters, 1966).

2.1.2. Orbiviruses

Since very few orbiviruses have yet been characterized with respect to the structure of their RNA or the polypeptide constitution of their capsids, and since they are serologically very diverse (Borden *et al.*, 1971), the principal criterion for admission to this genus is morphology (Murphy *et al.*, 1971): orbiviruses are about the same size as reoviruses, but they possess very characteristic, large capsomers which have the appearance of rings (hence the name, *orbis*, ring) (Borden *et al.*, 1971).

Orbiviruses multiply in and are transmitted by insects (Foster *et al.*, 1963; Jochim and Jones, 1966). Many orbiviruses have only been isolated from culicoid flies, mosquitoes, phlebotomines, or ticks; for that reason they were long regarded as arboviruses. However, unlike all other arboviruses, orbiviruses contain no lipid and are therefore resistant to lipid solvents (Borden *et al.*, 1971).

Orbiviruses fall into some 16 serologically completely distinct groups on the basis of complement fixation (Table 1) (see also Borden *et al.*, 1971). Individual members of the group, such as BTV or African horsesickness virus (AHSV), themselves comprise numerous serotypes which share complement-fixing antigens; but BTV and AHSV are genetically related to the extent of no more than 1% as judged by ability of their nucleic acids to hybridize with each other (Verwoerd and Huismans, 1969). Orbiviruses do not hemagglutinate erythroctyes of most species (Borden *et al.*, 1971), but AHSV hemagglutinates horse erythrocytes (Pavri, 1961).

Although only few orbiviruses have been isolated from vertebrates, antibodies to them are widely distributed. None cause serious clinical disease in man, though several may cause mild fevers. Several orbiviruses however cause serious disease in other mammals; the most important of these is BTV [see Howell and Verwoerd (1971) for a description of its pathology in sheep].

2.1.3. Cytoplasmic Polyhedrosis Viruses (CPV)

Cytoplasmic polyhedrosis disease of insects is characterized by the development in the midgut cells of some 80 species of insects (Smith,

1963) of unique cytoplasmic structures, termed polydedral inclusion bodies, which vary in size and shape (hexagonal, pentagonal, tetragonal, or triangular). This disease is caused by viruses, the most intensively studied of which is the CPV of the silkworm *Bombyx mori* (Aruga and Tanada, 1971). In this insect both tetragonal and hexagonal polyhedra occur, both of which, when dissolved in carbonate buffer of *p*H 10.7, yield almost pure suspensions of what appears to be the same virus, CPV. However, since both types of polyhedra can be cloned, polyhedral shape is in all likelihood controlled by the viral genome, and several different strains of this CPV most probably exist (Hukuhara, 1971). CPV of other insects, for example, that of *Malacosoma disstria*, are serologically distinct from that of *Bombyx mori* (Krywienczyk *et al.*, 1969). The silkworm CPV agglutinates chicken, sheep, and mouse erythrocytes (Miyajima and Kawase, 1969).

2.1.4.   The Plant Virus Genus

2.1.4(a).   Wound Tumor Virus (WTV)

Wound tumor virus, the most intensively studied member of this genus, multiplies in some 43 species of plants, comprising 20 different families, and in several species of the juice-sucking leafhopper *Agallia* (Black, 1965). In plants such as sweet clover it causes tumors on roots and stems; infection is initiated either by accidental wounds on leaves and stems or by leafhoppers. The virus can also be transmitted by grafting tumors or tissues from infected plants, although cuttings from diseased plants can develop into healthy plants. Mechanical transmission, even with large amounts of virus, is highly inefficient. In leafhoppers the virus multiplies primarily in the cytoplasm of fat body, muscle, midgut, Malpighian tubule, tracheal, salivary gland, and epidermal cells (Shikata and Maramorosch, 1965, 1967a), but it is also found in ganglion and glial cells (Hirumi *et al.*, 1967) and hemocytes (Granados *et al.*, 1968). Once infected, insects remain so; the virus causes no overt disease in insects, although degeneration of ganglion, intestinal, and fat body cells has been observed (Maramorosch *et al.*, 1969). Systemically infected insects contain some 10^9 virus particles per milligram of body weight (Gamez and Black, 1967). Prolonged passage in plants leads to the stepwise emergence of virus strains unable to multiply in insects (Black *et al.*, 1958; Liu *et al.*, 1973).

2.1.4(b).   Rice Dwarf Virus (RDV)

Rice dwarf virus causes a natural infection in rice plants and other Gramineae which results in stunting (Fukushi and Kimura, 1959). It is transmitted by leafhoppers in which it is capable of multiplying and in which it is transmitted transovarially (Fukushi, 1933).

2.1.4(c).   Fiji Disease Virus (FDV)

Fiji disease virus causes a disease of sugar cane characterized by the development, along the vascular bundles on the lower surface of leaves, of galls which arise by the proliferation of young phloem cells (Teakle and Steindl, 1969). Like the other members of this group of viruses it can also multiply in an insect, the leafhopper *Perkinsiella saccharina* Kirk., which acts as its vector (Wood, 1973).

2.1.4(d).   Maize Rough Dwarf Virus (MRDV)

Maize rough dwarf virus multiplies in some 16 species of the Gramineae and causes a severe disease in maize which is characterized by the development of small galls on the veins on the undersurface of leaves, restriction of root development, and dwarfing (Lovisolo, 1971; Harpaz, 1972). It also multiplies in several species of plant hoppers which transmit the disease. It is serologically closely related to rice black-streaked dwarf virus (Luisoni *et al.*, 1973); the two viruses are therefore to be regarded as strains of the same virus (Wood, 1973).

Two further candidates for inclusion in this genus are pangola stunt virus (Schank and Edwardson, 1968; Kitajima and Costa, 1970) and oat sterile dwarf virus (Brcak and Kralik, 1969). Very little work has yet been carried out on either of these viruses.

2.2.   Measurement

2.2.1.   Reovirus

2.2.1(a).   Plaque Formation

Reoviruses replicate and produce cytopathic effects in human, monkey, hamster, and mouse cells, among others. For plaquing, monkey kidney cells (Rhim and Melnick, 1961) were used at first, but more recently mouse L fibroblasts are preferred. The plaque size is characteristic of both the virus and the cell strain (McClain *et al.*,

1967). Among the commonly used strains of reovirus strains, Dearing and Abney (both type 3) produce plaques which are about 3 mm across after 4–5 days of incubation at 37°C, while those produced by strain Carter (type 3), D5 Jones (type 2), and Lang (type 1) are about 1–2 mm in diameter after 5–10 days. Heating and cooling infectious culture fluids in $2 M$ Mg^{2+} causes an enhancement of the titer of reovirus (Wallis et al., 1964); the mechanism involved is not known. Nor is it understood why the addition of pancreatin to cell monolayers sometimes increases the size of plaques and therefore decreases the time before they can be counted (Wallis et al., 1966). On the one hand, the enzyme may act on the cells: mild proteolytic digestion of the plasma membrane may facilitate virus uptake, accelerate the replicative cycle, and facilitate virus release. On the other hand, it is known that reovirus has a strong tendency to remain cell-associated, and pancreatin might not only release progeny virus more efficiently from cells, thereby enabling it to start further infection cycles more rapidly, but it might also free it from combination with cellular constituents or inhibitors which might actually prevent it from reinitiating infection.

The titer of unpurified preparations of some strains of reovirus, for example strain Lang (type 1), is sometimes increased markedly (10–50-fold) by treatment with proteolytic enzymes such as chymotrypsin; the particles which become activated in this manner have been called "potentially infectious virus" (Spendlove et al., 1966). The diameter of the virus particles appears to decrease at the same time, but they retain their hemagglutinating activity (Spendlove et al., 1970); it is likely therefore that under certain conditions chymotryptic digestion of some strains of reovirus removes part of the outer capsid shell, thereby giving rise to particles with a specific infectivity higher than that of virions (see below for a discussion of the mode of action of chymotrypsin on reovirus). This enhancement of infectivity may be mistaken for virus multiplication; an interesting example of this type has been described by Whitcomb and Jensen (1968) who, in attempting to determine whether reovirus could multiply in leafhoppers, found that its titer increased following injection, but traced this effect to enhancement of infectivity by proteolytic enzymes present in insects, rather than to multiplication.

2.2.1(b). Hemagglutination

Virions of all three reovirus serotypes agglutinate human erythrocytes of all four ABO blood groups, the order of reactivity being

A > AB > O > B (Brubaker *et al.*, 1964). Agglutination proceeds at both low (4°C) and elevated (37°C) temperatures. Serotype 3 strains also agglutinate bovine erythrocytes, but only at low temperatures (Eggers *et al.*, 1962). Reovirus does not possess a neuraminidase; but virions of serotypes 1 and 3 do elute from group O erythrocytes on prolonged incubation, leaving the cell receptors intact (Lerner *et al.*, 1963). Treatment of virions with p-chlormercuribenzoate inhibits the ability of the virus to agglutinate erythrocytes; the inhibition is reversed by reduced glutathione, which suggests that the configuration that is essential for causing agglutination contains free −SH groups (Lerner *et al.*, 1963). Treatment with periodate (Tillotson and Lerner, 1966), β-glucosidase (Lerner *et al.*, 1966), and N-acetyl- D -glucosamine (Gelb and Lerner, 1965) prevents hemagglutination, and it has therefore been suggested that reovirions contain a glycoprotein; all attempts to label reovirions with glucosamine or fucose, however, have been unsuccessful (Hand and Tamm, 1971), and there is no evidence that any of the seven known reovirus capsid polypeptides are glycopolypeptides. As for the reovirus receptors on the surface of erythrocytes, those on human erythrocytes are resistant to neuraminidase (Stanley, 1961), while those on bovine erythrocytes are destroyed by it (Gomatos and Tamm, 1962). The effect of sodium borohydride and carbohydrases on the interaction of reovirus type 2 and cellular receptors has been studied by Lerner and Miranda (1968).

Hemagglutination can be used for the assay of reovirus: one bovine erythrocyte HA unit is equivalent to about 6×10^6 plaque-forming units (PFU) on L-cell monolayers (Gomatos and Tamm, 1962). This number is subject to great variation since it depends on the actual conditions under which both hemagglutination and plaquing are performed. The hemagglutination assay is much more rapid than the plaque assay, and is useful for the quantitation of new strains before a plaquing technique has been developed and for the quantitation of strains which form only very small plaques, and during the development of a purification procedure; however, wherever possible, the far more sensitive plaque assay is preferred.

2.2.1(c). Enumeration of Virus Particles

For chemical and biochemical studies it is more relevant to know the total number of virus particles than the number of virus particles capable of initiating productive infection. The total number of virus particles is best measured by particle counting with the electron microscope; however once this has been done, a relationship between the number of virus particles and optical density at 260 nm can be established, and from then on virus concentration is most conveniently measured spectrophotometrically. The relationship between the optical density of a suspension of reovirus particles at 260 nm, the number of particles, and viral protein mass is 1 $ODU_{260\ nm}$ = 2.1 × 10^{12} particles = 185 μg protein (Smith *et al.*, 1969).

Under optimal conditions of plaquing the ratio of reovirus type 1 particles: PFU has been reported to be as low as 2:1 (Wallis *et al.*, 1964), and the ratio of chymotrypsin-activated reovirus particles: infectious units as measured by fluorescent cell counts as low as 1:1 (Spendlove *et al.*, 1970). However these ratios are 25–100 times lower than those commonly observed in routine assays of purified virus stocks.

2.2.2. Orbiviruses

Most orbiviruses are first isolated in the brain of suckling mice and then passaged in the brains of 1 to 4-day-old mice or hamsters. After several serial passages, the mortality generally rises to 100%; this provides a convenient and sensitive assay (Borden *et al.*, 1971). Some orbiviruses, like BTV, can also be propagated in the yolk sac of fertile hens' eggs; in fact, BTV can only be adapted to growth in mouse brain after passage in eggs (Howell and Verwoerd, 1971).

Orbiviruses multiply in a variety of cultured mammalian cells, particularly BHK21 and KB cells and mouse L fibroblasts, with the production of cytopathic effects; they can therefore be assayed by the serial end-point-dilution method. Plaque assays on BHK 21 or L cells have been developed for BTV (Howell *et al.*, 1967) and African horsesickness virus (Oellermann, 1970). Colorado tick fever virus may be plaqued similarly on Vero cells.

Orbivirus antigens can be quantitated by measuring complement fixation (Casals, 1967), which also provides the most convenient and widely used test for serologic relatedness.

2.2.3. Other Reoviridae

There are three basic approaches to the detection and measurement of these viruses. First, infectivity may be measured by serial end-point-dilution methods in susceptible hosts. In the case of

CPV, this is the silkworm (Aruga and Tanada, 1971); in the case of the plant viruses the method involves injecting or feeding vectors with suspensions containing virus, allowing the virus to multiply in them, and then testing them for ability to infect and cause symptoms in susceptible plants (Toyoda *et al.,* 1964; Black, 1972; Milne *et al.,* 1973). These methods are both crude and time consuming. The second approach is similar; however, end points are not determined by the presence or absence of symptoms, but by the presence or absence, after a certain interval of time, of viral antigens which are detected by their ability to react with antiviral antiserum in precipitin, complement-fixation, or immunofluorescence reactions. This method is more rapid than the first and has permitted the accumulation of basic information concerning virus spread and multiplication (Reddy and Black, 1966). The third approach, so far available only for WTV, involves the enumeration of clones of infected cells, or foci, in monolayers of cultured vector cells (Chiu *et al.,* 1966; Kimura and Black, 1971). This technique, which provides the equivalent of a plaquing technique, has now replaced earlier techniques based on the enumeration of infected cells by immunofluorescence (Chiu and Black, 1969) and by direct particle counting (Gamez and Black, 1968). The ratio of WTV particles: cell infecting units has been reported as being below 5:1 (Kimura and Black, 1972*a*; Hsu and Black, 1973; Reddy and Black, 1973*a*).

Kimura and Black (personal communication) have established the following relationship between the optical density at 260 nm of RNA extracted from WTV and the number of virus particles: $1 \text{ ODU}_{260 \text{ nm}} = 0.96 \times 10^{12}$ virus particles. Measurement of viral RNA provides a rapid and convenient estimate of virus concentration.

2.3. Morphology

Reoviridae resemble each other in morphology: there is a unique and distinctive structure, some 70 nm in diameter, quasispherical, with clearly discernible capsomers, which is usually referred to as "reovirus-like." On closer examination however, it becomes apparent that there are really at least four clearly distinguishable structural patterns within this family. Some of the basic properties of the virions of reoviridae are listed in Table 2.

2.3.1. Reovirus

The first pattern is that of reovirions (Fig. 1). They possess two capsid shells, each composed exclusively of protein arranged in discrete

TABLE 2

Properties of the Virions of Members of the Family Reoviridae

Virus	Diameter, nm	Sedimentation coefficient, S	Density in CsCl, g/ml	RNA, %	RNA, dalton $\times 10^6$	Protein dalton $\times 10^4$
Reovirus	76[a]	630[b]	1.36[c]	14.6[b]	15[d]	88
Core	52[a]	470[c]	1.43[c]	33[c]	15[d]	31
BTV (L particle)	69[e]	550[e]	1.36–1.38[e]	20[f]	12[e]	48
(D particle)	~60[e]	470[e]	1.38–1.42[e]	30[e]	12[e]	28
CPV	65[g]	440[h]	1.43[g]	23[l]	14.6[i]	49
WTV	66[j,g]	514[h]	1.41[l]	23[h]	15[m]	50
RDV	~70[n]	512[o]		12[o]	15[i]	110
FDV	~70[p]					
MRDV	65–70[q]					

[a] Luftig et al. (1972).
[b] Gomatos and Tamm (1963a).
[c] Zweerink (personal communication).
[d] Shatkin et al. (1968); Joklik (1970).
[e] Martin and Zweerink (1972); Verwoerd et al. (1972).
[f] Verwoerd (1969).
[g] Lewandowski and Traynor (1972).
[h] Kalmakoff et al. (1969).
[i] Fujii-Kawata et al. (1970).
[j] Streissle and Granados (1968).
[l] Gomatos and Tamm (1963b).
[m] Reddy and Black (1973b).
[n] Fukushi and Shikita (1963a).
[o] Suzuki and Kimura (1969).
[p] Teakle and Steindl (1969); Francki and Grivell (1972).
[q] Leseman (1972), Milne et al. (1973).

morphological subunits or capsomers (Gomatos et al., 1962; Jordon and Mayor, 1962; Loh et al., 1965). The outside diameters of the outer and inner shells are about 76 nm and 52 nm, respectively; the diameter of the central cavity is about 38 nm (Luftig et al., 1972). The particle which lacks the outer shell is known as the core; it comprises some 30–35% of the virion's volume and protein complement. The outer shell is stable at high and physiological salt concentrations, but its capsomers tend to be lost on storage at low ionic strength (Amano et al., 1971); under certain conditions it is also disrupted by heating (Mayor and Jordon, 1968). It is completely digestible by chymotrypsin, to which the core is resistant (Shatkin and Sipe, 1968a; Smith et al., 1969). Virions and cores are readily separated by density gradient centrifugation: their sedimentation coefficients are about 630 and 470 S,

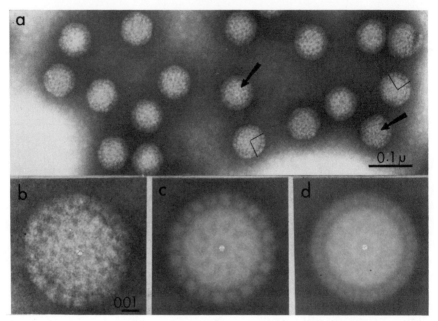

Fig. 1.   (a) Reovirus, stained with 4% PTA ($\times$98,000). (b), (c), and (d) represent
n = 0-, 10-, and 12-fold rotations, respectively, of a selected particle ($\times$327,000). From
Luftig *et al.* (1972).

and their buoyant densities in CsCl are 1.36 and 1.43 g/ml, respectively (Smith *et al.,* 1969). Virions contain 14–15% RNA (Gomatos
and Tamm, 1963*a*).

Although the capsomers on both the outer as well as on the inner
capsid shell are easily discernible, it has so far not been possible to determine their spatial interrelationships with certainty. The original interpretation was that the outer shell consists of 80 hexagonal and 12
pentagonal hollow columnar capsomers arranged according to 5:3:2
icosahedral symmetry (T = 9, 4 capsomers along each edge) (Vasquez
and Tournier, 1962). A later interpretation (Vasquez and Tournier,
1964) favored the view that there are 92 holes on the virion surface, 12
of them surrounded by five structural subunits and the rest by 6, which
are shared in such a manner that the total is 180. Studies on virions
stored in distilled water provide support for the latter view since this
treatment causes loosening and disruption of the outer capsid shell with
the generation of structures which on 6-fold rotation clearly reveal six
subunits arranged hexagonally in the form of rosettes (Amano *et al.,*
1971). Recently, however, evidence has been obtained which is difficult

to reconcile with this model (Luftig *et al.*, 1972): this is that the outer shell appears to possess 20 peripheral capsomers, and not 18, as demanded by either of the two interpretations described above. If there are 20 peripheral capsomers, then there must be a total of $400/\pi$, or 127, capsomers if they are all aligned exactly on a meridian, or slightly fewer if, as is likely, this is not the case. As for their shape, the capsomers appear to be either cylinders or truncated pyramids, 9 nm in length, and separated by about 1 nm from their neighbors (Luftig *et al.*, 1972). It is not clear how they relate to the hexagonal rosettes observed by Amano *et al.*, (1971), which are 18–20 nm in diameter and have a hole 4–6 nm in diameter.

In contrast to the rather labile outer shell, the core shell is an extremely stable structure which cannot be disrupted except by high concentrations of urea, guanidine, dimethyl formamide, dimethyl sulfoxide, sodium dodecyl sulfate, and the like. Its most obvious morphological feature is its 12 projections or spikes which are located as if on the 12 fivefold vertices of an icosahedron (Luftig *et al.*, 1972) (Fig. 2). They are about 10 nm in diameter, possess central channels about 5 nm wide, and project about 5.5 nm beyond the core surface, that is, about half the way through the outer capsid shell. Cores also exhibit capsomers which are smaller than those of the outer shell (4 nm in diameter). Their spatial arrangement cannot be discerned directly; but they can also be visualized clearly at the periphery, and again there are 20 peripheral capsomers rather than 12 or 18 (Luftig *et al.*, 1972).

Thus, both the outer and inner shells of reovirions are composed of capsomers which appear to be arranged according to similar if not identical symmetry principles. The icosahedral distribution of the core spikes indicates that they are arranged according to icosahedral symmetry principles, but it is not yet clear which symmetry system is actually involved. The two pieces of evidence which must be accounted for in assigning a symmetry system are the fact that there are 20 and not 18 peripheral capsomers, and that disruption of the outer capsid shell yields rosettes made up of six identical subunits located around a central hole. At the moment, these two facts are incompatible since the capsomers seen at the periphery are clearly distinct entities while capsomers composed of hexagonal and pentagonal rosettes require extensive sharing of subunits. The former structure is compatible with a total of 122 morphological units arranged as on an icosahedral deltahedron for which $P = 3$ and $T = 12$; the latter, with 92 morphological units arranged as on an icosahedral deltahedron for which $P = 1$, $T = 9$. The former arrangement belongs to the same symmetry class to

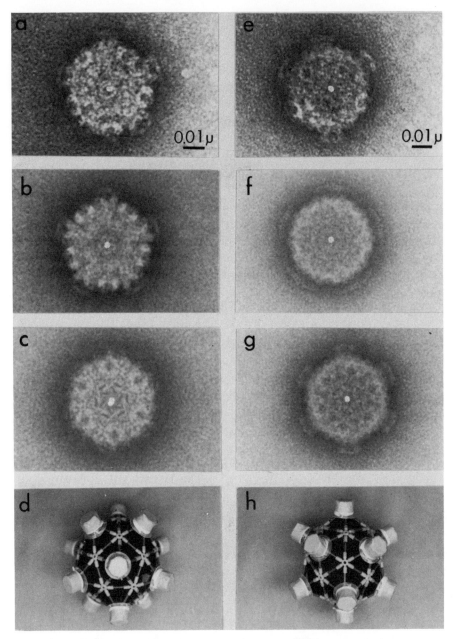

Fig. 2.   Two reovirus core particles whose central axis is either on a presumptive 5-fold (a) or 3-fold vertex (e). Enhancement of the five peripheral spikes of (a) is achieved with a $n = 5$ (b), but not with a $n = 6$ rotation (c). Enhancement of the six peripheral spikes of (e) is exhibited with a $n = 6$ (g), but not with a $n = 5$ rotation (f). A model depicting the appropriate aspect of each particle is shown in (d) and (h) ($\times 487,000$). From Luftig *et al.* (1972).

which the orbiviruses also belong (P = 3, T = 3, 32 morphological units); the latter is part of a series to which the herpesviruses (P = 1, T = 16, 162 morphological units) and the adenoviruses (P = 1, T = 25, 252 morphological units) belong.

Reovirus yields usually contain a small proportion of empty capsids, generally termed top component (Smith *et al.*, 1969). The structure of these particles, which lack all RNA, appears to be identical to that of virions.

2.3.2. Orbiviruses

The particles generally regarded as characteristic of orbiviruses clearly display 32 large ring-shaped capsomers which appear to consist of cylinders about 8 nm long, 10–12 nm wide, with a central cavity or hole about 4 nm in diameter, and which are arranged with icosahedral symmetry (P = 3 and T = 3) (Fig. 3) (Murphy *et al.*, 1968, 1971; Els and Verwoerd, 1969; Bowne and Ritchie, 1970; Oellermann *et al.*, 1970; Martin and Zweerink, 1972; Verwoerd *et al.*, 1972). The size of this type of orbivirus particle has been reported as to be in the range of 54–80 nm. Although sometimes lack of precise calibration and varia- tion in what is taken to represent the outer particle surface may have contributed to this surprisingly large spread, one careful comparative study of some 10 orbiviruses has confirmed that their diameters range from 65 to 80 nm (Murphy *et al.*, 1971). The particles have a central cavity some 35–40 nm in diameter, which is the same as that in reo- virions; this is in agreement with the fact that the reovirus and or- bivirus genomes are similar in size (see below). Lecatsas and Erasmus (1973) have reported that in the case of XBM/67 virus this cavity possesses a substructure, and they have proposed that its "icosahedral core" consists of twelve spherical subunits.

It is now clear that, at least as far as BTV is concerned, this type of particle (diameter about 60 nm) is far less infectious than another, the diameter of which is 6–10 nm larger and in which the ring-shaped capsomers, although still discernible, are much less prominent (Bowne and Ritchie, 1970; Martin and Zweerink, 1972; Verwoerd *et al.*, 1972) (Fig. 3). These larger particles contain two additional polypeptides which are located at their surface, seemingly in the form of a fea- tureless layer which is formally analogous to the outer capsid shell of reovirions. Since they contain more protein (about 43% more, Ver- woerd *et al.*, 1972), these particles are less dense than those described above; they have therefore been designated as L and D particles,

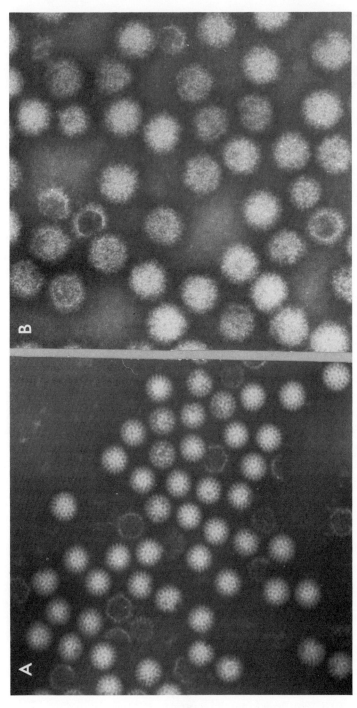

Fig. 3. Bluetongue virus, negatively stained. (A) D particles lacking the outer capsid layer; (B) L particles possessing the outer capsid layer (×14,000). Courtesy of Drs. D. W. Verwoerd and H. J. Els.

respectively (Martin and Zweerink, 1972). BTV L particles are not converted to D particles either by heat or by chymotrypsin, both of which damage or destroy the outer shell of reovirus; but they are converted to D particles by exposure to CsCl at pH values below 8 (Verwoerd *et al.*, 1972), to which reovirions are perfectly stable. The polypeptides removed from L particles by CsCl can apparently reassociate with D particles *in vitro* since on mixing the infectivity increases greatly (Verwoerd *et al.*, 1972).

The fact that L particles are far more infectious than D particles suggests that they represent the virion form of BTV. Similar particles have so far been described for SA 11 (Els and Lecatsas, 1972), Corriparta, Eubenangee, D'Aguilar, Warrego, Mitchell R, Wallal and M9/71, viruses (Lecatsas and Gorman, 1972). Presumably similar particles will be found for other orbiviruses as well; the reason why they have been overlooked so far may be that their appearance is much less striking than that of the D-type particles, or that D particles are generally produced in excess.

Several orbivirions occur not only in the two "naked" forms just described, but also surrounded by membranes (Murphy *et al.*, 1968; Schangl *et al.*, 1969; Bowne and Ritchie, 1970), which are acquired as they are liberated from cells by a process formally analogous to budding; sometimes several virus particles are found within a single membranous sac. However, such enveloped particles are generally in the minority since orbiviruses are usually liberated by lysis (Murphy *et al.*, 1971). The pseudoenvelopes can be removed by nonionic detergents or lipid solvents without diminishing infectivity and are, therefore, not regarded as essential components of orbivirions.

2.3.3. CPV

CPV particles have a diameter of 60–65 nm (Hosaka and Aizawa, 1964; Miura *et al.*, 1969; Asai *et al.*, 1972; Lewandowski and Traynor, 1972). Their most prominent morphologic feature (Fig. 4) is 12 large pyramidal projections or spikes which, as in the case of the reovirus core projections, are located as if on the 12 fivefold vertices of an icosahedron and which are flanked at their base by rings which are denser than the remainder of the capsid. The CPV spikes are larger than those of reovirus cores; they project about 20 nm, whereas the reovirus core spikes only project 5–6 nm. Like the latter, they appear to have central channels (about 10 nm in diameter).

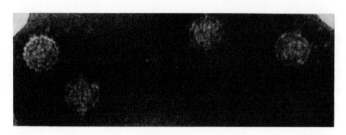

Fig. 4. CPV particles, negatively stained. Note pyramidal projections (×215,000). Courtesy of Drs. L. J. Lewandowski and B. L. Traynor.

It has so far been impossible to discern capsomers on the surface of CPV particles; as in the case of reovirus, 20 capsomers are often visible along the circumference (Lewandowski and Traynor, 1972). The existence of an inner shell has been postulated (Hosaka and Aizawa, 1964) but not convincingly demonstrated. In fact, CP virions exhibit properties characteristic of reovirus cores: the possession of the icosahedrally situated spikes, a rather simple polypeptide constitution (see below), resistance to chymotrypsin, and transcriptase activity.

2.3.4. The Plant Virus Genus

2.3.4(a). WTV

WTV particles are slightly smaller than reovirions (65–70 nm in diameter) and possess slightly smaller capsomers (7.5 nm in diameter), but like them they possess a central cavity 35–40 nm in diameter which accommodates a genome of about the same size (Fig. 5) (Bils and Hall, 1962; Streissle and Granados, 1968; Lewandowski and Traynor, 1972). WT virions sometimes appear distinctly hexagonal.

Just as the number of reovirus capsomers is a matter of some uncertainty, so is the number of capsomers on WT virions: the commonly accepted number is 92 (Bils and Hall, 1962), but recently Kimura (personal communication) has proposed a model based on 32 capsomers, each 18 nm in diameter and composed of 5 or 6 structural units about 7.5 nm in diameter.

In spite of this uncertainty, it seems that the structure of WTV is more similar to that of reovirus than that of any other member of the

Reoviridae family (Wood, 1973). There are however several significant differences. First, although WTV seems to possess two shells (Streissle and Granados, 1968), its polypeptide constitution is simple enough to be compatible with only one (see below); further, the density of WTV is 1.41 g/ml, 0.05 g/ml higher than that of reovirus. Second, whereas reovirions are quite stable in high concentrations of CsCl, WT virions are markedly unstable, being converted to "cores" with a density of about 1.44 g/ml (Lewandowski and Traynor, 1972). However, these "cores" bear no resemblance to reovirus cores (or to the D particles of BTV); they differ from WT virions primarily in being more permeable to phosphotungstate, not in polypeptide constitution. Third, WT virions are not noticeably affected by chymotrypsin (Lewandowski and Traynor, 1972), although treatment with trypsin, sodium pyrophosphate, and urea has been reported to remove the outer capsid shell, leaving an inner shell about 44 nm in diameter (Streissle and Granados, 1968). Finally, whereas reovirus particles only display transcriptase activity after modification of the outer capsid shell, WT virions themselves exhibit this enzymic activity (see below).

2.3.4(b).   RDV and FDV

Little fine-structure work on these two viruses has been published. Their morphology appears to be similar to that of WTV (Fukushi and Shikata, 1963a; Teakle and Steindl, 1969, Francki and Grivell, 1972). Kimura and Shikata (1968) have proposed a model for RDV based on 32 capsomers.

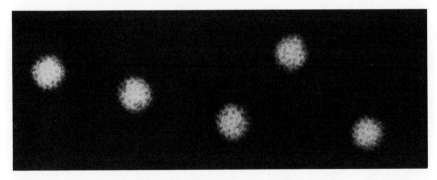

Fig. 5.   WTV particles, negatively stained (×135,000). Courtesy of Drs. L. J. Lewandowski and B. L. Traynor.

2.3.4(c). MRDV

This virus provides yet another variation on the "reovirus-like" morphological pattern (Leseman, 1972; Milne *et al.,* 1973). The particles are about 66 nm in diameter and possess a double capsid shell, the outer shell displaying "probably 92" morphological units (Fig. 6). In addition, each particle possesses 12 projections or spikes (A spikes) about 11 nm in length, one at each fivefold-symmetry axis. Storage at 4°C, heating at 50°C for 10 minutes, freeze-thawing, or shaking with chloroform (Wetter *et al.,* 1969) strips off the outer capsid shell to yield subviral particles some 53 nm in diameter which possess 12 B spikes which are coaxial with the A spikes. These B spikes are about 6 nm long and therefore penetrate through the outer capsid shell into the A spikes. Each B spike is implanted on a differentiated part of the inner capsid shell (the baseplate) which resembles the corresponding portion of the CP virion. Treatment with 1-percent neutral potassium phosphotungstate strips the B spikes from the subviral particles; on prolonged treatment, empty ghosts are produced. Detached B spikes are composed of five morphological subunits which surround a central hole (Milne *et al.,* 1973).

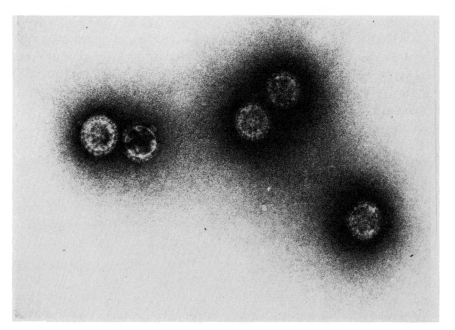

Fig. 6.   MRDV particles, negatively stained. The spikes are clearly visible on the particle with the partially degraded outer shell (×161,000). Courtesy of Dr. R. G. Milne.

2.4. Purification

2.4.1. Reovirus

Reoviruses grow well in many types of cultured cells; those most commonly used for the preparation of large amounts of virus are mouse L fibroblasts growing in suspension culture. Since infection at 37°C results in extensive cytopathic damage, infected cells are usually incubated at 33°C, where cytopathic effects are much less marked and virus yields are therefore 3- to 5-fold larger (Smith *et al.*, 1969). Reovirus is not liberated readily from cells but remains cell associated until well after the virus has ceased to multiply; early purification procedures therefore employed chymotryptic digestion in order to dissociate virus from cellular components (Gomatos and Tamm, 1963*a*). However, since it was subsequently found that the outer shell of reovirions is sensitive to chymotrypsin (Shatkin and Sipe, 1968*a*), this practice has been replaced by homogenization with Freon 113 (Shatkin, 1965*a*; Bellamy *et al.*, 1967; Smith *et al.*, 1969). Final purification is achieved by zone sedimentation in 20–40% sucrose density gradients, followed by equilibrium centrifugation in CsCl density gradients. As a rule, two bands are obtained: a major band with a buoyant density of 1.36 g/ml which contains virions, and a minor band with a buoyant density of 1.30 g/ml which contains empty virus particles (top component). Yields of purified virus as high as 30 mg/10^9 cells (300,000 virus particles/cell) can readily be obtained.

2.4.2. Orbiviruses

The most intensively studied orbivirus, BTV, is generally grown either in BHK 21 cells or in mouse L fibroblasts (Verwoerd, 1969; Verwoerd *et al.*, 1972; Martin and Zweerink, 1972). Like reovirus, it is purified by homogenizing infected cells with Freon, followed by zone sedimentation in sucrose density gradients. When it is then subjected to equilibrium centrifugation in CsCl density gradients, care must be taken to adjust the *p*H to values around 8 since otherwise not one but two bands result; unlike reovirus, BTV is unstable in neutral or slightly acid CsCl, readily losing its outer capsid shell. The particles in the denser band [variously reported at 1.38 g/ml (Martin and Zweerink, 1972) or at 1.42 g/ml (Verwoerd *et al.*, 1972)] are referred to as BTV D, those in the less dense [at 1.36 g/ml (Martin and Zweerink, 1972) or at 1.38 g/ml (Verwoerd *et al.*, 1972)] as BTV L. The L particles possess two capsid shells, the D particles only one (see above); L particles contain two more polypeptides than D particles (see below). Their sedimentation coefficients are 550 S and 470 S, respectively (Martin and Zweerink, 1972). Since the specific infectivity of L particles is some 100 to 10,000 times greater than that of D particles, L particles probably correspond to BT virions.

The yield of BTV is only about $0.1 \text{ mg}/10^9$ cells; it is not increased by maintaining cells in monolayer rather than in suspension culture, lowering the temperature, or omitting or inactivating serum (Martin and Zweerink, 1972). Increasing the multiplicity above 1 reduces the yield still further, possibly because BTV severely inhibits host cell protein synthesis (Huismans, 1971).

2.4.3. CPV

CPV is generally grown in silkworms (Miura *et al.*, 1968). Polyhedral bodies can be isolated in very large amounts from the midgut of infected insects; after repeated washing with distilled water, they are suspended in carbonate buffer pH 10.8 which dissolves the polyhedral matrix without destroying the infectivity of the released virions. On equilibrium density gradient centrifugation in CsCl, two bands are obtained: a major band at 1.435 g/ml which contains virions, and a minor band at 1.30 g/ml which contains empty virus particles (top component) (Lewandowski and Traynor, 1972). A further minor band at about 1.42 g/ml which contains particles that lack some of the smaller genome RNA segments is also sometimes obtained. CP virions sediment with 415–440 S.

2.4.4. The Plant Virus Genus

2.4.4(a). WTV

WTV is usually prepared from fresh root tumors produced in sweet clover plants (*Melilotus officinalis*), which are its richest source; but it may also be purified from viruliferous leafhoppers (Black, 1965). Extracts of triturated tumor or insect tissue are clarified by several cycles of low-speed centrifugation and then precipitated with polyethylene glycol (Reddy and Black, 1973*a*); exposure to halogenated hydrocarbons, such as Freon 113 and carbon tetrachloride, is avoided because they tend to convert virions to empty capsids (Black and Knight, 1970). The virus is then purified by zone centrifugation in sucrose density gradients. It is interesting to recall in this connection that zone sedimentation, now a widely used technique in every field of experimental biology, was pioneered by Brakke in the early 1950s with the object of purifying WTV [although potato yellow-dwarf virus was actually used as the model virus in developing the technique (Brakke, 1951, 1953, 1955)]. Like BTV, WTV is unstable in high concentrations of CsCl, and when centrifuged to equilibrium in CsCl density gradients gives rise to several bands which contain particles that differ slightly in structure and polypeptide constitution (Lewandowski and Traynor, 1972). Structures resembling empty virus particles (top component) are also formed, apparently as the result of the partial breakdown of virus particles; this is in contrast to the top-component particles of reovirus and CPV, which are not derived from virions.

WTV also multiplies in cultured insect vector cells (see above); no doubt such cells will prove useful for the preparation of radioactively labeled virus.

2.4.4(b). RDV and FDV

RDV is purified by chromatographing the sap of leaves and leaf sheaths of symptomatic plants on DEAE-cellulose columns, followed by zone sedimentation in sucrose density gradients (Toyoda *et al.,* 1965; Miura *et al.,* 1966). No information concerning the behavior of RDV in CsCl density gradients is available.

No detailed method for purifying FDV has been published.

2.4.4(c). MRDV

This virus is rather unstable and all operations involved in its purification are generally carried out as rapidly as possible in the cold. The optimal source of the virus consists of the roots or leaf enations of maize plants. The infected tissue is triturated and shaken with Freon 113; the use of carbon tetrachloride is avoided since it yields noninfectious virus. The virus in the aqueous phase is then isolated by repeated zone centrifugation in sucrose density gradients (Milne *et al.,* 1973).

TABLE 3

Stability of Members of the Family Reoviridae to Physical and Chemical Agents

Virus	Reagent	Stability	Reference
Reovirus	Heat	Stable; stabilized by Mg^{2+}	Wallis *et al.* (1964)
Orbivirus (BTV)		Labile; not stabilized by Mg^{2+}	Svehag (1963)
CPV		—	—
WTV		—	—
Reovirus	pH	Stable from pH 3–10	Stanley *et al.* (1953)
Orbivirus (BTV)		Very unstable; inactivated below pH 6.3	Owen (1964)
CPV		—	
WTV		Labile	Kimura and Black personal communication
Reovirus	High salt concentrations, particularly CsCl	Stable	—
Orbivirus (BTV)		Labile; outer capsid shell removed, infectivity decreased	Verwoerd *et al.* (1972); Martin and Zweerink (1972)
CPV		Stable	—
WTV		Labile	Lewandowski and Traynor (1972)
Reovirus	Chymotrypsin	Outer capsid shell removed	Shatkin and Sipe (1968*a*); Joklik (1972)
Orbivirus (BTV)		Stable	—
CPV		Stable	—
WTV		Stable	—
Reovirus	Centrifugal force, pelletting	Stable	—
Orbivirus (BTV)		Labile	Verwoerd (1970)
CPV		Stable	—
WTV		Labile	Black *et al.* (1967)
Reovirus	Halogenated hydrocarbons (Freon, carbon tetrachloride)	Stable	—
Orbivirus (BTV)		Stable	—
CPV		—	—
WTV		Converted to empty capsids	Black and Knight (1970)
MRDV		Inactivated; converted to cores by carbon tetrachloride	Milne *et al.* (1973)

2.5. Stability

The members of the four genera differ markedly in their stability to various physical and chemical reagents. The relevant data are summarized in Table 3. All reoviridae are stable toward lipid solvents and nonionic detergents.

3. THE NATURE OF THE RNA

All reoviridae contain double-stranded RNA. The amount of RNA per virion, $12-15 \times 10^6$ daltons, is roughly the same for all members of the family; this RNA is present not in the form of one double-stranded molecule, but in the form of 10 or 12 segments which range in molecular weight from 0.3 to 2.7×10^6. Details concerning the nature and the sizes of these segments are summarized in Table 4 and Fig. 7. In addition, reovirions contain a large number of single-stranded oligoribonucleotides which collectively amount to $4-5 \times 10^6$ daltons.

3.1. Reovirus

3.1.1. Double-Stranded RNA

The fact that reovirus contains double-stranded RNA was discovered by Gomatos and collaborators who observed that cytoplasmic inclusions in L cells infected with reovirus fluoresced pale green when

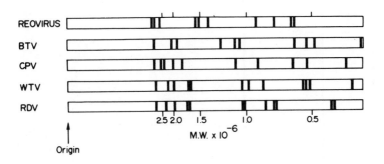

Fig. 7. Chart depicting the relative sizes of the individual segments of the genome RNAs of various members of the family Reoviridae.

TABLE 4

Properties of the Double-Stranded RNA of Members of the Family Reoviridae

Virus	Percent in virion	Number of segments	Total mol. wt., daltons $\times 10^6$	Size range, daltons $\times 10^6$	GC, %	5' terminus	3' terminus
Reovirus	14.6[a]	10[b]	15.0[b,c]	2.8–0.6[b,c]	43.8[a]	(p)ppG[d]	C_{OH}[e]
Orbivirus (BTV)	20[f]	10[g]	12.1[h]	2.7–0.3[h,i]	42.4[f]		
CPV	23[m]	10[k]	14.6[k]	2.8–0.35[k]	43.0[i]		C_{OH} and U_{OH}[l]
WTV	23[m]	12[m,n]	15.1[n,o]	2.8–0.3[n,o]	38[p]		C_{OH} and U_{OH}[q]
RDV	12[r]	12[k]	15.3[k]	2.8–0.4[k]	44[s]		

[a] Gomatos and Tamm (1963a).
[b] Shatkin et al. (1968).
[c] Bellamy et al. (1967).
[d] Banerjee and Shatkin (1971).
[e] Banerjee and Grece (1971).
[f] Verwoerd (1969).
[g] Verwoerd et al. (1970).
[h] Martin and Zweerink (1972).
[i] Verwoerd et al. (1972).
[j] Miura et al. (1968).
[k] Fujii-Kawata et al. (1970).
[l] Furiuchi and Miura (1973). Each segment contains one strand terminating in C_{OH} and another terminating in U_{OH}.
[m] Kalmakoff et al. (1969).
[n] Reddy and Black (1973b).
[o] Lewandowski and Traynor (1972).
[p] Black and Markham (1963).
[q] Lewandowski and Leppla (1972). The distribution of the C_{OH} and U_{OH} termini on the individual segments has not yet been determined.
[r] Suzuki and Kimura (1969).
[s] Miura et al. (1966).

treated with acridine orange (Gomatos *et al.*, 1962). This is indicative of double-stranded nucleic acids which bind only a small amount of the dye and therefore stain orthochromatically; single-stranded nucleic acids, which bind more dye, stain metachromatically and fluoresce bright red. The inclusions proved to be resistant to deoxyribonuclease but susceptible to ribonuclease at low salt concentrations; and it was soon shown that the nucleic acid isolated from purified virions was indeed double-stranded RNA (Gomatos and Tamm, 1963*a*). The evidence rests on the following facts among others: (1) The RNA exhibits very sharp melting profiles, with the T_m depending on the ionic strength (Shatkin, 1965*a*; Bellamy *et al.*, 1967). (2) It is resistant to ribonuclease, the resistance depending on the concentration of both monovalent and divalent cations as well as on the concentration of ribonuclease (Shatkin, 1965*a*; Bellamy *et al.*, 1967). (3) It is susceptible to ribonuclease III which is specific for double-stranded RNA. (4) Formaldehyde fails to induce hyperchromicity (Gomatos and Tamm, 1963*a*). (5) Its density in Cs_2SO_4 is 1.61 g/ml rather than 1.65 g/ml which is characteristic of single-stranded RNA (Shatkin, 1965*a*; Iglewski and Franklin, 1967). (6) Its base compositon indicates equality of A and U, as well as of G and C (Gomatos and Tamm, 1963*a*; Bellamy *et al.*, 1967). (7) X-ray diffraction patterns are consistent with double-strandedness (Langridge and Gomatos, 1963; Arnott *et al.*, 1966).

A unique feature of the double-stranded RNA in reovirions is that it exists not in the form of a single molecule, but as a collection of discrete and unique segments. The first indication of this was the demonstration that reovirus RNA consists of a heterogeneous population of molecules which exhibit a trimodal length distribution with maxima at 1.1, 0.6, and 0.35 μm, corresponding to about 2.5, 1.4, and 0.8 $\times$ 10^6 daltons (Dunnebacke and Kleinschmidt, 1967; Vasquez and Kleinschmidt, 1968). Even the largest of these clearly corresponded to only a portion of the genome, since reovirions had already been shown to contain about 14.6% RNA, corresponding to a molecular weight of at least 10 $\times$ 10^6 daltons (Gomatos and Tamm, 1963*a*). It was then shown that regardless of the means used to liberate it, reovirus RNA displays three size classes of molecules when analyzed in sucrose density gradients: these are the *L, M,* and *S* species of molecules which sediment with 14, 12, and 10.5 S, corresponding to molecular weights of about 2.7, 1.4, and 0.7 $\times$ 10^6 daltons, or about 4500, 2300, and 1200 nucleotide base pairs (Shatkin, 1965*a*; Bellamy *et al.*, 1967; Watanabe and Graham, 1967). The molecules in these three size classes were shown to be discrete segments rather than random fragments of larger molecules by the fact that they did not hybridize with each other and that they were transcribed into specific species of mRNA molecules within infected cells (Bellamy and Joklik, 1967a; Watanabe *et al.*, 1967b). These three size classes were then further separated by polyacrylamide gel electrophoresis into 10 discrete and unique molecular species (Fig. 8) which are present in equimolar amounts and possess an aggregate molecular weight of about 15×10^6 daltons (Shatkin *et al.*, 1968) (Table 4). The 5′ and 3′ termini of all these segments are (p)ppGpPyp- and -pPypApApC$_{OH}$, respectively (Banerjee and Shatkin, 1971; Banerjee *et al.*, 1971b; Banerjee and Grece, 1971), which again provides strong evidence that they are completely double-stranded molecules which arise as the result of independent synthetic events. Final proof of the segmented nature of the reovirus genome came with the demonstration that even prior to extraction there are approximately as many 3′ termini in the RNA within each reovirion as in the RNA released from it (Millward and Graham, 1970).

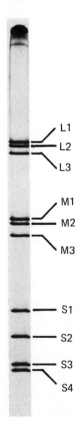

Fig. 8. Reovirus genome RNA electrophoresed in a polyacrylamide gel. Direction of electrophoresis is from top to bottom. Autoradiogram of RNA labeled with ^{14}C-uridine. Courtesy of Dr. A. R. Schuerch.

The nature of the arrangement of the RNA segments within reovirions is not known. Originally it was conjectured that they might be linked by weak noncovalent bonds, since when virions are disrupted very gently, strands that could conceivably correspond to the entire reovirus genome have occasionally been seen (Dunnebacke and Kleinschmidt, 1967; Granboulan and Niveleau, 1967); however it is now known that all ten segments can be transcribed into single-stranded RNA at the same time (see below), and this is difficult to envision if they are linked. It was also thought that linkage might provide a mechanism for ensuring that each progeny virion received a unique and complete set of all ten segments; but it is now know that such assortment proceeds at the level of single-stranded, not double-stranded, RNA molecules (see below), so that the *raison d'être* for linkage of double-stranded segments has disappeared.

3.1.2. Reovirus Oligonucleotides

In addition to double-stranded RNA, reovirions also contain single-stranded RNA of low molecular weight; up to 20–25% of the total amount of RNA in reovirions may be of this type (Bellamy and Joklik, 1967b; Shatkin and Sipe, 1968b; Koide et al., 1968). It comprises a mixture of oligoribonucleotides from 2 to about 20 nucleotides long (Bellamy and Hole, 1970; Bellamy et al., 1970) which are present within the central virion cavity, but rapidly leak out once the outer capsid shell begins to be degraded (Joklik, 1972). When fractionated first on DEAE-Sephadex and then by two-dimensional electrophoresis-homochromatography this mixture is resolved into its components, most of which have been sequenced (Bellamy et al., 1972; Nichols et al., 1972a; Stoltzfus and Banerjee, 1972). This work has shown that reovirus single-stranded RNA comprises two classes of molecules. First, there is a series of molecules in which the only nucleic acid base is adenine; they range in length from 2 to about 20 nucleotides, and have either ppp, pp, or p (in decreasing order) at their 5′ termini.* Their

---

* Stoltzfus and Banerjee (1972) found only 5′-p at the ends of oligoadenylates. It is conceivable that the cause of the discrepancy betweeen their results and those of the other group lies in the relative nucleoside triphosphate phosphohydrolase activities of the virus strains used by the two groups (see below). It is noteworthy in this respect that whereas Banerjee et al. (1971a) found predominantly 5′-pp at the ends of reovirus transcripts synthesized by cores in vitro, Nichols et al. (1972b) found predominantly 5′-ppp (see following text).

formula can thus be represented by $(p)(p) p(A)_{1-19}A_{OH}$. There are about 850 such molecules present in each virion and they account for some 55% of the total oligonucleotides; they are now known as the reovirus *oligoadenylates*. Second, there is a series of oligonucleotides $(p)ppGC_{OH}$, $(p)ppGCU_{OH}$, $(p)ppGCUA_{OH}$, $(p)ppGCUA(A)_{1-3}A_{OH}$, and $(p)ppGCUA(U)_{1-4}U_{OH}$, which are now known as the reovirus 5′-G-terminated oligonucleotides. There are about 2000 of these molecules in each reovirion. In addition, there are some 350 other molecules from 2–8 nucleotides long (about 10% of the total), the sequence of which has not yet been determined. Altogether there are some 3200 oligonucleotide molecules in each reovirion, with a combined molecular weight of 4–5 × 10⁶ daltons (Table 5).

Since most of these oligonucleotides have 5′-ppp or -pp groups, they cannot represent random breakdown products of larger molecules; rather, they must be initiated and transcribed by an RNA polymerase, and presumably by that which is present within reovirions (see below). It has been proposed that reovirus oligonucleotides are the products of abortive transcription by this enzyme during the final stages of morphogenesis (Bellamy *et al.*, 1972; Nichols *et al.*, 1972a); this is discussed further below. There is no evidence that they are either essential for infectivity or for the expression of any other viral function. The fact that the composition of the oligonucleotide population is not constant but is influenced by the temperature at which the virus is propagated (Lai and Bellamy, 1971) is in accord with the notion that they have little if any biological function.

TABLE 5

The Oligonucleotides Present in Reovirus Particles[a]

Oligonucleotide(s)	Sequence	Chain length	Approximate number of molecules per virion
Oligoadenylates	$(p)(p)p(A)_{1-19}A_{OH}$	2–20	850
5′-G-terminated oligonucleotides	$(p)ppGC_{OH}$	2	50
	$(p)ppGCU_{OH}$	3	900
	$(p)(p)pGCUA_{OH}$	4	775
	$(p)ppGCU(A)_{1-3}A_{OH}$	5–7	130
	$(p)ppGCUA(U)_{1-4}U_{OH}$	6–9	130
	Unknown	2–8	350

[a] From Nichols *et al.* (1972a).

3.2. Orbiviruses

Since few orbiviruses have been purified, proof that their genomes consist of double-stranded RNA is available for only few, although work with suitable metabolic inhibitors has established that several contain RNA. Those which have been shown to possess double-stranded RNA, according to criteria such as, melting behavior, resistance to RNase, and base composition, are BTV (Verwoerd *et al.,* 1970, 1972; Martin and Zweerink, 1972), African horsesickness virus (Oellermann *et al.,* 1970), Colorado tick fever virus (Green, 1970), and Wallal virus (Huismans, personal communication).

The only orbivirus RNA to have been characterized in any detail is that of BTV. This RNA, which accounts for about 20% of the virion mass (Verwoerd, 1969), consists of 10 segments which, like those of reovirus, fall into three size classes (although the spread within each class is greater than in the case of reovirus) (Martin and Zweerink, 1972; Verwoerd *et al.,* 1972) (Table 4 and Fig. 7). The largest BTV segment (molecular weight 2.7×10^6 daltons) is almost exactly the same size as the largest reovirus segment, but all three BTV M segments are smaller than the three reovirus M segments, and three of the four BTV S segments are smaller than the smallest reovirus S segment. The aggregate molecular weight of the 10 BTV segments is about 12×10^6 daltons, compared with about 15×10^6 for the 10 reovirus segments. Oellerman (1970) has shown that the RNA of African horsesickness virus is very similar, as is that of Wallal virus (Huismans, personal communication).

No information is available as yet concerning the nature of the 5′ and 3′ termini of BTV RNA. BTV contains no oligonucleotides.

3.3. Cytoplasmic Polyhedrosis Viruses

CPV can be prepared in very large amounts; when several grams of virus are shaken with 90% phenol and the aqueous layer is made 1 M with respect to NaCl and added to 3 vol. of cold ethanol, a jellylike precipitate forms which may be spooled onto a glass rod (Miura *et al.,* 1968). This material is double-stranded RNA as evidenced by its base composition (A = U and G = C, 43% G+C), sharp thermal denaturation profile, inability to react with formaldehyde, resistance to ribonuclease, and by circular dichroism, optical rotatory dispersion, and X-ray diffraction studies. The RNA content of CPV particles is 23%.

When viewed with the electron microscope, a heterogeneous population of strands with a bimodal size distribution is seen, with peaks at 0.4 and 1.3 μm corresponding to molecular weights of about 1 and 3 $\times$ 10^6 daltons, respectively (Miura *et al.*, 1968; Nishimura and Hosaka, 1969). In the analytical ultracentrifuge two boundaries are obtained, the $s_{20,w}$ at infinite dilution of which are 15.4 and 12.1 S, respectively.

Analysis by polyacrylamide gel electrophoresis reveals that CPV RNA consists of equimolar amounts of 10 distinct species of double-stranded RNA which range in molecular weight from about 2.8 to 0.3 $\times$ 10^6 (Fujii-Kawata *et al.*, 1970; Lewandowski and Leppla, 1972; Lewandowski and Traynor, 1972). Their size distribution is bimodal rather than trimodal as in the case of reovirus and orbivirus (Fig. 7). The molecular weights of 5 of the 10 segments are larger than 1.8 $\times$ 10^6, while those of the remainder are between 1.2 and 0.3 $\times$ 10^6. Their aggregate molecular weight is about 14.6 $\times$ 10^6, almost the same as that of the 10 reovirus segments (Table 4). As in the case of reovirus, it has been shown, by labeling 3′ termini *in situ,* that all 10 segments exist as such within virus particles (Lewandowski and Millward, 1971).

The nature of the 3′ termini of CPV RNA has been investigated by oxidizing them with periodate, reducing with tritiated borohydride, and analyzing the radioactive tri-alcohols released after hydrolysis with ribonuclease T2 or alkali (Furiuchi and Miura, 1972; Lewandowski and Leppla, 1972). Whereas reovirus RNA contains only C_{OH} termini, CPV RNA contains equal numbers of C_{OH} and U_{OH} termini. Very recently, Furiuchi and Miura (1973) have found that all segments of CPV RNA possess identical 3 termini: each consists of one strand that terminates in $PypC_{OH}$ and an antiparallel strand that terminates in $PypU_{OH}$.

It has been reported that some non-nucleoside material which is released by alkali and does not adsorb to charcoal is associated with all CPV RNA segments (Furiuchi and Miura, 1973), but its nature and significance remain to be elucidated. CPV contains no oligonucleotides (Fujii-Kawata *et al.*, 1970).

3.4. The Plant Virus Genus

The RNA of both WTV and RDV is double-stranded as judged by the same criteria as were used in the case of reovirus, BTV, and CPV

RNA (e.g., Gomatos and Tamm, 1963b; Black and Markham, 1963; Sato *et al.*, 1966; Miura *et al.*, 1966; Samejima *et al.*, 1968; Wood and Streissle, 1970). The RNA contents of WTV and RDV have been reported as being 23% RNA (Kalmakoff *et al.*, 1969) and 12% (Toyoda *et al.*, 1964), respectively, and their G+C contents as 38% (Toyoda *et al.*, 1964) and 44% (Miura *et al.*, 1966); however, direct comparative studies are required to determine whether these very large differences are real or not.

Electron microscopic examination of extracted WTV and RDV RNA indicates that each consists of a heterogenous population of RNA molecules from 0.1 to 1.5 μm long, which exhibits 4 or 5 weak size maxima (Kleinschmidt *et al.*, 1964; Fujii-Kawata *et al.*, 1970). Polyacrylamide gel electrophoresis resolves these populations in each case into 12 components, which range in molecular weight from 2.8 to 0.3×10^6 for WTV RNA and from 2.8 to 0.44×10^6 in the case of RDV (Reddy and Black, 1973b; Fujii-Kawata *et al.*, 1970). Some of the segments, however, migrate very close together, and Lewandowski and Leppla (1972) are of the opinion that WTV RNA consists of 13 segments. As can be seen from the electrophoretic migration patterns (Fig. 7), the sizes of most of the segments of WTV and RDV RNA, except some of the smaller ones, are virtually identical. In both cases the segment sizes are rather uniformaly distributed over their entire range, without the clustering into the three size classes characteristic of the reovirus RNA segments. The aggregate molecular weights of the WTV and RDV RNA segments are about 15.0 and 15.3×10^6, respectively (Table 4). Neither virus contains oligonucleotides.

Like CPV RNA, WTV RNA possesses approximately equal numbers of C_{OH} and U_{OH} residues at its 3′ termini (Lewandowski and Leppla, 1972). It is not yet known whether these are distributed in the same manner as those on CPV RNA. Minor amounts of G_{OH} and especially A_{OH} are also present in WTV RNA. Control experiments indicate that these are not introduced spuriously and they must, therefore, preexist in the virus preparation used (since the analyses were carried out on whole virus, not on extracted RNA).

The RNA of FDV and MRDV has not yet been characterized. The evidence that FDV is double-stranded is immunochemical (Francki and Jackson, 1972); the double-strandedness of MRDV RNA was demonstrated by Redolfi and Pennazio (1972).

4. THE NATURE OF THE CAPSID POLYPEPTIDES

4.1. Reovirus

4.1.1. The Nature of Reovirus Polypeptides

Reovirions are dissociated into their component polypeptides by treatment with sodium dodecyl sulfate (SDS) and 2-mercaptoethanol (2-ME). Electrophoresis in polyacrylamide gels of the resulting mixture of SDS-polypeptide complexes reveals that reovirions are composed of seven species of polypeptides which, like the double-stranded RNA segments, fall into three size classes (Fig. 9) (Loh and Shatkin, 1968; Smith *et al.*, 1969). Their molecular weights, number per virion, and relative frequencies on a mass as well as on a molar basis are listed in Table 6. The polypeptide complement of top component is identical to that of virions (Smith *et al.*, 1969).

The sizes of the three groups of capsid polypeptides correspond to the coding capacities of the three genome RNA segment groups: the λ, μ, and σ polypeptides comprise some 1400–1500, 700–800, and 350–400 amino acids, while the *L, M,* and *S* RNA segments comprise about 4500, 2300, and 1000–1300 nucleotide base pairs, respectively (Joklik, 1970). This relationship suggests that the capsid polypeptides are coded by messenger RNAs transcribed from entire genome RNA segments; evidence that this is actually the case has recently been obtained as a result of studies on *in vitro* transcription and translation of reovirus messenger RNA (see below). The only exception is

TABLE 6

Capsid Polypeptides of Reovirus[a]

Species	Mol. wt., daltons	Percent in virion	Approximate number of molecules per virion	Molar ratio	Location
$\lambda 1$	155,000	15	110	5.5	Core
$\lambda 2$	140,000	11	90	4.5	Core
$\mu 1$	80,000	2	20	1.0	Core
$\mu 2$	72,000	36	550	29.5	Outer shell
$\sigma 1$	42,000	1	30	1.5	Outer shell
$\sigma 2$	38,000	7	200	10.5	Core
$\sigma 3$	34,000	28	900	47.5	Outer shell

[a] From Smith *et al.* (1969).

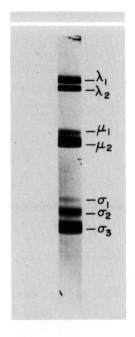

Fig. 9. Reovirus capsid polypeptides electrophoresed in a SDS-urea-polyacrylamide gel. Direction of electrophoresis is from top to bottom. Stained with Coomassie Brilliant Blue.

polypeptide $\mu2$, which is not a primary gene product, but is derived by cleavage of a precursor, polypeptide $\mu1$, which is itself present in virions in small amounts (see below). Polypeptide $\mu2$ probably exists within the virus as a disulfide-bonded dimer since dissociation of virions with SDS in the absence of 2-ME results in the disappearance of $\mu2$ and the appearance of a new band close to $\lambda1$ and $\lambda2$ (Smith *et al.*, 1969).

Reovirus capsid polypeptides can be separated by chromatography on several types of columns (Pett *et al.*, 1973). When virions are solubilized in urea, their constituent polypeptides can be separated on DEAE-Sephadex into three fractions which contain $\mu2$, $\lambda1 + \lambda2 + \sigma2$, and $\sigma3$, respectively; on CM-Sephadex none of the polypeptides are retarded except $\mu2$. When virions are solubilized with 2-ME and SDS, the polypeptide-SDS complexes can be separated on agarose columns into three fractions, according to their size, which comprise polypeptides $\lambda1$ and $\lambda2$, $\mu1$ and $\mu2$, and $\sigma1$, $\sigma2$, and $\sigma3$, respectively. These three chromatographic systems permit the large scale (in quantities of 10–100 mg) isolation of all major species of reovirus capsid polypeptides with the exception of $\lambda1 + \lambda2$, which have not yet been separated.

The amino acid compositions of the reovirus capsid polypeptides present no unusual features (Pett *et al.*, 1973). All polypeptides, with the exception of $\mu2$ possess blocked amino-terminal groups, the nature of which is not yet known; the amino-terminal amino acid sequence of $\mu2$ is Pro-Gly-Gly-Val-Pro- (Pett *et al.*, 1973). This implies that when polypeptide $\mu1$ is cleaved to $\mu2$, it is the amino-terminal portion of the molecule which is removed. The carboxyl-terminal amino acids of several of these polypeptides have also been determined by sequential degradation with carboxypeptidase A and B. They are: polypeptide $\sigma3$, -(val-val-leu)-COOH; $\mu2$, -leu(arg,tyr,tyr)-Arg-COOH; and either one or both of $\lambda1$ and $\lambda2$ terminate(s) in -Arg-COOH, with a different adjacent amino acid sequence from that of $\mu2$ (Pett *et al.*, 1973). These data demonstrate that all the major reovirus capsid polypeptides are unique molecular species, and it is very likely that this is true for the minor species $\sigma1$ also. This conclusion is at variance with that reached by Roy *et al.* (1972), who found that the λ, μ, and σ polypeptides separated by SDS-polyacrylamide gel electrophoresis all possessed the N-terminal amino acid sequence Pro-Gly-Gly-Val-, which suggested the possibility of gene duplication. However, it is likely that this result was due to contamination of the λ and σ polypeptide bands with derivatives of $\mu2$, which has the above N-terminal amino acid sequence; thus, if polypeptide $\mu2$ is not completely reduced, its dimer comigrates with the λ polypeptide band, and, as will be discussed below, certain proteolytic breakdown products of $\mu2$ which may arise on storage and remain associated with virions have electrophoretic migration rates close to those of the σ polypeptides.

4.1.2. The Polypeptides of the Reovirus Outer Capsid Shell

Three of the seven reovirus capsid polypeptides, namely $\sigma3$, $\mu2$, and $\sigma1$, which together make up about 65% of the total virion protein, constitute the outer capsid shell (Smith *et al.*, 1969). Both $\sigma3$ and $\mu2$ are at the virion surface since they are efficiently iodinated by the lactoperoxidase technique (Lewandowski and Traynor, 1972; Martin *et al.*, 1973).* It is however still quite uncertain how $\sigma3$ and $\mu2$ are associated with each other, and whether the clearly discernible capsomers are composed of both or of only one. Most of the information concerning these questions comes from studies of the effect of chymotrypsin on the outer capsid shell. Under suitable conditions this shell is digested by chymotrypsin according to a precisely defined series of reactions (Joklik, 1972): polypeptide $\sigma3$ is digested first via

---

* Polypeptide $\sigma1$ is present in amounts too small to be detected reliably by iodination.

several intermediates, some of which remain transiently associated with the virus particles; then, polypeptide $\mu 2$ is removed in the same manner; finally $\sigma 1$ is digested. The resultant particles, the cores, are resistant to chymotrypsin. However chymotrypsin does not always convert reovirions to cores; whether it does so depends on the virus strain, the concentration of virus and the concentration of chymotrypsin (Joklik, 1972; Shatkin and LaFiandra, 1972), and the nature of the monovalent cations that are present (Borsa *et al.*, 1973*a,b,c*). Under some conditions digestion of the outer capsid shell does not proceed to completion, and particles are formed that although still intermediate in their physical and biological properties between virions and cores, are nevertheless quite resistant to chymotrypsin. Two of these particles are of particular interest. The first is formed when the chymotrypsin concentration exceeds 100 $\mu g/ml$ for strain Carter and 1000 $\mu g/ml$ for strains Abney and Dearing, and when the monovalent cation is sodium: under these conditions particles are formed that lack polypeptide $\sigma 3$ and a 12,000-dalton fragment of $\mu 2$ (Joklik, 1972). These particles resemble reovirions in morphology (although the capsomers appear more distinct, as though $\sigma 3$ were located between capsomers), their density is 0.01 g/ml higher, they are still fully infectious, they possess their full oligonucleotide complement, and they exhibit no transcriptase activity (see below). Owing to their close similarity to virions in their physical, biological, and enzymatic properties, in spite of lacking about one-third of the capsid polypeptide complement, these particles have been termed "paravirions" (Joklik, 1972). The second type of intermediate particle is formed when strain Dearing virions are digested with chymotrypsin at a concentration of about 200 $\mu g/ml$ in the presence of sodium ions (Shatkin and LaFiandra, 1972). These particles appear to have the same polypeptide composition as paravirions, but they lack the majority of their oligonucleotides, their density is 0.03 g/ml higher than that of virions, they are fully infectious, and they display full transcriptase activity. These particles, which have been designated SVP_i (infectious subviral particles, Shatkin and LaFiandra, 1972), represent a form that is slightly closer to cores than to paravirions. They closely resemble the SVP that are formed *in vivo* following infection: these particles are also digestion end products, they lack $\sigma 3$ and an 8000-dalton rather than a 12,000-dalton fragment of $\mu 2$, and they possess reovirus morphology with prominent capsomers, an active transcriptase, and a relatively high specific infectivity (see below).

In summary, it appears that the capsomers of the outer shell are composed primarily of polypeptide $\mu 2$, and that $\sigma 3$ is either located between capsomers or is associated with them in such a way that removing it does not alter the gross appearance of the virus particle. The location of the third outer-shell polypeptide, $\sigma 1$, which is only present to the extent of some 20 molecules, is not known. It is conceivable that it is a component of special structures which may be postulated to overlie the 12 core spikes; as pointed out above, those spikes penetrate halfway through the outer capsid shell, and to accommodate them the outer shell must presumably be specially modified.

4.1.3.   The Polypeptides of the Reovirus Core

Cores differ from virions in the following properties: they contain only about 35% of the virions' protein complement; they contain all double-stranded genome RNA in nuclease-resistant form, but no oligonucleotides; their density is 0.08 g/ml higher than that of virions (1.44 rather than 1.36 g/ml, Smith *et al.*, 1969); their sedimentation coefficient is 400 S as compared with the virions' 630 S; their specific infectivity is some 4–5 logs lower than that of virions (Smith *et al.*, 1969; Banerjee and Shatkin, 1970; Joklik, 1972); and they contain the transcriptase in its active form (Shatkin and Sipe, 1968a; Skehel and Joklik, 1969).

The arrangement of the polypeptides in the core presents several problems. One is the question of whether one of the core polypeptides is intimately associated with the RNA segments within the core cavity. There are several indications that this is not the case. First, as pointed out above, reovirus top-component particles are composed of exactly the same polypeptides as virions. If the RNA segments were normally associated with a certain protein, one would expect this protein as well as the RNA to be missing from top component. Second, there is insufficient space: the volume of the core cavity is only 16% of the virion volume (Luftig *et al.*, 1972), and the RNA accounts for about 14.5% of the virion mass. Even taking into account the fact that the partial specific volume of RNA is less than that of protein, it is very doubtful whether all of any core polypeptide except $\mu 1$ (of which there are only about 20 molecules) could be associated with the genome RNA segments. The possibility that only some, but not all $\lambda 1$, $\lambda 2$, or $\sigma 2$ molecules are associated with RNA is probably very small.

Little is known concerning the location of the various polypeptides in the actual structure of the core, which clearly has two components: the shell proper, which accounts for about 80–85% of the core's mass, and the spikes, which account for 15–20% of the mass. These figures should be considered in relation to the overall polypeptide composition of cores, which is λ1 and λ2, each 30–40%, σ2, 20%, and μ1, about 5%. The only piece of evidence available so far is that the most readily iodinated of the three major core polypeptides is λ2 (Martin *et al.*, 1973). On the assumption that no one polypeptide can be a major component of *both* shell and spikes, the most plausible conclusion at this time is that the core shell is composed of polypeptides λ1 and λ2, the latter occupying most of its outer surface, and that the spikes are composed predominantly of σ2. The minor polypeptide μ1 is also iodinated readily and may also be a spike component. Much further work will be necessary to determine whether this model is correct.

4.2. Orbiviruses

The only orbivirus of which the polypeptide composition has been studied is BTV (Martin and Zweerink, 1972; Verwoerd *et al.*, 1972). BTV L particles comprise 7 polypeptide species, the same number as reovirions; but their relative sizes and frequencies differ markedly from those of reovirus polypeptides (Table 7, Fig. 10). There are four major polypeptides, namely polypeptides 2, 3, 5, and 7 (molecular weights 110,000; 100,000; 58,000; and 32,000, respectively); and three minor polypeptides, polypeptides 1, 4, and 6 (molecular weights, 155,00; 72, 000; and 38,000, respectively). As in the case of reovirus, the molecular weights of the BTV capsid polypeptides are consistent with their being

TABLE 7

Capsid Polypeptides of BTV[a]

Polypeptide	Mol. wt., daltons	Percent in BTV L particles	Approximate number of molecules per BTV L particle	Molar ratio	Location
1	155,000	2	7	0.7	BTV D particle
2	110,000	22.8	98	10.4	Outer shell
3	100,000	16.2	76	8.0	BTV D particle
4	72,000	1	6	0.6	BTV D particle
5	58,000	20.1	156	16.5	Outer shell
6	38,000	2.8	32	3.4	BTV D particle
7	32,000	34.9	570	60.3	BTV D particle

[a] From Martin and Zweerink (1972) and Verwoerd *et al.* (1972).

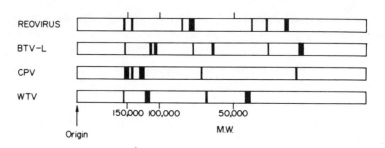

Fig. 10. Chart depicting the relative sizes and molar frequencies of the capsid polypeptide species of various members of the family Reoviridae.

coded by seven of the ten genome RNA segments. Preliminary studies indicate that capsid polypeptides of Wallal virus closely resemble those of BTV (Huismans, personal communication).

The polypeptide constitution of BTV D particles is the same as that of the L particles except that they lack the two major polypeptides 2 and 5, which together comprise about 43% of the total. Particles intermediate between L and D particles that lack polypeptide 2 but still possess polypeptide 5 have been described (Verwoerd et al., 1972). These two polypeptides are therefore presumably located on the outer surface of BTV L particles as the components of the diffuse and featureless outer shell (see above). This conclusion is supported by the fact that they are the two polypeptides which are most intensely labeled with ^{125}I and lactoperoxidase (Martin et al., 1973). Polypeptides 1, 3, and 4 are the most intensively labeled BTV D-particle components.

Unlike the outer capsid shell of reovirus particles, the diffuse outer layer of BTV L particles is resistant to chymotrypsin; like reovirus cores, BTV D particles are also resistant to this enzyme (Verwoerd et al., 1972).

4.3. Cytoplasmic Polyhedrosis Viruses

The polypeptide composition of CPV particles has been investigated by dissociating them with urea-SDS, labeling the resulting polypeptide mixture with ^{125}I, and separating it by electrophoresis on polyacrylamide gels (Lewandowski and Traynor, 1972). This procedure reveals the presence of five polypeptide bands which range in molecular weight from 151,000 to 33,000; their molecular weights and frequencies in virions on a mass and molar basis are listed in Table 8 (also see Fig.

10). About 10% of the protein-bound label migrates very rapidly, where small peptides would be expected; the significance of this material is not clear. Similar material is found in reovirions (Smith *et al.*, 1969); it is generally assumed that it is not an integral or essential part of virions.

Iodination of whole CP virions shows that polypeptides I and III are iodinated most extensively, while polypeptides II, IV, and V are iodinated little, if at all. The surface of CP virions is thus most probably composed mainly of polypeptides I and III.

CPV preparations usually contain small amounts of particles that lack some of the smaller RNA segments (satellite virions) and top-component particles devoid of all RNA. Both contain, in addition to capsid polypeptides, polypeptide fragments; in particular, their largest polypeptide is some 5000 daltons smaller than that of virions. Both types of particles are therefore probably virion breakdown products (Lewandowski and Traynor, 1972).

The molecular weights of the five CPV capsid-polypeptide species are such that they could be coded by monocistronic mRNA species transcribed from five of the ten genome segments. The other five genome segments may code for five polypeptides that make up the polyhedral bodies. There are two lines of evidence in favor of this hypothesis: first, the shape of polyhedral bodies does indeed appear to be controlled by the virus strain which they contain (Hukuhara, 1971); second, polyhedral bodies consist predominantly of two species of polypeptides with molecular weights of 29,500 and 19,550 which account for some 90% of their total protein, and three minor polypeptide components with molecular weights of 122,000; 100,000; and 48,000 (Lewandowski and Traynor, 1972). These sizes are very close to those

TABLE 8

Capsid Polypeptides of CPV

Polypeptide	Mol. wt., daltons	Percent in virion[a]	Molar ratio
I	151,000	36	25
II	142,000	16	12
III	130,000	34	28
IV	67,000	2	3
V	33,000	10	32

[a] Based on distribution of ^{125}I following iodination of dissociated whole virus. From Lewandowski and Traynor (1972).

TABLE 9

Capsid Polypeptides of WTV[a]

Polypeptide	Mol. wt., daltons
I	156,000
II	122,000
III	63,000
IV	44,000

[a] From Lewandowski and Traynor (1972).

expected of the gene products of the 5 genome RNA segments that do not appear to code for capsid polypeptides.

4.4.   The Plant Virus Genus

The only member of this genus whose polypeptide constitution has been examined is WTV (Lewandowski and Traynor, 1972). Using the same technique as described above for CPV particles, it was shown that WT virions consist of two major components, polypeptides II and IV, and two minor ones, I and III; in addition, there are three or four components present in such small amounts that their significance is doubtful. WTV top component lacks polypeptides I and III. The molecular weights of these polypeptides are listed in Table 9 (see also Fig. 10).

In intact WT virions polypeptides II and III are iodinated most efficiently (Lewandowski and Traynor, 1972); polypeptide II is therefore the principal WT virion surface component, while the other major polypeptide, IV, is apparently an internal component.

5.   THE TRANSCRIPTASE

The double-stranded (DS) genome RNA of reoviridae cannot serve as messenger RNA. Such single-stranded (SS) messenger RNA is provided by the action of a transcriptase, or rather a DS→SS RNA polymerase, which is part of their capsids.

5.1. Reovirus

Intact reovirions display no transcriptase activity; in order to activate the enzyme, the outer capsid shell must be partially or completely removed. This may be achieved by either of two procedures. First, the virus may be heated at 70°C for periods as brief as 20 seconds (Borsa and Graham, 1968). Heating is known to remove outer shell capsomers (Mayor and Jordan, 1968), but it is not known how many capsomers must be removed before activation occurs since the polypeptide composition of particles the transcriptase of which has been activated by heating has not yet been determined. Presumably the number is not large. However, it is known that activation is dependent on capsomer removal since antibody, which stabilizes the outer shell, prevents activation. Second, treatment of reovirions with chymotrypsin, which digests their outer shell, also activates the enzyme (Shatkin and Sipe, 1968a). Once again it is not necessary to remove the entire outer shell: removal of polypeptide $\sigma3$ is not sufficient to activate the enzyme, but subsequent cleavage of polypeptide $\mu2$ is (see above). Apparently cleavage of only a few $\mu2$ molecules is sufficient, for enzyme activity appears while most $\mu2$ molecules are still intact (Joklik, 1972). Among the more or less completely characterized particles which possess transcriptase activity are paravirions and SVP_i (see above), SVP generated within the cell following infection (Levin *et al.*, 1970b; Chang and Zweerink, 1971; Silverstein *et al.*, 1972), cores, and immature virus particles that are formed during the later stages of the infection cycle (see below).

The reason why modification or removal of the outer capsid shell activates the transcriptase is not clear. Among the possible explanations are that such modification or removal may uncover the central channels of the core spikes through which nucleoside triphosphates may be admitted and transcripts released, or that it may release conformational constraints and thereby permit the polypeptide chains that constitute the enzyme to assume the configuration essential for activity.

The nature of the polypeptide chains on which the catalytic site of the transcriptase is located is not known. It has so far been impossible to separate the enzyme from cores since their disruption or dissociation invariably leads to complete loss of enzyme activity. Until recently, it was not even clear whether there is only one enzyme molecule or catalytic site in each particle, or several. This question has now been partially answered by direct visual observation, for cores from which up to nine individual strands of single-stranded RNA are simultaneously extruded, each apparently from a different source—possibly through the spike channels—have been observed (Gillies *et al.*, 1971). This evidence suggests that there is at least one catalytic site for each genome segment, and that all ten segments can be transcribed simultaneously. It also makes it very unlikely that a polypeptide other than one or more of the four known core polypeptides is a transcriptase component since the presence of as many as ten such polypeptide molecules per virion is very unlikely to have escaped detection. Most probably the catalytic sites exist on the inside of the core shell (there are no catalytic sites on the outside since cores transcribe exogenous double-stranded RNA very poorly if at all (Schuerch and Joklik, unpublished observations), possibly near the base of the spikes and therefore close to the putative release channels; but it is not clear on which of the four core polypeptides the catalytic sites are located. It has already been pointed out in this connection (Joklik, 1970) that the three major components of reovirus cores, polypeptides $\lambda 1$, $\lambda 2$, and $\sigma 2$, bear a remarkable resemblance to the three polypeptides which comprise the *E. coli* core DNA-dependent RNA polymerase, namely β', β, and α (Burgess, 1969), both with respect to size and molar ratio. This comparison has been extended to the other reoviridae and their transcriptases, all of which possess basically similar polypeptide constituents (Lewandowski and Traynor, 1972).

Transcriptase activity has been detected in infected cells and partially purified from them (Gomatos, 1968, 1970). Although it was not fully characterized, there is little doubt that the enzyme preparation comprised a mixture of parental virion-derived SVP and progeny immature particles (see below).

Reovirus cores also catalyze an exchange reaction between the four ribonucleoside triphosphates and inorganic pyrophosphate (Wachsman *et al.*, 1970). The only single triphosphate to support this exchange is GTP, with which the rate is about half of that with all four. The fact that the optimal conditions for pyrophosphate exchange are similar to those for polymerization, and that individually only GTP, which is known to be present at the 5′ termini of reovirus RNA strands, supports it suggests that the exchange reaction represents part of the overall transcriptase reaction; however, the degree of participation of individual nucleoside triphosphates in the exchange reaction is not related to the overall base composition of reovirus RNA.

Reovirus cores also possess a nucleoside triphosphate phosphohydrolase activity which liberates inorganic phosphate from all common ribo- and deoxyribonucleoside triphosphates (Kapuler *et al.*,

1970; Borsa *et al.*, 1970). Apparently the same catalytic site is responsible for all four activities; the relative rates of hydrolysis are ATP > GTP > CTP > UTP. The enzyme differs in its response to metal cations and in the nature of the mutual competitive inhibitions among nucleoside triphosphates from all other known nucleoside triphosphate phosphohydrolases. Its function and the advantage that its presence confers on reovirions are not clear. Presumably it is responsible for converting some of the terminal 5′-triphosphate groups of both genome RNA strands (Banerjee and Shatkin, 1971), its transcripts (Banerjee *et al.*, 1971*a*; Nichols *et al.*, 1972*b*), and oligonucleotides (Nichols *et al.*, 1972*a*; Stoltzfus and Banerjee, 1972) to diphosphates (see above).

5.2. Orbiviruses

Like reovirions, BTV L particles display no transcriptase activity (Verwoerd *et al.*, 1972; Martin and Zweerink, 1972); like reovirus cores, BTV D particles do. The BTV transcriptase closely resembles the corresponding reovirus enzyme in its properties with two notable exceptions: it has a preference for Mn^{2+} over Mg^{2+}, and its optimum temperature is 28°C rather than about 45°C (Verwoerd and Huismans, 1972). This property of the BTV transcriptase, coupled with the fact that BTV yields in mammalian cells are low and that it multiplies in insect cells, has led to the suggestion that BTV may be primarily an insect virus (Verwoerd *et al.*, 1972).

While transcripts are probably released from reovirus cores via the channels located in the centers of the spikes, it is not at all clear how BTV transcripts are released. The possibility that the 32 ring-shaped capsomers possess channels extending through the entire capsid shell is not supported by electron micrographs of sectioned particles.

5.3. Cytoplasmic Polyhedrosis Viruses

The presence of a transcriptase in CPV was first demonstrated by Lewandowski *et al.*, (1969) who found that CP virions exhibited enzyme activity without having to be activated. By contrast, Shimotohno and Miura (1973) reported that CPV isolated by differential centrifugation of solubilized polyhedra displays transcriptase activity only after extraction with difluorodichloromethane (Diflon). The manner in which this treatment activates the enzyme is not clear.

The likeliest explanation is that Diflon does not act on CP virions directly, but removes impurities that for some reason or other prevent the enzyme from acting or that degrade the transcripts; it may be significant that CPV preparations often contain ribonucleases, as judged by the fact that transcripts tend to be small unless bentonite is added to reaction mixtures (Lewandowski *et al.,* 1969; Shimotohno and Miura, 1973). The particles currently regarded as CP virions, therefore, most probably possess transcriptase activity without having to be degraded ("activated") in any way (see also Donaghue and Hayashi, 1972).

The CPV transcriptase, like the reovirus enzyme, prefers Mg^{2+} over Mn^{2+}; however, like the BTV enzyme, it possesses a low optimum temperature of only 27°C. Its transcripts have been resolved by sucrose density gradient centrifugation into two fractions, the larger of which hybridizes only with the larger genome RNA segments, and the smaller only with the smaller (Shimotohno and Miura, 1973). The synthesis of both groups of transcripts was shown to start at the same time.

5.4. The Plant Virus Genus

WTV particles also display transcriptase activity without requiring any form of activation (Black and Knight, 1970), as do the "core" particles of slightly higher buoyant density (Lewandowski and Traynor, 1972). The properties of the enzyme are analogous to those of the corresponding reovirus, BTV, and CPV enzymes. Its optimum temperature is 28–30°C; it prefers Mg^{2+} over Mn^{2+}.

The presence of a transcriptase in other members of this genus does not yet appear to have been explored.

6. THE REPLICATION OF REOVIRUSES

6.1. Morphological Studies

There have been numerous microscopic and electron microscopic studies of the cytological changes that accompany reovirus multiplication and morphogenesis. The cytopathology of reovirus infection has been reviewed by Rosen (1968). Its most characteristic feature is the development in the cytoplasm of inclusions or "factories" which may be visualized by a variety of techniques: staining for RNA with acridine orange (Gomatos *et al.,* 1962), which provided the first clue that reovirus contains double-stranded RNA; staining with fluorescein-coupled antibody to double-stranded RNA (actually poly I:C) (Silverstein and Shur, 1970); staining for viral protein with fluorescein-coupled antibody (Drouhet, 1970; Rhim *et al.*, 1962; Spendlove *et al.*, 1963a; Oie *et al.*, 1966; Fields *et al.*, 1971);direct electron microscopic observation (Gomatos *et al.*, 1962; Dales, 1963; Spendlove *et al.*, 1963b; Dales *et al.*, 1965; Jenson *et al.*, 1965; Anderson and Doane, 1966; Fields *et al.*, 1971); and autoradiography and staining with ferritin-conjugated antibody coupled with electron microscopy (Dales *et al.*, 1965). These inclusions, which appear after 6–8 hours at 37°C, are at first particularly prevalent in the perinuclear region, where they tend to be associated with the spindle fibers of the mitotic apparatus; at later stages of the infection cycle they coalesce into a reticular network which gradually spreads throughout the entire cytoplasm. However, in line with the observation that not all foci of morphogenesis are associated with the mitotic apparatus, reovirus replication is not absolutely dependent upon the presence of mitotic tubules; it proceeds at the normal rate in cells treated with colchicine (Dales, 1963; Spendlove *et al.*, 1963a, 1964), and in such cells the reticular network of viral antigen seen normally is replaced by large clumped masses.

As infection progresses, microtubules coated with newly formed virus-specified protein appear within the factories, followed by virus aggregates interspersed with fine dense threads (Dales *et al.*, 1965). Occasionally, crystalline arrays of full or empty capsids are formed (Rhim *et al.*, 1962; Fields *et al.*, 1971). Intermediate stages of morphogenesis are rarely seen; these are best observed using ts mutants under nonpermissive conditions (Fields *et al.*, 1971).

6.2. The One-Step Growth Cycle

Reoviruses are capable of infecting cells of many animal species, as is to be expected on the basis of their very wide distribution in nature; several aspects of their multiplication cycles have been studied at one time or another in a variety of mammalian cells. However, most of the studies on which our knowledge concerning the molecular biology of reovirus multiplication is based have been performed on mouse L fibroblasts infected with the Dearing strain of reovirus type 3. The reason for this is that L cells are readily available in large amounts since they grow readily in suspension culture and that the Dearing strain multiplies particularly well in them (see above). Most of the following discussion of the reactions which proceed during the reovirus multiplication cycle are therefore based on studies of the Dearing strain of reovirus multiplying in mouse L fibroblasts. Other systems that have been examined are reovirus type 2 growing in human amnion cells (Oie *et al.,* 1966), reovirus type 1 in L cells (Prevec *et al.,* 1968), and reovirus type 1 (strain Lang), type 2 (strain D-5 Jones), and type 3 (Abney) in L cells (Shatkin and Rada, 1967*a*; Shatkin *et al.* 1968; Loh and Shatkin, 1968; Shatkin and Sipe, 1968*b*; Banerjee and Shatkin, 1970).

The one-step growth cycle of reovirus can be divided into two distinct phases (Gomatos and Tamm, 1963*c*; Kudo and Graham, 1965; Shatkin and Rada, 1967*a*; Bellamy and Joklik, 1967*a*; Watanabe *et al.,* 1967*a*) (Fig. 11). First, there is an early phase which can itself be divided into a period when the infecting virus particles are being uncoated (period a) and a period when early messenger RNA is being transcribed from parental genomes at a relatively low rate (period b); this early transcription is not inhibited by preventing protein synthesis. It was therefore thought initially that the enzyme responsible for it was a cellular DNA-dependent RNA polymerase or DNA polymerase; however, it was then found that just like vaccinia virus, which had just been shown to contain a DNA-dependent RNA polymerase (Kates and

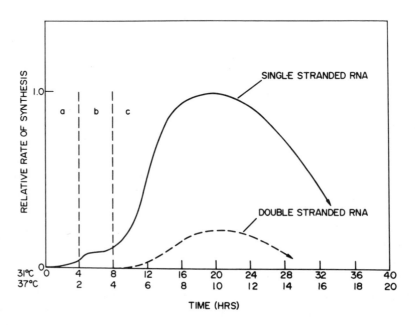

Fig. 11.   Time course of synthesis of reovirus RNA during a one step growth cycle.

McAuslan, 1967), so too reovirus contains an RNA-dependent RNA polymerase or transcriptase (Borsa and Graham, 1968; Shatkin and Sipe, 1968a). The duration of the first phase of the one-step growth cycle depends primarily on two variables, namely the multiplicity of infection and the temperature of incubation: at multiplicities of 10–20 PFU adsorbed/cell (generally almost 1000 particles/cell) it lasts for about 3–4 hours at 38°C and 8–10 hours at 31°C.

The second phase of the one-step growth cycle (period c) (Fig. 11) commences with the formation of progeny double-stranded RNA which is identical with genome RNA (Kudo and Graham, 1965; Shatkin and Rada, 1967a; Shatkin et al., 1968). At the same time there occurs a large increase (5- to 10-fold) in the rate of transcription of single-stranded RNA (late mRNA). The enzymes responsible for both are synthesized de novo since both processes are inhibited by inhibitors of protein synthesis (Kudo and Graham, 1965; Shatkin and Rada, 1967a; Watanabe et al., 1967a). If protein synthesis is inhibited after RNA synthesis has commenced, single-stranded RNA synthesis continues at a linear rate, indicating that the corresponding enzyme is stable; by contrast synthesis of double-stranded RNA ceases. The rates of both double- and single-stranded RNA synthesis reach a peak at 6–8 hours at 38°C and 16–20 hours at 31°C, and then decline. Progeny virus is formed throughout this phase, after first becoming detectable 1–2 hours after the first progeny genome RNA is formed. In spite of the severe cytopathic effects caused at 37°C, very little progeny virus is released (although cell constituents such as ribosomes readily leak out of infected cells); most of the virus yield remains cell-associated until well after virus formation has ceased.

We will now consider the reovirus one-step growth cycle in functional terms, focusing primarily on adsorption and uncoating, the transcription of mRNA both in vitro and in vivo, the translation of mRNA both in vitro and in vivo, the formation of progeny double-stranded RNA, and morphogenesis.

6.3. Adsorption and Uptake

Reovirus adsorbs readily to a wide variety of cells, both in monolayer and in suspension culture. Its rate of adsorption to L cells is very similar to that of vaccinia virus under comparable conditions; at a cell concentration of 10^7 cells/ml in Puck's solution containing 0.02M Mg^{2+} and 1% fetal calf serum at 37°C, 38, 52, and 65% of added virus adsorbs in 7.5, 15, and 30 minutes, respectively (Joklik, 1972). From these figures, an adsorption rate constant of about 2.5×10^{-9} cm^3/min/cell can be calculated. Very large numbers of virus particles, up to about 50,000, can adsorb per cell; this approaches close packing of virus particles on the cell surface.

The uptake of reovirus has been studied primarily by electron microscopy (Dales *et al.*, 1965; Silverstein and Dales, 1968). Reovirions enter cells by means of a process of invagination and become engulfed within phagocytic vacuoles which move into the interior of the cell and there fuse with lysosomes. Within 30 minutes after adsorption more than half of the adsorbed virus is present in lysosomes, most of which contain several virus particles. Within the lysosomes virions are degraded to subviral particles (SVP) (see below), which are then transferred, during the next 2–4 hours, to dense perinuclear inclusions that develop into the "factories" which are the sites of accumulation of progeny viral RNA and protein, and of morphogenesis (see above).

6.4. Uncoating

Reovirus is unique among viruses in that its genome is not uncoated, i.e., it is not separated physically from its capsid following infection; instead, infecting reovirions are converted to SVP (Silverstein *et al.*, 1970, 1972; Chang and Zweerink, 1971). The conversion of reovirions to SVP is very efficient and virtually complete by one hour after infection; it is apparently effected by lysosomal enzymes and involves the digestion of about one-half of the protein in the outer capsid shell (about one-third of total virion capsid protein). The protein which is lost is all of polypeptide $\sigma3$ and an 8000-dalton fragment of polypeptide $\mu2$; SVP thus correspond closely to one of the stages of digestion of reovirus by chymotrypsin *in vitro* (Joklik, 1972; Shatkin and LaFiandra, 1972) (see above). The SVP differ from virions in morphology: their diameter is smaller (but larger than that of cores) and the capsomers on their surface are more clearly discernible (Silverstein *et al.*, 1972). Their density is 0.02 g/ml greater than that of virions. As would be expected from the fact that the inner capsid shell is intact, the genome is still completely resistant to nucleases, but, as would be expected from the fact that degradation of the outer shell has progressed beyond loss of polypeptide $\sigma3$, they exhibit full transcriptase activity (Levin *et al.*, 1970b; Chang and Zweerink, 1971; Silverstein *et al.*, 1972).

Most SVP are not degraded further; very little, if any, naked double-stranded RNA is liberated (Silverstein and Dales, 1968; Chang and Zweerink, 1971). Instead, SVP persist throughout the infection cycle (Silverstein *et al.*, 1970), and during its later stages they are found to be combined with newly synthesized polypeptide σ3; this causes their density of 1.38 g/ml to change back to 1.365 g/ml, very slightly more than that of virions (1.36 g/ml) (Chang and Zweerink, 1971; Silverstein *et al.*, 1972), and their transcriptase activity to be abolished (Astell *et al.*, 1972). These reconstituted particles, which are distinguishable from virions only by their lack of the 8000-dalton fragment of polypeptide μ2, are then liberated along with the progeny. Their presence among the progeny, especially after infection at high multiplicity and when the yield is relatively low, is detectable by the appearance of their 64,000-dalton μ2 fragment among the polypeptide complement of the viral yield (unpublished observation). It is not known whether they are infectious.

6.5.   The Transcription of Reovirus mRNA

The single-stranded reovirus RNA that is synthesized in infected cells hybridizes very efficiently to reovirus genome RNA; it does not self-anneal, which indicates that it is transcribed from only one of the two strands of genome RNA (Shatkin and Rada, 1967*a*). It is messenger RNA (see below) and most of it is associated with polyribosomes (Prevec and Graham, 1966; Shatkin and Rada, 1967*a*; Bellamy and Joklik, 1967*a*). There are two classes of reovirus mRNA, as defined by when it is synthesized and what particles synthesize it: early mRNA is transcribed from parental genomes by parental SVP, while late mRNA is transcribed from progeny genomes by immature virus particles (see below). The principal question concerning the transcription of these two mRNA populations is whether they contain the same genetic information, i.e., whether they comprise the 10 individual mRNA species in the same relative proportions. In order to assess the information available concerning this and related questions it is necessary to examine first how the reovirus transcriptase transcribes single-stranded RNA *in vitro*.

6.5.1.   Transcription *In Vitro*

A variety of particles derived from reovirions as a result of the more or less complete removal of the outer capsid shell transcribe reovirus genome RNA into single-stranded RNA *in vitro*; among these are SVP isolated from infected cells (Levin *et al.*, 1970*b*; Chang and Zweerink, 1971; Silverstein *et al.*, 1972) and the cores produced as the result of chymotryptic digestion (Shatkin and Sipe, 1968*a*; Skehel and Joklik, 1969; Banerjee and Shatkin, 1970; Joklik, 1972). The reaction catalyzed by all these particles is the same: it is the completely asymmetric transcription of all ten genome RNA segments into single-stranded RNA molecules which, as shown by competitive hybridization analysis, possess the same polarity (plus) as reovirus messenger RNA molecules isolated from the polyribosomes of infected cells (Hay and Joklik, 1971). The 5′-terminal nucleotide of all transcripts synthesized both *in vitro* and *in vivo* is G (Levin *et al.*, 1970*a*; Banerjee *et al.*, 1971*a*; Ward *et al.*, 1972), bearing either ppp- (Nichols *et al.*, 1972*b*) or pp groups (Banerjee *et al.*, 1971*a*; Ward *et al.*, 1972); the presence of the latter is most probably due to the presence within the virion of the nucleoside triphosphate phosphohydrolase (see footnote p. 261). All transcripts have C_{OH} at their 3′ termini (Banerjee *et al.*, 1971*b*).

The transcripts are of the same length as their double-stranded templates; this is indicated by the fact that their sedimentation coefficients are the same as those of denatured double-stranded RNA segments (Skehel and Joklik, 1969; Banerjee and Shatkin, 1970) and by the fact that double-stranded hybrids formed by them and minus-strands (derived from virion RNA) possess exactly the same electrophoretic mobilities as the double-stranded genome RNA segments which are present in virions, which indicates the absence of even short, unpaired, single-stranded tails (Skehel and Joklik, 1969; Ito and Joklik, 1972*a,b*). By the same criteria, the transcripts are exactly the same length as the ten species of mRNA molecules formed *in vivo* (Watanabe *et al.*, 1968*b*; Zweerink and Joklik, 1970; Hay and Joklik, 1971), which are known to be exactly the same length as the genome RNA segments; in fact, they *are* the plus strands of progeny genome RNA (see below).

Transcription is generally measured either by determining the amount of labeled nucleoside triphosphates incorporated into acid-insoluble material (Shatkin and Sipe, 1968*a*; Skehel and Joklik, 1969) or by optical techniques. The most sensitive optical technique involves fluorimetric measurement of RNA-ethidium bromide (EtBr) complexes; at low concentrations EtBr does not inhibit the transcriptase, but it binds to reovirus single-stranded RNA, thereby producing an increase in fluorescence which can be measured constantly so as to provide a continuous measure of transcription (Kapuler, 1971). The fact that EtBr binds to reovirus mRNA demonstrates that it has a complex secondary structure; in fact, the *s* and *m* reovirus RNA species appear to possess almost as much secondary structure as MS2, R17, and f2 phage RNA, and the *l* RNA species appears to possess about one-half as much (Warrington *et al.*, 1973). This structure is also indicated by the fact that unless special precautions are taken to eliminate all traces of ribonuclease from transcriptase reaction mixtures, the sedimentation coefficients of the transcripts are indeed 25, 18, and 14 S in plain sucrose density gradients, but become considerably less in sucrose in 90% dimethylsulfoxide–sucrose density gradients, in which RNA strands are unfolded so that the presence of nicks in portions of the molecules normally present as hydrogen-bonded double-stranded regions is revealed (Hay and Joklik, unpublished results). The secondary structure of reovirus mRNA can, therefore, be thought of in terms of alternating looped and helical regions as formulated in the flower model proposed for MS2 RNA by Min Jou *et al.*(1972).

The transcription catalyzed by the transcriptase is fully conservative, i.e., neither strand of the double-stranded template appears among the products (Skehel and Joklik, 1969; Levin *et al.*, 1970*b*). Its action is therefore analogous to that of the classical DNA-dependent RNA polymerases. It is, however, not inhibited by actinomycin D, presumably because this compound fails to bind to reovirus double-stranded RNA (Gomatos *et al.*, 1964; Kudo and Graham, 1965; Shatkin, 1965*b*; Loh and Soergel, 1965; Shatkin and Rada, 1967 *a,b*).

Under optimal conditions all ten template segments are transcribed at the same rate, i.e., equal masses of all ten transcripts are formed; as a consequence, the number of molecules of the various transcripts formed is inversely proportional to their molecular weight (Skehel and Joklik, 1969). However, this holds only for conditions under which the overall rate of transcription is optimal; this requires high concentrations of the four nucleosides triphosphates and of Mg^{2+}. If these concentrations are decreased, the overall rate of polymerization decreases, but the rate of transcription of the various segments does not decline to the same extent. If, for example, the Mg^{2+} concentration is decreased from 10 mM to 1 mM, the ratio of the relative rates of synthesis of *s* and *l* transcripts changes from 1 to 5; and when the concentration of one of the nucleoside triphosphates is decreased from 2 mM, to 2 μM, only one *s* transcript is formed, the *s*4, a fact which was utilized in sequencing its 5′ end (Nichols *et al.*, 1972*b*) (see below). The transcription pattern *in vitro*, i.e., the uncontrolled transcription pattern, is thus a function of the substrate and Mg^{2+} concentration.

There is no transcription at all if any one of the nucleoside triphosphates is omitted altogether. The ability of the transcriptase to use nucleoside triphosphates is not limited to those of A, G, U, and C; 5-BrUTP and 5-BrCTP also serve as substrates (Kapuler, 1970). Its optimum temperature is very high, between 47°C and 52°C, but it is rapidly inactivated at 55°C (Skehel and Joklik, 1969; Kapuler, 1970). Its temperature coefficient between 34°C and 44°C is an extraordinarily high 14.

The rate of nucleotide addition, under optimum conditions, has been estimated at about 7–8 nucleotide residues per second on the basis of intact transcripts of the s and l classes appearing between 1 and 2 minutes and 4 and 8 minutes, respectively, after the addition of label (Skehel and Joklik, 1969). Using nucleoside triphosphates of higher specific activity, Banerjee and Shatkin (1970) found l transcripts being formed within one minute; this corresponds to a rate of nucleotide residue addition of over 60 per second. Strangely enough, the mass of transcripts formed in 60 minutes generally no more than equals the mass of template; this corresponds to a rate of nucleotide addition no more than one-fifth of even the lesser of these two estimates (Skehel and Joklik, 1969). The reason for the difference is not known. It is conceivable that the interval between completion and reinitiation of transcription is long in relation to the time necessary for transcription; however, not only does the first round of transcription appear to be initiated efficiently on all templates, but such a mode of transcription would not lead readily to the formation of equal masses of all transcripts in unit time without some rather unlikely *ad hoc* assumptions. In addition, it is not likely that only a small fraction of cores are active in transcription since the density of all cores increases by about 0.02 g/ml when transcription is initiated (Skehel and Joklik, 1969). Yet another explanation would be that each particle only synthesizes one transcript at a time; however, this is not so since cores from which up to 9 transcripts protrude have been visualized by electron microscopy, strongly suggesting that all ten genome RNA segments can be transcribed simultaneously (Gillies *et al.*, 1971). Further work is clearly required to explain why the overall rate of RNA synthesis is slower than expected. In spite of this phenomenon, very large amounts of reovirus mRNA can be synthesized *in vitro* because reovirus is easily prepared in quantity and because the transcriptase is active for very long periods of time (more than 48 hours, see for example Levin *et al.*, 1970b). As a result, reovirus cores represent one of the most convenient sources of pure mRNA.

6.5.2. Transcription *In Vivo*

Early mRNA plays a unique role in reovirus multiplication: since parental genomes are not uncoated, it is the sole carrier of genetic information from parent to progeny. It is transcribed by the SVP, to which parental virions are uncoated, but only after a curious lag. Infecting reovirus particles are converted to SVP that possess the transcriptase in its active form within 60 minutes (Silverstein *et al.*, 1970; Chang and Zweerink, 1971), but sensitive hybridization techniques have shown that almost no viral mRNA is detectable in infected cells for about 2 hours (Wiebe and Joklik, unpublished results) (see Fig. 11). The reason for this is probably that SVP are only slowly liberated from the lysosomes within which they are formed (see above); although SVP within lysosomes might well be capable of transcribing their RNA, only very few transcipts are in fact formed, either because lysosomes contain no nucleoside triphosphates or because the transcripts that are formed are immediately degraded, or for some other reason.

Late reovirus mRNA is transcribed by immature progeny virus particles (see below). The amount of late mRNA that is formed greatly exceeds that of early mRNA. Estimates of the relative amounts come from two types of approaches: cells in which infection is allowed to proceed in the presence of cycloheximide so as to prevent the formation of progeny particles (Watanabe *et al.*, 1967a,b), and cells infected with *ts* mutants negative for double-stranded RNA synthesis (Ito and Joklik, 1972a). Both approaches agree that 80–95% of reovirus mRNA is synthesized by transcriptase present in immature progeny virus particles and is thus late mRNA. There is little doubt that the transcriptase that was isolated some time ago from infected cells and that resisted purification owing to its insolubility (Gomatos 1968, 1970) comprised predominantly a population of immature progeny virus particles (see above).

The enzyme that transcribes both early and late reovirus mRNA is the same: it is the virion-associated transcriptase. As pointed out above, the substrates for this enzyme are nucleoside triphosphates; nucleoside diphosphates are completely inactive. Recently however an enzyme system has been found in the larger-particle fraction of infected mouse L fibroblasts which appears to support the synthesis of reovirus mRNA and double-stranded RNA (see below) from nucleoside diphosphates (Schochetman and Millward, 1972). The mechanism of this synthesis apparently involves a nucleoside diphosphokinase that is active only in infected cells (since incubation of the corresponding fraction from normal cells with cores and the four nucleoside diphosphates fails to support RNA transcription). There is no evidence to suggest that such an enzyme might be virus-coded.

It is of considerable interest that reovirus mRNA does not contain a sequence of poly A at its 3′ terminus (Stoltzfus et al., 1973). The only other messenger RNA families known to share this property are histone mRNAs (Adesnik and Darnell, 1972) and the "scarce" herpesvirus mRNA species (Silverstein et al., 1973). The translation of reovirus mRNA has so far shown no unusual features (apart from its high efficiency) (see below); this argues against a function of mRNA-associated poly A in the control of translation.

6.5.3. Relative Rates of Transcription of Individual Species of mRNA Molecules Throughout the Infection Cycle

We come now to the question of whether the reovirus genome expresses itself freely throughout the multiplication cycle, or whether the transcription and translation of some of its segments is suppressed during certain phases of the cycle.

Information concerning the rate of synthesis of the individual species of reovirus mRNA is readily obtained by hybridizing pulse-labeled viral mRNA to unlabeled double-stranded RNA, separating the resulting hybrids by polyacrylamide gel electrophoresis, and determining the amount of radioactivity in each hybrid species (Watanabe et al., 1968b; Zweerink and Joklik, 1970). Suitable controls to correct for differences in the hybridization efficiencies among the various mRNA species must of course be carried out. Since the stability of all species of mRNA is approximately the same for labeling periods up to about 2 hours (Watanabe et al., 1968b), the amount of label incorporated into each is a valid measure of the frequency with which it is transcribed.*

Analysis along these lines has led to interesting results. Zweerink and Joklik (1970) found that the relative transcription frequencies of the ten species of mRNA were constant throughout the infection cycle, from the earliest time that they could be measured (from 2 to 4 hours after infection, under conditions when progeny double-stranded RNA

---

* The reason for quantitating reovirus mRNA in this manner is that double-stranded RNA yields much tighter bands on electrophoresis in polyacrylamide gels than single-stranded RNA. However, techniques for separating all 10 species of single-stranded RNA by polyacrylamide gel electrophoresis have recently been developed (Floyd et al., 1974; Schuerch and Joklik, unpublished results).

TABLE 10

Approximate Relative Transcription
Frequencies of Reovirus mRNA Species
In Vitro and *In Vivo*[a]

mRNA species	*In vitro*	*In vivo*
s4	1.0	1.0
s3	1.0	1.0
s2	0.88	0.5
s1	0.88	0.5
m3	0.5	0.5
m2	0.5	0.3
m1	0.5	0.15
l3	0.275	0.05
l2	0.275	0.05
l1	0.275	0.05

[a] From Zweerink and Joklik (1970).

synthesis began just before 4 hours) to the end of the cycle. These relative frequencies were not the same as those with which the various reovirus mRNA species were transcribed by cores *in vitro* (Skehel and Joklik, 1969). The relative transciption frequencies *in vivo* and *in vitro* are listed in Table 10. It is doubtful, however, whether the differences are evidence for regulation of transcription *in vivo;* it is more likely that their explanation is as follows: The *in vitro* pattern, in which nucleotides are added to all ten transcript species at the same rate, applies to "optimal" conditions, i.e., high concentrations of nucleoside triphosphates and Mg^{2+}, when the transcription rates are maximal. As pointed out above, when the concentration of either Mg^{2+} or of one of the nucleoside triphosphates is decreased, the overall rate of transcription declines, and the frequencies with which the individual mRNA segments are then transcribed begin to diverge markedly. Thus, although all genome RNA segments are transcribed equally rapidly when transcription proceeds at its maximum rate, the fact that this is not so *in vivo* may merely reflect the fact that the Mg^{2+} and/or nucleoside triphosphate concentrations within the cell are lower than those required to support the maximal rate of transcription *in vitro*.*

* It has recently been found that progeny genome RNA segments are synthesized sequentially, S segments being formed first and L segments last; and that, once formed, they are transcribed into mRNA (Zweerink, 1974) (see below). This reaction sequence could give rise to a steady state in which cells contain more S than M or L templates, which may result in greater amounts of s than m or l transcripts being synthesized, as is actually observed. However, it is unlikely that this state could account for the considerable variations in transcription frequencies within size classes (see Table 10).

Watanabe *et al.* (1968*b*) reported results which differ from these. They found that during the early stages of the infection cycle, prior to the formation of double-stranded RNA, only four species of mRNA were transcribed, namely *s*4, *s*3, *m*3, and *l*3; furthermore, in the presence of cycloheximide the same four species of mRNA, and only these four, were formed. Thus, whereas Zweerink and Joklik (1970) found no specific controls over the transcription of either early or late reovirus mRNA, Watanabe *et al.* (1968*b*) found that early reovirus mRNA comprised only four RNA species, while late mRNA comprised all ten. These two sets of results have not yet been reconciled. The following findings from related investigations are relevant in this connection. First, *ts* mutants that are unable to synthesize more than 1% of normal amounts of double-stranded RNA synthesize all ten species of messenger RNA at the nonpermissive temperature (Ito and Joklik, 1972*a*; Cross and Fields, 1972). This implies that the particles which synthesize only four mRNA species are precursors of SVP. Second, when reovirions are digested with chymotrypsin *in vitro*, the earliest degradation products to display transcriptase activity, namely those that lack polypeptide $\sigma 3$ and an 8000-dalton fragment of $\mu 2$ and correspond exactly in polypeptide constitution to SVP that are formed in infected cells, transcribe all ten segments of genome RNA (Joklik, unpublished results). Third, SVP isolated from infected cells transcribe all 10 segments of genome RNA (Levin *et al.*, 1970). Fourth, the SVP$_i$ characterized by Shatkin and LaFiandra (1972) (see above) transcribe all ten segments of genome RNA *in vitro*; they also do so when they infect cells. However, when they infect cells in the presence of cycloheximide, only RNA species *s*4, *s*3, and *m*3 (as well as a small amount of *l* species RNA) are formed (Shatkin and LaFiandra, 1972). Thus, the same particles that *in vitro* and *in vivo* catalyze the transcription of all ten species of genome RNA, transcribe only four *in vivo* in the presence of cycloheximide. If this effect is indeed due to inhibition of protein synthesis, then some cellular protein which pre-exists in uninfected cells actively represses the transcription of six species of reovirus mRNA, and *de novo* protein synthesis (cell or virus-coded) is required *after* infection in order to reverse its effect (in other words, to derepress their transcription). Fifth, it may be significant that the species of mRNA that are formed in the presence of cycloheximide, in particular *s*4, *s*3, and *m*3, are those that are formed in greatest amount in its absence (Zweerink and Joklik, 1970). This suggests that the "cycloheximide" effect may be an artifact in the sense that when the overall rate of mRNA transcription is low (as the rate of early mRNA transcription always is), those mRNA species that are only formed in small amounts may tend to be lost during the manipulations involved in mRNA isolation and hybridization, thus giving the illusion that the species that are formed in largest amounts are the only ones formed. Careful further work will clearly be required to determine whether early reovirus mRNA really only comprises four of the ten possible species.

6.6. The Translation of Reovirus mRNA

6.6.1. The Translation of Reovirus mRNA *In Vitro*

The translation of the RNA synthesized by the reovirus transcriptase has been studied *in vitro* in two types of systems. The first employed extracts of infected L cells that contained virus-specific polyribosomes and supported the completion (rather than the initiation) of reovirus-specified polypeptides (McDowell and Joklik, 1971). In these extracts amino acids were incorporated predominantly into eight polypeptides (Fig. 12B): six of these possessed electrophoretic mobilities in SDS-polyacrylamide gels identical with six of the seven reovirus capsid polypeptides, namely $\lambda 1$, $\lambda 2$, $\mu 1$, $\sigma 1$, $\sigma 2$, and $\sigma 3$, while the other two, which migrated just behind $\mu 1$ and between $\sigma 2$ and $\sigma 3$, were designated $\mu 0$ and $\sigma 2A$, respectively; they proved to be identical in electrophoretic mobility with two "essential nonstructural" polypeptides that are formed in infected cells (see below). No $\mu 2$, the principal virion capsid component, was formed in this cell-free system; instead large amounts of $\mu 1$, a minor virion constituent which is the precursor of $\mu 2$ (see below), were synthesized.

The second type of systems consisted of those in which initiation occurs. It was first found that reovirus mRNA transcribed by cores *in vitro* stimulated amino acid incorporation into polypeptides some 10,000–15,000 daltons in size when incubated with supplemented L-cell S 150 extracts and ribosomes, and that pretreatment of the mRNA with formaldehyde increased the extent of incorporation severalfold (Levin *et al.*, 1971). Subsequently it was reported that a cell-free protein-synthesizing system from L cells was capable of translating *m* species of reovirus mRNA molecules into polypeptides which coelectrophoresed with μ polypeptides, and that *s* species of mRNA molecules were translated into σ-sized polypeptides (Graziadei and Lengyel, 1972). More recently, *in vitro* protein-synthesizing systems

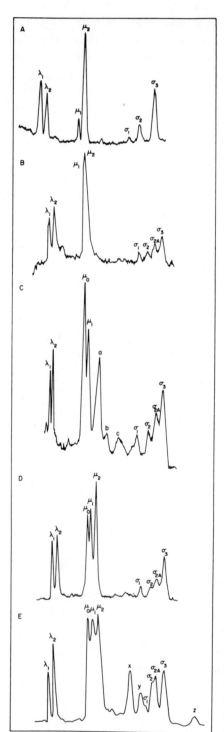

Fig. 12. Reovirus-specified polypeptides synthesized *in vitro* and *in vivo*. Tracings of autoradiograms of polyacrylamide gels. Direction of electrophoresis is from left to right. (A) Capsid polypeptides of reovirions; (B) polypeptides synthesized *in vitro* by a cell-free protein-synthesizing extract of cells infected with reovirus; (C) polypeptides synthesized *in vitro* by a cell-free protein-synthesizing extract of rabbit reticulocytes in response to reovirus RNA transcribed *in vitro* by reovirus cores; (D) polypeptides synthesized *in vivo* from 17.5 to 19.5 hours after infection at 31°C; (E) polypeptides synthesized *in vivo* from 5 to 7 hours after infection at 37°C. From McDowell and Joklik, (1971), McDowell *et al.* (1972), and Zweerink *et al.* (1971).

have been developed from several types of cells in which the majority of reovirus mRNA species formed by cores *in vitro* is translated into polypeptides seemingly identical to those synthesized in infected cells (McDowell *et al.*, 1972). The most efficient of these systems were derived from rabbit reticulocytes and Krebs II ascites tumor cells, but systems from L cells, HeLa cells, and CHO cells were also active. In the latter systems from 5 to 7 complete viral polypeptides were synthesized; in the former two the synthesis of eight species of polypeptides which possessed electrophoretic mobilities in SDS-polyacrylamide gels identical with those synthesized in the extracts of infected L cells described above could be clearly detected (Fig. 12C). Once again, large amounts of $\mu1$ and of the two nonstructural polypeptides $\mu0$ and $\sigma2A$ were synthesized along with the other structural polypeptides, but $\mu2$ was again not formed.

Thus, in both *in vitro* systems the ten species of reovirus mRNA are translated into eight polypeptides. When the distance migrated by these eight polypeptides in SDS-polyacrylamide gels is plotted against the distance traveled by the genome RNA segments, a straight line is obtained when the following assignments are made: polypeptide $\lambda1$ is coded by genome RNA segment *L1*; $\lambda2$ by either *L2* or *L3*; $\mu0$ by *M1*; $\mu1$ by *M2*; $\sigma1$ by *S1*; $\sigma2$ by *S2*; $\sigma2A$ by *S3*; and $\sigma3$ by *S4* (Zweerink *et al.*, 1971). Evidence that $\mu1$ is coded by *M2* has been obtained by the use of *ts* mutants (Ito and Joklik, 1972c) (see below); but proof that all these pairings are correct will require characterization of the polypeptides into which individual species of mRNA are translated *in vitro*. The polypeptides corresponding to one of the *L* segments and to *M3* have not yet been found, probably because they are formed in small amounts only and possess electrophoretic mobilities close to those of other λ and μ polypeptides.

The fact that reovirus mRNA is translated faithfully, combined with its availability in large amounts, has caused systems in which it is translated to be very advantageous for the study of the mechanism of protein synthesis in mammalian systems. This work is only just beginning since the advantages of reovirus RNA as mRNA have only recently been realized. However, it has already been shown that all three size classes of mRNA, especially when treated with low concentrations of HCHO, form initiation complexes with ribosomal subunits, Met-tRNA$_F$ and GTP; that the Pur-acceptor reaction leading to the formation of Met-Pur proceeds readily; and that fusidic acid in concentrations which have no effect on the utilization of Met-tRNA$_F$ completely inhibits the utilization of Met-tRNA$_M$ (Levin *et al.*, 1972).

These results suggest that reovirus mRNA contains AUG initiator
codons that form complexes with Met-tRNA$_F$ at a puromycin-sensitive
site on the ribosome.

6.6.2. Translation of Reovirus mRNA *In Vivo*

The overall rate of protein synthesis does not decrease for several
hours following infection with reovirus (Gomatos and Tamm, 1963c;
Kudo and Graham, 1965; Ensminger and Tamm, 1969a). Reovirus-
specified proteins are synthesized very slowly during the early period,
but when late mRNA begins to be formed rapidly, virus-specified protein synthesis very soon replaces that specified by the host (Zweerink
and Joklik, 1970). The overall rate of virus-specified polypeptide synthesis closely parallels that of virus-specified mRNA synthesis and is
influenced in the same manner by the multiplicity of infection and the
temperature of incubation (see above).

Virus-specific polypeptides may be conveniently concentrated
from extracts of infected cells by precipitation with antiviral antiserum
(Fields *et al.*, 1972). Both complement-fixing, group-specific and
serotype-specific antigenic determinants can be detected.

About two-thirds of the reovirus mRNA formed in infected cells
cosediments with polyribosomes (Prevec and Graham, 1966; Shatkin
and Rada, 1967a; Ward *et al.*, 1972). All species of mRNA are
associated with polyribosomes in approximately the same proportions
in which they are transcribed (Ward *et al.*, 1972). As a rule this would
be taken as evidence that all species of mRNA have roughly the same
affinity for ribosomes. There are, however, some unusual features
about the physical state of this RNA; in particular, RNA from both
heavy (> 30 ribosomes) and light (5–8 ribosomes) polyribosomes
consists of similar relative amounts of the *l, m,* and *s* classes of
reovirus mRNA (Ward *et al.*, 1972). This evidence suggested that the
RNA species may be linked; this theory was confirmed when it was
found that on disruption of polyribosomes with EDTA some of the
RNA from the heavy, though not from the light, polyribosome region
existed in the form of nucleoprotein complexes that contained reovirus
capsid polypeptides of all three size classes, with those of the μ class
predominating (Ward and Shatkin, 1972). Intracellular reovirus
mRNA that sediments between about 100 and 600 S thus occurs in two
forms, discrete mRNA molecules in polyribosomes and ribonucleoprotein complexes. The significance of the latter is not clear. On the one
hand, they may have no function in protein synthesis and may

represent the most immature form of virion precursors, which Zweerink et al. (1972) have shown to possess sedimentation coefficients ranging from 250 500 S (see below); on the other hand, they may have some function in regulating viral polypeptide synthesis (Ward and Shatkin, 1972). They are clearly quite different from the ribonucleo-protein particles that accumulate as a result of the breakdown of polyribosomes when infected cells are deprived of essential amino acids (Christman et al., 1973). These particles sediment with about 50 S, possess a density of 1.40 g/ml, and collectively contain all ten species of reovirus mRNA, but no viral (or ribosomal) protein. They are rapidly mobilized into functional polyribosomes when the cells are restored to normal growth medium.

The nature of the reovirus-specified polypeptides that are synthesized in infected cells can be readily determined by polyacryl-amide gel electrophoresis of infected cell extracts followed by autora-diography. During the early stages of the infection cycle, when virus-specified polypeptides make up only a small proportion of the total protein that is formed, it is necessary to use actinomycin D and a profile subtraction technique (Zweerink and Joklik, 1970) or immune precipitation (Fields et al., 1972) in order to discern the pattern clearly; later on, when infected cells synthesize reovirus-specified polypeptides almost exclusively, this is not necessary. A typical gel profile of the polypeptides synthesized during the interval 17.5–19.5 hours after infection at 31°C is shown in Fig. 12D (Zweerink et al., 1971). It is very similar to that of the translation products of reovirus mRNA in vitro. In vivo, nine polypeptides are synthesized; six are identical with the six capsid polypeptides $\lambda1$, $\lambda2$, $\mu1$, $\sigma1$, $\sigma2$, and $\sigma3$, two are the noncapsid polypeptides $\mu0$ and $\sigma2A$, and $\mu2$ is formed as well. Just as in vitro, no polypeptides corresponding to mRNA species L2 or L3 and M3 have yet been detected. This pattern is found at all stages of the infection cycle (Zweerink and Joklik, 1970), indicating that the frequency with which the individual reovirus-specified polypeptides are translated is either uncontrolled, or if it is controlled, that this control does not change during the cell cycle. As a result, the populations of early and late polypeptides are the same, as is demonstrated also by the fact that ts mutants that are negative for the synthesis of double-stranded RNA form all capsid polypeptides (see below). Further, not only are the same nine polypeptides synthesized at all stages of the infection cycle, but they are also always synthesized in about the same relative proportions which approximate those of their in vitro translation; it seems, therefore, that the translation of individual species of reovirus mRNA is not subject to any controls that operate only in infected cells. It is interesting in this regard that capsid polypeptides are formed in infected cells in approximately the same relative proportions as those in which they occur in virions.

The only difference between the patterns of polypeptides formed *in vitro* and *in vivo* is that polypeptide $\mu 2$ is formed *in vivo* in large amounts. Polypeptide $\mu 2$ is not a primary gene product: This is shown by (1) the fact that whereas the relative amount of label incorporated into all other polypeptides is independent of the duration of the labeling period, the amount of label incorporated into $\mu 2$ increases with increasing time (Zweerink and Joklik, 1970), and (2) pulse-chase experiments which demonstrate that as the amount of label in $\mu 2$ increases, that in $\mu 1$ decreases (Zweerink *et al.*, 1971). The enzyme that effects the cleavage of $\mu 1$ to $\mu 2$, which apparently removes an 8000-dalton fragment of the molecule from its amino-terminus (Pett *et al.*, 1973) (see above), has not yet been characterized. It does not operate *in vitro* when endogenous reovirus mRNA is translated in cell-free protein-synthesizing systems derived from infected cells (see above).

The polypeptide pattern shown in Fig. 12D is obtained when the infection cycle proceeds at 31°C; if infected cells are incubated instead at 37°C, the profile shown in Fig. 12E is obtained (Zweerink *et al.*, 1971). It reveals the presence of three additional polypeptides, which are designated x, y, and z. They are breakdown products of either $\mu 1$ or, more likely, $\mu 2$; they are very similar in size to certain intermediates of $\mu 2$ breakdown which appear when virions are digested with chymotrypsin *in vitro* (Joklik, 1972) (see above). Since they do not appear in cells infected at 31°C, in which virus yields are considerably greater than in cells infected at 37°C, they are obviously not essential; they have, therefore, been termed "nonessential non-capsid polypeptides." It is noteworthy in this connection that cytopathic effects are much more marked at 37°C than at 31°C, which no doubt accounts for the higher virus yields at the lower temperatures. The likeliest explanation for the genesis of polypeptides x, y, and z is that at the higher temperature damage to lysosomes causes proteolytic enzymes to spill out into the cytoplasm or that proteolytic enzymes then become activated by some other mechanism, and that these enzymes attack those viral polypeptides that are most susceptible to them, in particular $\mu 1$ and $\mu 2$.

Reovirus capsid polypeptides isolated following solubilization of virions are very insoluble when they are separated from the protein denaturants that were used to prepare them (see above). It is not remarkable, therefore, that the majority of intracellular capsid polypeptides exist in the form of particulate structures or aggregates which range in size and complexity from simple complexes of $\mu2$ and $\sigma3$ (the outer capsid shell components) to full and empty capsids (Huismans and Joklik, unpublished results). However, there is also a sizeable pool of free capsid polypeptides within the cell, the size of which is probably determined by the affinity of each individual polypeptide for the others and for the various morphogenetic intermediates.

6.6.3. Relation between the Frequencies of Transcription and Translation of Individual Species of Reovirus mRNA

Since not all polypeptide species are formed in equimolar amounts, the question arises whether there is any correlation between the amount of each that is formed and the relative abundance of each corresponding mRNA species, that is, whether each mRNA species is translated with equal frequency. The data listed in Table 11, which are calculated from the profiles shown in Fig. 12, show that this is not the case (Joklik, 1973a,b): the ratios of the translation to the transcription

TABLE 11

Approximate Relative Frequencies of Transcription and Translation of the Ten Species of Reovirus mRNA *In Vivo*[a]

mRNA species	Transcription frequency	Polypeptide species	Translation frequency	$\left(\dfrac{\text{Translation frequency}}{\text{Transcription frequency}}\right)$
s4	1.0	$\sigma3$	0.7	0.7
s3	1.0	$\sigma2A$	0.3	0.3
s2	0.5	$\sigma2$	0.2	0.4
s1	0.5	$\sigma1$	0.05	0.1
m3	0.5	?	<0.01	<0.02
m2	0.3	$\mu1(\mu2)$	1.0	3.3
m1	0.15	$\mu0$	0.5	3.3
l3	0.05 }	$\lambda2 + ?$	0.15 and <0.01	3.0 and <0.2
l2	0.05 }			
l1	0.05	$\lambda1$	0.1	2.0

[a] From Zweerink and Joklik (1970) and Zweerink *et al.* (1971).

frequencies range, on a molar basis, all the way from more than 3 for
$\mu 1/m2$, $\mu 0/m1$, and $\lambda 2/l3$ or $l2$, down to 0.1 for $\sigma 1/s1$, and even less
for $m3$, the most frequently transcribed m species, the corresponding
polypeptide of which has not yet even been detected. The conclusion is
that the various mRNA species are translated with very different frequencies. The reason for this is not clear. Most probably, the elements
that control translation frequency reside in the nucleotide sequences
between the 5′ termini of the mRNA molecules and the initiation
codons. Reovirus offers several advantages for studying their nature.
The first is the fact that reovirus mRNA molecules can be obtained in
large amounts and that techniques for sequencing them are available;
indeed, the first 25 nucleotides of one s species, have already been
shown to be

$$(p)ppGCCAUUUUUGCU(C,U)UCCAGACGUUG$$

(Nichols *et al*., 1972*b*). This sequence does not contain the initiation
codon AUG, the presence of which would be expected on the basis of
ribosome- and Met-tRNA$_F$-binding studies (Levin *et al*., 1972) (see
above). This indicates that just as in the case of R17, MS2, and Qβ
RNA, an untranslated region, presumably with regulatory functions,
precedes the coding portion of the mRNA molecule. A second advantage is that the reovirus system provides an unusual opportunity for
studying a family of mRNA molecules, the relative translation frequencies of which can be measured, thereby providing a convenient
correlation between structure and function. The reovirus system,
therefore, offers the hope that with it information of general applicability can be obtained concerning the manner in which the
untranslated 5-terminal nucleotide sequences of mRNAs regulate frequency of translation.

6.7. The Formation of Progeny Double-Stranded RNA

The fact that the replication of reovirus RNA proceeds by a
mechanism which is totally dissimilar from that by which double-
stranded DNA replicates became evident with the realization that
parental double-stranded RNA is not uncoated, but conserved (Silverstein *et al*., 1970), and that the only way in which genetic information
is passed on from parent to progeny is via plus-stranded transcripts.
The function of these transcripts must therefore be twofold: They must
be translated into polypeptides, and they must also serve as the tem-

plates for the transcription of minus strands. If these minus strands remained associated with their plus strands, progeny double-stranded RNA would be generated. Evidence for the validity of this mechanism was provided by Schonberg *et al.* (1971), who investigated the time in the infection cycle when each of the two strands of progeny double-stranded RNA was synthesized. This was achieved by labeling cells at various stages of the infection cycle, and then hybridizing the progeny double-stranded RNA with excess unlabeled plus-stranded RNA. If progeny plus and minus strands are formed simultaneously and both are labeled equally, half of the label should appear in the hybrid; if only the plus strands are labeled, none should appear; and if only the minus strands are formed while label is present, all of the label should appear in the hybrids. It was found in this way that the plus and minus strands of progeny double-stranded RNA are not formed simultaneously, but that a significant portion of the plus strands are formed during the early stages of the infection cycle, while minus strands are only formed later, when double-stranded RNA actually appears. The enzyme catalyzing the formation of plus strands is presumably the transcriptase; the enzyme catalyzing the formation of minus strands is an enzyme often referred to as the "replicase," but more accurately described as the SS→DS RNA polymerase (Zweerink *et al.*, 1972).

The synthesis of reovirus minus strands, and the concomitant formation of progeny genomes, has been studied extensively in extracts of infected cells. The following information concerning this reaction and the structures with which it is associated has been obtained:

1. The newly synthesized minus strands do not separate from their plus-stranded templates. Minus strand synthesis results in the formation of double-stranded RNA and is detected as such. The double-stranded RNA product is indistinguishable from reovirus-genome RNA (Watanabe *et al.*, 1968a; Acs *et al.*, 1971; Sakuma and Watanabe, 1971; Zweerink *et al.*, 1972)

2. Equivalent numbers of all species of double-stranded RNA are formed (Watanabe *et al.*, 1968a; Acs *et al.*, 1971). Structures which contain intact plus strands and incomplete minus strands (that is, the synthesis of which has been initiated *in vivo*) are intermediates in the formation of species of each of the three size classes of double-stranded RNA; this is consistent with the hypothesis that each plus strand has an individual initiation site for minus-strand synthesis (Sakuma and Watanabe, 1972a). Minus-strand synthesis proceeds in the 5′ to 3′ direction (Sakuma and Watanabe, 1972a).

3.   Under optimal conditions synthesis of minus strands proceeds for very short periods of time only (less than 10 minutes) (Sakuma and Watanabe, 1971; Zweerink *et al.*, 1972). If the concentration of any one of the nucleoside triphosphates is reduced, the rate of the reaction decreases and the time for which RNA is polymerized is correspondingly increased, but the total amount of RNA formed never exceeds the amount of template (Zweerink *et al.*, 1972). This information suggests that plus strands are transcribed into minus strands once and once only, and that no new structures in which minus-strand synthesis can be initiated are formed in *in vitro*.

4.   The template for minus-strand synthesis is destroyed by treatment with ribonuclease, demonstrating not only that it is accessible to the enzyme but also that it is single-stranded (Acs *et al.*, 1971).

5.   The structures within which double-stranded RNA is formed and with which the SS→DS RNA polymerase is therefore associated are normally associated with large particles.* When separated from them by treatment with deoxycholate or NP40, they sediment heterogeneously from 300 to 600 S; their density in CsCl is about 1.34 g/ml (Zweerink *et al.*, 1972). Double-stranded RNA is not released from these particles but remains associated with them. Transcription of minus strands appears to be associated with or closely followed by a change in their protein complement since the newly formed double-stranded RNA is not accessible to ribonuclease at low ionic strength and, therefore, appears to reside in enzyme-impermeable structures (Acs *et al.*, 1971). The protein complement of these "product particles" which contain 10 segments of double-stranded RNA appears to be remarkably similar to that of virions since, when treated with chymotrypsin, they give rise to particles which have the same density (1.43 g/ml) as cores (Zweerink *et al.*, 1972; see also Sakuma and Watanabe, 1972*b*). Recently, evidence has been obtained that the double-stranded molecules of the three size classes are formed sequentially in particles with progressively increasing sedimentation coefficients: Thus, molecules of the *S, M,* and *L* classes are formed in particles that sediment with about 300, 450, and 550 S, respectively (Zweerink, 1974). Analysis of the polypeptide composition of these particles indicates that they contain the core polypeptides (with the smallest parti-

---

* This is consistent with the observation of Gomatos (1967) that reovirus double-stranded RNA never occurs free in the cytoplasm, but that it is always either associated with the large-particle fraction or present in immature or mature virus particles.

cles being deficient in $\lambda2$) and varying amounts of $\mu0$, $\mu1$, and $\mu2$. None except the very largest contain any $\sigma3$.

6. The three classes of particles in which progeny S-, M-, and L-genome segments are formed are intermediates in viral morphogenesis. All appear to possess DS→SS RNA polymerase activity (Sakuma and Watanabe, 1971; Zweerink et al., 1972); they are responsible for synthesizing the major portion (90% or more) of the plus-stranded RNA that is formed in infected cells (see above).

7. The weight of available evidence indicates that the assortment of RNA segments into sets proceeds at the stage of single-stranded rather than double-stranded RNA. The most plausible model is that the structures within which double-stranded RNA arises consist of one molecule of each of the ten plus-stranded RNA species and several virus-specified polypeptides of both the structural and nonstructural variety. Nothing is known yet concerning the mechanism which ensures that each structure receives one, and one only, of each of the ten plus-stranded RNA molecules. At least two possibilities may be envisaged here. The first is that of a recognition mechanism based on RNA–RNA interactions; plus strands may possess anywhere along their length brief sequences that are complementary to sequences on other strands and that can be used for recognition purposes. The second possibility is that of a recognition mechanism based not on RNA–RNA, but on RNA–protein (that is, reovirus-specified capsid or noncapsid protein) interactions. Of these two alternatives, the second is perhaps the more likely.

6.8. Morphogenesis

Little is known as yet concerning the manner in which reovirus particles are assembled. The most immature virion precursors are the particles within which double-stranded RNA is formed (see above): They are RNase-sensitive complexes of the 10 single-stranded RNA species and some virus-specified polypeptides which have not yet been fully characterized. Apparently there are several classes of these complexes which differ in the nature of the RNA species that is transcribed in them as well as in size, the smaller being the precursors of larger: complexes which sediment with about 250 S transcribe the four S species, those which sediment with about 450 S transcribe the three M species, and those that sediment with about 550 S transcribe the three L species (Zweerink, 1974). At the same time, a series of as yet uncharacterized changes in their polypeptide complements occurs, giving rise to a variety of subviral particles, the most stable of which resemble cores in many of their properties. These particles contain RNA in nuclease-resistant form (Acs *et al.*, 1971); their density is that of cores (Sakuma and Watanabe, 1972*b*; Morgan and Zweerink, 1974), but their sedimentation coefficient is 400 S rather than 470 S (Morgan and Zweerink, 1974); they are composed principally of the four core polypeptides $\lambda 1$, $\lambda 2$ (in diminished amount), $\mu 1$, and $\sigma 2$ (Morgan and Zweerink, 1974); they possess transcriptase activity (Zweerink *et al.*, 1972); and they resemble cores morphologically (Morgan and Zweerink, 1974). These particles are present in very low amounts in cells infected at 31°C, but they accumulate in cells infected at 39°C, when they are evidently converted to virions less rapidly than they are formed. They are the final products of infection in cells infected at 39°C with mutants of groups B and G (Fields *et al.*, 1971; Morgan and Zweerink, 1974) (see below).

The manner in which these particles gradually mature into virions is not known; however, it is likely that one of the final steps, if not the final step, is the addition of polypeptide $\sigma 3$ which, as has been described above, finally abolishes their transcriptase activity (Astell *et al.*, 1972).

In addition to virions, empty capsids (or top-component particles) usually accumulate late in infection to the extent of some 5% of the total yield. This proportion is increased by omitting lysine from the medium (Loh and Oie, 1969) or by adding ethidium bromide (Lai *et al.*, 1973). Both treatments inhibit the formation of virions, particularly the latter, which permits the isolation of pure top component. Other incomplete virus particles are also sometimes found, especially in cells infected with certain *ts* mutants. Two examples are (1) segments of outer capsid shells, which presumably accumulate because their principal components, $\mu 2$ and $\sigma 3$, are the two polypeptides that are formed in largest amounts in infected cells and therefore the most likely to aggregate into morphologic subunits (Ito and Joklik, unpublished results); and (2) empty virus particles that, while possessing intact outer capsid shells and therefore morphologically identical with virions, lack the two innermost core components, namely $\lambda 1$ and $\sigma 2$ (Matsuhisa and Joklik, 1974). Characterization of such incomplete virus particles may well throw light on the morphogenetic pathway.

6.9. The Genesis of Reovirus Oligonucleotides

The presence of large numbers of oligonucleotides in reovirions has long provided a puzzle. Within the cell they are not found free, but only in association with particulate fractions; they are synthesized in all reovirus-infected cells, irrespective of their type; and they are known to be formed at about the same time as double-stranded RNA (Bellamy and Joklik, 1967*b*; Shatkin and Sipe, 1968*b*). Since some of the virion precursors described in the previous section do not contain oligonucleotides although they do contain double-stranded RNA (Zweerink, personal communication), the question arises as to when in the maturation sequence they are formed. There is no firm answer to this question yet, but a hypothesis which fits the available evidence is that the reovirus oligonucleotides are the products of abortive transcription which arise during the terminal stages of morphogenesis and which become sealed into the nascent virions (Bellamy *et al.*, 1972; Nichols *et al.*, 1972*a*). The arguments in favor of this hypothesis are as follows: As discussed above, the transcriptase is inactive in mature virions; it is activated by the removal from virions of polypeptide $\sigma 3$ and a small portion of $\mu 2$, and it is inactivated by the reassociation of $\sigma 3$ with SVP. Further, transcription of the double-stranded RNA segments is presumably brought about by their movement relative to the catalytic sites of the transcriptase. It is conceivable that when transcription ceases during the final stages of morphogenesis the movement of template relative to enzyme may be inhibited slightly before its ability to form phosphodiester bonds. There may then be a brief period of time when initiation of transcription is abortive so that the enzyme may only be able to transcribe very short stretches of template; these short transcripts may then be sealed into the virus particles which would be maturing at the same time.

If this hypothesis is correct, the nucleotide base sequence of the oligonucleotides would be expected to resemble the 5′-terminal regions of reovirus mRNAs. This is indeed the case: the basic sequence common to all 5′-G-terminated oligonucleotides, GCUA-, is strikingly similar to the 5′-terminal region of one of the *s* strands, which is GC-CUA- (Nichols *et al.*, 1972*a,b*; Bellamy *et al.*, 1972; Stoltzfus and Banerjee, 1972), as well as compatible with the sequence GPy- which appears to be common to the 5′ ends of all reovirus RNA strands (Banerjee and Shatkin, 1971).

Abortive transcription is thus capable of accounting for the origin of the 5′-(p)ppG-terminated oligonucleotides. The presence of the oligoadenylates poses a slightly different problem which has been complicated by the recent discovery that most eukaryotic mRNAs possess long stretches of poly A at their 3′ ends. The possibility has therefore been considered that reovirus plus strands also terminate in poly A sequences, that these sequences mark them as templates for transcription into minus strands, and that in the process they are cleaved and encap-sidated (Stoltzfus and Banerjee, 1972). However this is very unlikely since (1) the amount of poly A per virion (about 850 oligoadenylates of average chain length 10 nucleotide residues (Nichols *et al.*, 1972*a*)) greatly exceeds the amount expected on this hypothesis; (2) the oligoadenylates often terminate in ppp- or pp- (see above), which suggests that they are the products of independent synthetic events; and (3) recent evidence strongly suggests that reovirus plus strands contain no poly A sequences (Stoltzfus *et al.*, 1973) (see above). It is likely, therefore, that the reovirus oligoadenylates are also the products of abortive transcription, the sequences transcribed in this case being se-quences of U. It is known in this connection that a sequence of 5 U residues occupies positions 5–9 inclusive from the 5′ terminus of one of the *s* plus strands (Nichols *et al.*, 1972*b*), and transcription of such a se-quence by a slippage mechanism similar to that described by Chamberlin and Berg (1965) could generate the reovirus oligo-adenylates. Alternatively, the reovirus transcriptase may possess tem-plate-independent poly A polymerase activity.

If the oligonucleotides are abortive transcription products trapped within virions as the result of an idiosyncracy of the final stages of reovirus morphogenesis, they would presumably not be essential for in-fectivity, nor would any other biological function be expected of them. Indeed, several types of particles produced by chymotryptic digestion of reovirions *in vitro* possess high infectivity and little or no oligonu-cleotides (Joklik, 1972; Shatkin and LaFiandra, 1972). The "reovirus" reported by Krug and Gomatos (1969) to be infectious but devoid of oligonucleotides, and which had been purified by treatment with chymotrypsin, may well have consisted of particles of this type.

6.10. Reovirus Temperature-Sensitive Mutants

Temperature-sensitive mutants of reovirus have been sought with the hope that elucidation of the functions that they are unable to perform at the restrictive temperature would contribute to our overall understanding of the series of reactions that constitute multiplication. Cells infected with *ts* mutants at restrictive temperatures are also often used as sources of intermediates on the morphogenetic pathway that only occur in minute amounts in cells infected with wild-type virus.

Two sets of *ts* mutants of reovirus have been isolated. Since they were characterized according to different criteria and used for the study of different portions and aspects of the multiplication cycle, they will be treated separately. It would be very desirable to compare them directly in the same laboratory.

6.10.1.   The Mutants of Fields and Joklik (1969)

A set of about 60 stable *ts* mutants was isolated by mutagenizing virions of the Dearing strain with nitrous acid (NA) or N-methyl-N′-nitroso-nitroguanidine (MNNG) or treating infected cells with proflavine (PRO), and then using the plaque-enlargement technique. These mutants vary in reversion frequency, leakiness, and the temperature which is nonpermissive for them.

6.10.1(a).   Genetic Characterization

Since the reovirus genome consists of a set of ten individual RNA segments, sets of intact segments can be generated by genome-segment reassortment from two or more sets, each containing different mutant segments. In practice, the frequency with which such reassortment occurs reaches very high values; up to 50% of the yield of cells infected with pairs of single mutants may be wild-type virus (Fields and Joklik, 1969). This is not surprising in view of the currently accepted mode of reovirus multiplication (see above); the fact that the frequency of wild-type recombinants is often as low as 1–3% is presumably due to the differing relative growth characteristics of the two sets of mutants and of wild-type virus. The generation of wild-type virus by genome-segment reassortment is usually referred to as recombination, but true recombination involving breakage and reunion of covalent bonds within genome segments has so far not been demonstrated.

Using genome-segment reassortment analysis by infecting cells at the permissive temperature with pairs of *ts* mutants and scoring for the presence or absence of wild-type recombinants among the yields, reovirus mutants have been ordered into seven groups, A–G. Twenty-eight mutants fall into group A, 3 into group B, two into group D, and 1 each into groups C, E, F, and G.

Complementation of the ability to multiply is weak among reoviruses; complementation indices rarely exceed two (Fields and Joklik, 1969). However, complementation of the ability to form single-stranded RNA, which, since most reovirus mRNA is made by virion precursors (see above), requires all functions except very late ones, can readily be detected. Using this test, reovirus mutants can also be ordered into several groups. Although not all mutants have yet been tested, genome-segment reassortment and complementation groupings appear to coincide (Ito and Joklik, 1972*a*).

The frequencies with which pairs of reovirus mutants give rise to wild-type recombinants have been analyzed in detail in order to detect segment linkage or association (Fields, 1971; 1973). None was found.

6.10.1(b). Biochemical Characterization

Prototypes of all mutant classes have been examined for their ability to transcribe mRNA, translate mRNA, and form double-stranded progeny RNA at restrictive temperatures. The results, summarized in Table 12, are as follows:

1. Mutants of groups A, B, F and G are RNA-positive in the sense of synthesizing progeny double-stranded RNA at the nonpermissive temperature; mutants of groups C, D and E are essentially double-stranded RNA negative (less than 1% of normal amounts) (Ito and Joklik, 1972a; Cross and Fields, 1972). When double-stranded RNA is synthesized, the ten segments are always formed in the same relative proportions as in cells infected with wild-type (wt) virus. The group C mutant ts 447 is unable to form, at 39°C, the complexes within which DS RNA is synthesized, but complexes that are formed at 31°C are able to synthesize DS RNA in vitro at 39°C. However, the DS RNA-synthesizing complexes of ts 447 are more heat-labile than those of wild-type virus; this suggests that one of the structural core polypeptides is defective (Matsuhisa and Joklik, 1974). This hypothesis

TABLE 12

Summary of Properties of the Reovirus ts Mutants of Fields and Joklik[a]

Group	Relative amount synthesized at nonpermissive temperatures			Comments
	DS RNA	SS RNA	Protein	
A	100	100	100	Late mutants; mutation in genome segment L2
B	25–50	25–50	50–100	Accumulate corelike particles
C	<0.1	~5	~10	Accumulates outer capsid shells; fails to form DS RNA-synthesizing complexes; may contain mutated λ1 or σ2
D	<0.1	~5	~10	Contain mutated polypeptide μ2; DS RNA synthesis ceases on shift-up
E	<1	~5	5–10	Very early mutant; DS RNA synthesis continues on shift-up
F	50–100	50–100	50–100	Late mutant
G	~15	~20	~20	Possesses ts transcriptase and accumulates corelike particles

[a] For details, see text and the publications cited therein.

is supported by the finding that top-component particles that lack $\lambda 1$ and $\sigma 2$, the two innermost core components, are formed in cells infected with this mutant (Matsuhisa and Joklik, 1974). Mutant *ts* 447 may therefore possess defective $\lambda 1$ or $\sigma 2$. The mutant of group E is a very early mutant: if cells infected with it are exposed to the permissive temperature for as little as 30 minutes at the beginning of the infection cycle, they will subsequently produce normal amounts of double-stranded RNA (and virus yields) at the restrictive temperature. The mutants of group D are capsid polypeptide mutants (Ito and Joklik, 1972*c*).

2. The only mutant to possess a temperature-sensitive transcriptase is the group G mutant *ts* 453. This mutant synthesizes less mRNA *in vitro* than all other mutants, irrespective of the temperature, and its enzyme is more labile at 50°C than that of all others (Cross and Fields, 1972).

3. Mutants of groups A, B, F, and G transcribe 25–100% of normal amounts of mRNA *in vivo* at the nonpermissive temperature; mutants of groups C, D, and E only transcribe about 5–10% as much (Ito and Joklik, 1972*a*; Rise and Cross, 1972). This reflects the fact that mutants of the latter groups are incapable of synthesizing progeny double-stranded RNA. In all cases, all species of mRNA are transcribed in the same relative proportions as in cells infected at the permissive temperature.

4. Mutants of all groups synthesize all major species of capsid polypeptides at the nonpermissive temperature in the same relative proportions as at the permissive temperature, the total amount of capsid polypeptide synthesized being roughly proportional to the overall amount of mRNA transcribed (Fields *et al.*, 1972). Immunofluorescence studies indicate that mutants of groups A and E induce viral antigen distribution patterns similar to those induced by wild-type virus, that the mutants of group D produce smaller cytoplasmic fluorescent masses, and that the mutants of group B and C form discrete minute cytoplasmic masses (Fields *et al.*, 1971). Mutants of the various groups also differ widely with respect to the nature of the virus-specific structures that accumulate in cells infected by them at the nonpermissive temperature (Fields *et al.*, 1971). Mutants of groups A and F accumulate particles that are morphologically indistinguishable from wild-type virions but are not infectious. Mutants of groups B and G are blocked at an earlier stage; they accumulate "corelike" particles that possess the polypeptide composition of normal cores except for a partial deficiency of $\lambda 2$ and the presence of small amounts of $\mu 0$ and $\mu 2$ (Morgan and Zweerink, 1974). Mutants of groups C, D, and E ac-

cumulate particles that resemble empty capsids (Fields *et al.*, 1971). The group C mutant *ts* 447, which synthesizes less polypeptides than any other since it forms the least amount of double-stranded RNA, actually accumulates structures that comprise outer capsid shell components only (Ito and Joklik, unpublished results). This is understandable since on a molar basis polypeptides $\mu2$ and $\sigma3$ are formed in by far the largest amounts during the course of reovirus infection (see above).

5. An unexpected feature of hybrid double-stranded reovirus RNA molecules appears to provide a means of identifying the genome segments in which mutations causing temperature-sensitivity, and indeed any mutation, are located. Ito and Joklik (1972*b*) observed that certain species of hybrid double-stranded RNA molecules consisting of mutant plus strands and wild-type minus strands (forward hybrids, or "hybrids" for short) migrated slightly more slowly when electrophoresed in polyacrylamide gels than the reverse hybrids (that is, those in which the plus strand is wild type and the minus strand mutant), or any of the homologous mutant or wild-type double-stranded RNA molecules, all of which migrated at the same rate. Thirty-five mutants have been examined so far (Schuerch and Joklik, 1973), and almost half, irrespective of the mutagen used to induce them, have been found to yield such retarded hybrids in some segment or other (for example, see Fig. 13). Several spontaneous phenotypically temperature-insensitive revertants of mutants that yield retarded hybrids do not do so. The results obtained so far suggest that the mutation that leads to temperature sensitivity of the mutants in group A resides in genome segment *L2*, and that the corresponding mutation for the group E mutant is in genome segment *S3* (Schuerch and Joklik, 1973). Four mutants possess two genome segments that yield retarded hybrids and, therefore, appear to be double mutants; but since they do not exhibit abnormally low reversion frequencies, it is unlikely that both mutations cause temperature sensitivity. Evidence that retarded electrophoretic-migration behavior of hybrid molecules is indeed linked to a mutation (and therefore is mutant-group specific) is provided by the two mutants of group D, one of which yields retarded *L1* and *M2* hybrids. Both of these mutants possess an altered polypeptide $\mu2$, which is coded (via its precursor $\mu1$) by genome RNA segment *M2* (Ito and Joklik, 1972*c*). The reason why the electrophoretic migration rate of certain hybrid RNA molecules is retarded is not known with certainty. There is little doubt that the effect is caused by some feature of their secondary structure since the extent of retardation is greater in gels that contain urea or formamide, i.e., reagents that reduce the

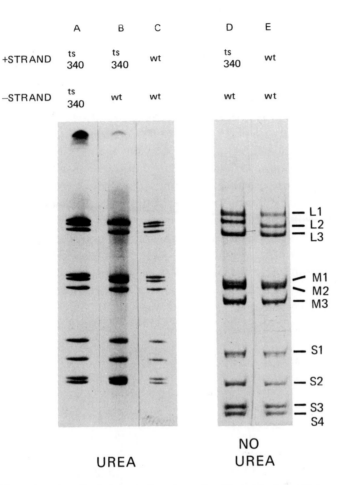

Fig. 13. Autoradiogram of polyacrylamide gels in which various homologous and heterologous double-stranded RNA hybrids had been electrophoresed. Note that the homologous hybrids *ts* 340/*ts* 340 and *wt*/*wt* migrate identically, but that the *L2* segment of the hybrid *ts* 340/*wt* is retarded both in the presence of urea (when it coelectrophoreses with the *L1* segment) and in its absence. From Schuerch and Joklik (1973).

extent of hydrogen-bond formation between nucleic acid bases, than in gels that do not (Schuerch and Joklik, 1973). Ito and Joklik (1972*b*) have proposed that retarded hybrids contain loops caused by mismatching of single base pairs in certain critical locations. This hypothesis accounts for the fact that not all mutations result in the formation of retarded hybrids, and that in all cases except one it is the forward and not the reverse hybrid which is retarded; the sole exception is a mutant induced with proflavine which may be a frame-shift rather than a point mutant. However, the basic feature of the hypothesis, namely the existence of loops, has not yet been proved experimentally.

6. The mutants of group B cause a different disease in rats than wild-type virus (Fields and Raine, 1972; Fields, 1972). Wild-type virus produces an acute necrotizing encephalitis with death generally occurring after one to two weeks. By contrast, many of the animals inoculated with mutants of group B survive but fail to grow normally; they also tend to assume a characteristic humped posture. The brains of such animals manifest marked thinning of the cerebral cortical mantle and dilation of the lateral ventricles, followed by gross cavitation of the cortex; overall, the condition resembles hydrocephalus *ex vacuo*. Attempts at virus isolation from such animals have failed so far. Fields has speculated that degenerative central nervous system disease and perhaps autoimmune disease also may be caused by mutant defective viruses, and suggested that *ts* mutants of reovirus may prove useful for testing this hypothesis.

6.10.2.   The Mutants of Ikegami and Gomatos

Ikegami and Gomatos (1968) isolated 6 *ts* mutants of the Dearing strain of reovirus type 3: two were spontaneous mutants, two were induced with nitrous acid, and two were isolated from virus yields formed in the presence of 5-fluorouracil. None were capable of multiplying at 37°C; their optimal growth temperatures were 30–33°C. None were heat-labile at 37°C. On the basis of their differential thermosensitivity at 52°C, the ratio of infectivity to hemagglutinating activity, and their response to temperature-shift, the six mutants were classified into two groups. Subsequently, eight further mutants were characterized in similar fashion (Ikegami and Gomatos, 1972). None contained a *ts* transcriptase; they formed immature virus particles and viral mRNA at the nonpermissive temperature and thus resembled the mutants of group A of Fields and Joklik (see above). All 14 mutants markedly inhibited both host- and virus-specific protein synthesis at late stages of the infection cycle at the nonpermissive temperature. The reason for the inhibition was not inability of viral mRNA to associate with ribosomes, but it has not yet been characterized further. It was suggested that reovirus may code for factors essential for the synthesis of virus-specific polypeptides and that these factors are temperature sensitive in the mutants studied here.

6.11.   Genome-Segment Deletion Mutants

Although the mechanism that ensures that each progeny reovirion contains a unique and complete set of ten genome RNA segments is very efficient, it is not perfect; most if not all stocks of reovirus appear to contain some particles which contain only nine rather than ten double-stranded RNA segments. Thus, Nonoyama *et al.* (1970) and Nonoyama and Graham (1970) found that stocks of the Dearing strain of reovirus produced after repeated serial passage at medium to high multiplicity consisted mostly of particles that were less dense than virions because they lacked the *L1* genome RNA segment. These particles, the L particles, were indistinguishable from virions (H particles) in their morphology; they were not infectious on their own, but required coinfection with complete virions for their propagation. In consequence, virus stocks could be freed of L particles by passage at multiplicities of less than 1. The L particles are thus deletion mutants that resemble the von Magnus particles of influenza virus, the T particles of vesicular stomatitis virus, the defective particles of poliovirus and of SV 40, etc.

A different kind of genome-segment deletion mutant is formed by the mutant *ts* 447 of group C (see above), stocks of which always contain about equal amounts of particles that contain and that lack the *L3* genome RNA segment (Schuerch *et al.*, 1974). It has also been observed that on brief passage at high multiplicity the mutant *ts* 556 of group F yields particles that are defective in *L1*, as well as particles that are defective in both *L1* and *L3* (Schuerch *et al.*, 1974).

6.12.   The Effect of Reovirus Infection on Host Cell Functions

Although infection with reovirus causes extensive cytopathic effects at late stages of the multiplication cycle, it does not rapidly switch off host-specific macromolecular synthesis at early stages.

6.12.1.   Protein Synthesis

Gomatos and Tamm (1963c) used autoradiography to show that reovirus infection did not inhibit protein synthesis in monolayer cells for about 8 hours; this was confirmed by Kudo and Graham (1965), who noted that protein synthesis was inhibited somewhat earlier in suspension culture cells. The primary reason for protein-synthesis inhibition late in infection was attributed to cell lysis (Ensminger and Tamm, 1969*a*). These studies related to total rather than to host-specific protein synthesis, which is inhibited some 3–6 hours earlier than total protein synthesis (Zweerink and Joklik, 1970) (Fig. 14). The precise time of onset of host-protein-synthesis inhibition depends on the multiplicity of infection and on the temperature of incubation; it correlates closely with the onset of the rapid phase of viral mRNA synthesis, thus suggesting that host protein synthesis is inhibited by direct competition between host and viral messenger RNA for some component of the protein-synthesizing system. Whether viral messenger RNA has more advantage than that of sheer numbers is not known.

6.12.2. DNA Synthesis

Host DNA synthesis is inhibited several hours before overall protein synthesis (Ensminger and Tamm, 1969*a*) (Fig. 14). Studies on synchronized cells have shown that, whereas DNA synthesis in the early part of the S phase is relatively unaffected by infection with reovirus, in late S phase it is inhibited strongly (Ensminger and Tamm,

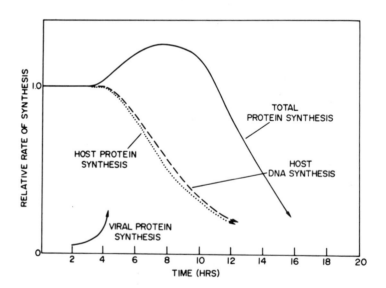

Fig. 14. The effect of infection with reovirus on the rate of total protein synthesis, host cell protein synthesis, and host DNA synthesis. Mouse L fibroblasts in suspension culture, multiplicity of infection 500 particles (5–10 PFU) per cell, 37°C.

1970). Inhibition is not due to breakdown of host DNA nor to inactivation of DNA polymerase (as far as can be tested *in vitro*), nor does DNA become less efficient a template for *in vitro* DNA synthesis; rather, DNA synthesis appears to be inhibited because the number of chromosomal regions involved in active DNA replication is reduced, i.e., because multifocal initiation of DNA replication is prevented (Ensminger and Tamm, 1969*b*; Hand *et al.*, 1971). This mode of inhibition is analogous to that by which inhibition of protein synthesis (by puromycin or cycloheximide) acts, thus suggesting that reovirus infection inhibits cellular DNA synthesis not by a specific inhibitory mechanism, but as a consequence of preventing host protein synthesis. The kinetics of DNA- and protein-synthesis inhibition are in accord with this hypothesis: Infection with reovirus inhibits host DNA synthesis 3–6 hours before inhibiting overall protein synthesis (Ensminger and Tamm, 1969*a*), and host protein synthesis is inhibited 3–6 hours before total protein synthesis (Zweerink and Joklik, 1970) (Fig. 14).

While this scheme accounts satisfactorily for both protein- and DNA-synthesis inhibition in cells infected with reovirus, several other mechanisms have also been considered. One is that the virus codes for proteins during the initial stages of the infection cycle which directly or indirectly inhibit host DNA and protein synthesis. This possibility has been intensively investigated for many viruses, but no really conclusive evidence for it has yet been obtained. Another possibility is that a protein component of infecting virions is the inhibitory molecular species. This possibility can be tested in the case of reovirus owing to the existence of the top-component particles (empty capsids) which contain exactly the same polypeptides as reovirions and which should, therefore, affect cells in exactly the same manner. It has been found that even high multiplicities (over 5000 particles per cell) of reovirus top component fail to inhibit L-cell RNA, protein, or DNA synthesis (Lai *et al.*, 1973; Hand and Tamm, 1973); hence, the inhibition of host cell macromolecular biosynthesis by reovirus appears to be caused not by capsid polypeptide components of infecting virions, but by the expression of some viral function after infection.

The effect of several other reovirion derivatives on host DNA replication has also been investigated. Reovirus irradiated with UV light, so as to abolish infectivity but not transcriptase activity, inhibits DNA replication (Hand and Tamm, 1973; Shaw and Cox, 1973) and still causes marked cytopathic effects (Lai and Joklik, 1973). Reovirus cores, on the other hand, which also possess very low infectivity but have transcriptase activity, do not inhibit DNA replication (Cox and Shaw, 1970; Hand and Tamm, 1973); presumably the fate of virions

and cores in infected cells is quite different. Finally, reovirus oligonucleotides, which can be adsorbed to cells in the presence of DEAE-
dextran, inhibit DNA replication weakly (Hand and Tamm, 1973).

6.13.   The Effect of Inhibitors on Reovirus Multiplication

There are no specific inhibitors of reovirus multiplication. The effect of various metabolic inhibitors has been summarized by Shatkin
(1969). Among the most immediately and potentially useful are:

Actinomycin D. At a concentration of about 0.5 μg/ml it inhibits
host cell ribosomal RNA synthesis completely and messenger RNA
very markedly, but has little effect on the synthesis of either single- or
double-stranded reovirus RNA (Shatkin, 1965b; Kudo and Graham,
1965; Loh and Soergel, 1965).

Cycloheximide and puromycin. These have little effect on the
extent of early viral mRNA synthesis (although, as discussed above,
they may affect the relative frequency of transcription of individual
RNA segments), but they completely inhibit the formation of progeny
double-stranded RNA and consequently, that of all late mRNA (Watanabe *et al.*, 1967b).

Ethidium bromide. At a concentration of 30 μg/ml, it completely
prevents the synthesis of double-stranded RNA, but has no effect on
the transcription and translation of early viral mRNA (Lai *et al.*,
1973).

Interferon. At 50 plaque reduction doses (PRD_{50}) per ml, it inhibits reovirus replication in suspension culture L cells by some 90%
(Wiebe and Joklik, 1973; Gupta *et al.*, 1974), the extent of inhibition depending on the multiplicity of infection. Only very little progeny double-
stranded RNA is formed in interferon-treated cells, and they contain
few if any virus-specific polyribosomes. During the early stages of infection, parental SVP transcribe 30–70% less viral mRNA in interferon-
treated than in normal cells; the possible reasons for this range from a
direct effect of the putative antiviral protein induced by interferon on the
SVP to an inhibition of the release of SVP from the phagocytic vesicles
and lysosomes in which they are generated (see above). Although this effect contributes to the overall inhibition, the primary effect of interferon
on reovirus multiplication is most probably the same as its proposed effect on vaccinia and EMC virus multiplication (Joklik and Merigan,
1966; Kerr, 1971; Metz and Esteban, 1972; Friedman *et al.*, 1972a,b),
namely, inhibition of the translation of the early mRNA that is
transcribed. Evidence for this view is provided by the finding that while

reovirus mRNA is translated efficiently in a cell-free protein-synthesizing system prepared from uninfected Krebs ascites tumor cells, it is not translated in such a system prepared from cells pretreated with interferon; by contrast, host cell mRNA is translated equally efficiently in both systems (Samuel and Joklik, 1974). It has also been claimed that reovirus mRNA species of abnormal size are synthesized in cells pretreated with interferon (Gauntt, 1972), but the molecular basis of this effect is obscure.

6.14. The Induction of Interferon by Reovirus

Reovirus is an excellent inducer of interferon (Long and Burke, 1971; Oie and Loh, 1971; Lai and Joklik, 1973). In roller cultures of suitably aged mouse L929 fibroblasts, interferon titers of over 100,000 PRD_{50}/ml are readily achievable (Wiebe and Joklik, unpublished results). Double-stranded reovirus RNA itself is also an efficient inducer of interferon formation (Tytell *et al.*, 1967; Long and Burke, 1971); and it was thought at first that the interferon inducer in cells infected with reovirus was uncoated, double-stranded RNA. However, neither is parental reovirus RNA uncoated, nor is progeny double-stranded RNA formed free in the cytoplasm: double-stranded reovirus RNA never exists in the free state in infected cells (see above). The question therefore arises whether the induction of interferon by reovirus can be ascribed to any of the limited number of functions known to be coded by its genome. Attempts to answer this question have been made using the *ts* mutants described above (Lai and Joklik, 1973). Strangely enough, none of the mutants belonging to six of the seven genome-segment reassortment groups which were examined were capable of inducing the formation of significant amounts of interferon at the nonpermissive temperature; this was true both of early mutants and of very late ones that were capable of supporting the synthesis of almost normal amounts of both single-stranded and double-stranded viral RNA and protein. The only parameter with which the amount of interferon that was induced could be correlated was the final yield of infectious virus, and even this correlation held only for the majority, not for all of the mutants examined. The conclusion drawn from this line of approach was that interferon induction by reovirus was dependent on a very late event in morphogenesis.

A totally different picture was obtained when the ability of UV-irradiated reovirus to induce interferon was examined, for reovirus inactivated well beyond complete loss of ability to multiply can still induce up to 30% of normal amounts of interferon (Long and Burke, 1971; Lai and Joklik, 1973). There are at least two types of mechanisms by which such virus might induce the formation of interferon. First, interferon induction could be the consequence of the expression of a very early viral function. In favor of this hypothesis is the fact that a small amount of early reovirus mRNA is synthesized in cells infected with UV-inactivated reovirus (Lai and Joklik, 1973; Hand and Tamm, 1973), and the fact that the UV sensitivity of the ability of reovirus to induce interferon formation coincides with that of the transcriptase (B. Dishman and Joklik, unpublished results). Against this hypothesis is the fact that if only expression of a very early viral function is required for the induction of interferon synthesis, most *ts* mutants should induce interferon well; but they do not.

The second mechanism is cell damage. The amount of interferon induced correlates roughly with the intensity of cytopathic damage: Thus, *wt* virus induces more cytopathic damage at 39°C than any *ts* mutant; UV-inactivated virus induces cytopathic damage; and ts 447, which causes little cytopathic damage and induces little interferon at 39°C, becomes markedly cytopathic and an excellent interferon inducer at 39°C when inactivated with UV irradiation (Lai and Joklik, 1973). The mechanism by which reovirus, *ts* mutants of reovirus, and UV-irradiated reovirus cause cytopathic damage is not known; but elucidating it may well provide the key to the problem of how reovirus, or indeed any virus, induces interferon.

7. THE REPLICATION OF ORBIVIRUSES

The only orbivirus the multiplication of which has been studied in any detail is BTV. This virus multiplies in a variety of cells including BHK 21 and L cells (Howell *et al.*, 1967), but its yield is always at least 100 times lower than that of reovirus; this has greatly hampered elucidation of the reactions involved in its multiplication. For example, it is not yet known whether in the initial stages of infection BTV L particles are converted to D particles, and whether the D particles are themselves degraded partially or completely; nor is it known whether the mode of BTV progeny double-stranded RNA formation is analogous to that by which progeny reovirus genome RNA is formed.

Both single- and double-stranded RNA are formed in cells infected with BTV. The kinetics of synthesis of both resembles that of reovirus-specific RNA synthesis: single-stranded BTV RNA is synthesized slowly at first, presumably by transcription of parental genome segments, and more rapidly after several hours, when progeny double-stranded RNA has presumably been synthesized and is then being transcribed (Huismans, 1970a).

Intracellular BTV single-stranded RNA comprises all ten possible species of transcripts. Their relative rates of transcription remain essentially constant throughout the entire multiplication cycle, and they are not affected by the presence of cycloheximide. These results indicate the absence of specific controls over BTV RNA transcription (Huismans and Verwoerd, 1973). Further, the relative frequencies with which individual mRNA species are transcribed *in vivo* are almost exactly the same as those with which they are transcribed *in vitro*. Strangely enough, one transcript, number 5 or *m2*, is formed more than twice as frequently as expected on the basis of completely uncontrolled transcription, and another, number 10 or *s4*, is formed less than half as frequently as expected (Huismans and Verwoerd, 1973). The reason for these discrepancies is not known.

The relative frequencies of translation of the individual BTV mRNA species are not yet known, but polyribosomes in infected cells contain all ten species in the same relative proportions as those in which they are synthesized (Huismans and Verwoerd, 1973).

BTV has a severe inhibitory effect on host cell protein synthesis which is particularly marked in suspension culture cells (Huismans, 1971). This inhibition is due to disruption of polyribosomes, which, remarkably enough, proceeds in the presence as well as in the absence of cycloheximide; this suggests that it is caused by a component of infecting BTV particles. Not surprisingly, and probably because protein synthesis is inhibited, infection with BTV also rapidly inhibits DNA synthesis (Huismans, 1970b).

The manners in which BTV and reovirus infection inhibit protein synthesis appear to be quite different. In cells infected with reovirus there occurs a smooth changeover from host- to virus-specific protein synthesis when viral mRNA begins to be transcribed in large amounts. In cells infected with BTV, viral mRNA is also transcribed very actively (Huismans and Verwoerd, 1973); however, not only is host protein synthesis strongly inhibited, but only very small amounts of viral protein are formed. Infection with BTV thus appears to cause severe damage to the protein-synthesizing system which may explain in part why BTV is highly cytopathogenic, why its yields are always low, and why even these are drastically reduced if the multiplicity exceeds 1 PFU/cell (Martin and Zweerink, 1972).

Numerous electron microscopic studies have been made of the

morphogenesis of orbiviruses (Bowne and Jones, 1966; Bowne and Jochim, 1967; Lecatsas and Erasmus, 1967; Lecatsas, 1968; Murphy *et al.*, 1968, 1971; Oshimo and Emmons, 1968; Schnagl *et al.*, 1969; Yunker and Cory, 1969; Breese and Osawa, 1969; Lecatsas *et al.*, 1969; Bowne and Ritchie, 1970; Cromack *et al.*, 1971; Emmons *et al.*, 1972; Lecatsas *et al.*, 1973). Their development does not display the intimate association with the spindle tubules of the mitotic apparatus that reovirus morphogenesis does; orbiviruses generally develop within intracytoplasmic granular inclusions with which filaments and tubules are often associated. At later stages of the infection cycle, viral particles may become associated with membranous structures and pass into cytoplasmic vesicles. Release appears to proceed predominantly via a process of extrusion across the plasma membrane. Although orbivirus particles sometimes appear to be surrounded by membranous sacs, these are by no means essential for infectivity, and orbivirus particles isolated by disruption of cells and density gradient centrifugation never possess membranes.

8. THE REPLICATION OF THE CYTOPLASMIC POLYHEDROSIS VIRUSES (CPV)

Biochemical investigations of the replication of CPV are in their infancy since no satisfactory tissue-culture system has yet been developed; what studies have been reported have been carried out with entire silkworm larvae (Watanabe, 1967; Furusawa and Kawase, 1971; Hayashi and Donoghue, 1971; Payne and Kalmakoff, 1973). Larvae were fed with mulberry leaves coated with CPV suspensions; they were then injected with ^{32}P- or ^{3}H-uridine and actinomycin D, and the RNA that was formed in the cells of the midgut was characterized. Both single- and double-stranded RNA was found to be synthesized; the former was shown to be CPV specific by virtue of its ability to hybridize with double-stranded CPV genome RNA (Hayashi and Donoghue, 1971; Payne and Kalmakoff, 1973).

9. THE REPLICATION OF MEMBERS OF THE PLANT VIRUS GENUS

Studies on the replication of members of the plant virus genus have been confined almost entirely to its morphologic aspects. The development of WTV has been studied with the electron microscope in plants (Shikata and Maramorosch, 1966, 1967*a*) as well as in viruliferous leafhoppers (Shikata and Maramorosch, 1965, 1967b) and insect nervous tissue (Hirumi et al., 1967) and hemocytes (Granados et al., 1968); the development of MRDV has been studied by Conti and Lovisolo (1971) and Vidano (1970) (see also Harpaz, 1972); that of FDV by Teakle and Steindl (1969) and Francki and Grivell (1972); and that of RDV by Fukushi and Shikata (1963b), among others. All these viruses multiply in the cytoplasm. In general, the following sequential stages in virus morphogenesis can be discerned: the development of a viroplasm, i.e., the accumulation of electron-dense aggregates; the appearance at the periphery of the viroplasm of a few fully formed virus particles; the formation of further virions not only at the periphery but also within the viroplasm; the engulfment of virions within membranous structures; and the formation of microcrystals or paracrystalline arrays of virus particles near the viroplasms.

The only one of these viruses the multiplication of which has been quantitated is WTV. Using an assay based on the measurement of the amount of virus-specific soluble antigen developed in leafhoppers after a standardized interval of time, Reddy and Black (1966) measured the rate of WTV multiplication in the leafhopper Agallia constricta (Van Duzee) and found that the amount of virus rose from the 7th to the 30th day, and then decreased 10-fold during the next 15 days. More recently, this multiplication pattern has been confirmed using the far more convenient focus-forming assay (on insect cell monolayers) (Reddy and Black, 1972): the virus multiplied about 100,000-fold between days 8 and 25. The multiplication of WTV in cultured leafhopper cells has been determined similarly (Kimura and Black, 1972b): progeny virus first appeared in the medium at 6 hours after infection, and during the course of the next 8 hours the titers of released virus increased about 100-fold, apparently without gross cell destruction. The multiplication of the virus was also assessed by following the appearance of foci of infection with the use of immunofluorescent staining: the first foci appeared at 4 hours after infection, thus indicating that the formation of virus-specific protein preceded the liberation of viral progeny by at least 2 hours. This type of system promises to be very useful for the study of the biochemical reactions involved in the multiplication of plant reoviridae since all are capable of multiplying in insect cells.

ACKNOWLEDGMENTS

I would like to express my thanks to numerous colleagues who generously provided reprints, preprints, and photographs; among them were Drs. Black, Fields, Lewandowski, Maramorosch, Milne, Miura, Shatkin, Traynor, and Verwoerd. I would also like to thank Drs. H. J. Zweerink and H. Huismans for critically reading the manuscript and stimulating discussions.

REFERENCES

Acs, G., Klett, H., Schonberg, M., Christman, J. K., Levin, D. H., and Silverstein, S. C., 1971, Mechanism of reovirus double-stranded ribonucleic acid synthesis *in vivo* and *in vitro, J. Virol.* **8,** 684.

Adesnik, M., and Darnell, J. E., Jr., 1972, Biogenesis and characterization of histone messenger RNA in HeLa cells, *J. Mol. Biol.* **67,** 397.

Amano, Y., Katagiri, S., Ishida, N., and Watanabe, Y., 1971, Spontaneous degradation of reovirus capsid into subunits, *J. Virol.* **8,** 805.

Anderson, M., and Doane, F. W., 1966, An electron-microscope study of reovirus type 2 in L cells, *J. Pathol. Bacteriol.* **92,** 433.

Arnott, S., Hutchinson, F., Spencer, M., Wilkins, M. H. F., Fuller, W., and Langridge, R., 1966, X-ray diffraction studies of double helical ribonucleic acid, *Nature (Lond.)* **211,** 227.

Aruga, H., and Tanada, Y. eds., 1971, The Cytoplasmic-Polyhedrosis Virus of the Silkworm, University of Tokyo Press, Tokyo.

Asai, J., Kawamoto, F., and Kawase, S., 1972, On the structure of the cytoplasmic-polyhedrosis virus of the silkworm, *Bombyx mori, J. Invertebr. Pathol.* **19,** 279.

Astell, C., Silverstein, S. C., Levin, D. H., and Acs, G., 1972, Regulation of the reovirus transcriptase by a viral capsomer protein, *Virology* **48,** 648.

Banerjee, A. K., and Grece, M. A., 1971, An identical 3′-terminal sequence in the ten reovirus genome RNA segments, *Biochem. Biophys. Res. Commun.* **45,** 1518.

Banerjee, A. K., and Shatkin, A. J., 1970, Transcription *in vitro* by reovirus-associated ribonucleic acid-dependent polymerase, *J. Virol.* **6,** 1.

Banerjee, A. K., and Shatkin, A. J., 1971, Guanine-5′-diphosphate at the 5′ termini of reovirus RNA: Evidence for a segmented genome within the virion. *J. Mol. Biol.* **61,** 643.

Banerjee, A. K., Ward, R. L., and Shatkin, A. J., 1971*a*, Initiation of reovirus mRNA synthesis *in vitro, Nat. New Biol.* **230,** 169.

Banerjee, A. K., Ward, R. L., and Shatkin, A. J., 1971*b*, Cytosine at the 3′-termini of reovirus genome and *in vitro* RNA, *Nat. New Biol.* **232,** 114.

Bellamy, A. R., and Hole, L. V., 1970, Single-stranded oligonucleotides from reoivirus type 3, *Virology* **40,** 808.

Bellamy, A. R., and Joklik, W. K., 1967*a*, Studies on reovirus RNA. II. Characterization of reovirus messenger RNA and of the genome RNA segments from which it is transcribed, *J. Mol. Biol.* **29,** 19.

Bellamy, A. R., and Joklik, W. K., 1967*b*, Studies on the A-rich RNA of reovirus, *Proc. Natl. Acad. Sci. USA* **58,** 1389.

Bellamy, A. R., Shapiro, L., August, J. T., and Joklik, W. K., 1967, Studies on reovirus RNA. I. Characterization of reovirus genome RNA, *J. Mol. Biol.* **29,** 1.

Bellamy, A. R., Hole, L. V., and Baguley, B. C., 1970, Isolation of the trinucleotide pppGpCpU from reovirus, *Virology* **42,** 415.

Bellamy, A. R., Nichols, J. L., and Joklik, W. K., 1972, Nucleotide sequences of reovirus oligonucleotides: Evidence for abortive RNA synthesis during virus maturation, *Nat. New Biol.* **238**, 49.

Bils, R. F., and Hall, C. E., 1962, Electron microscopy of wound tumor virus, *Virology* **17**, 123.

Black, D. R., and Knight, C. A., 1970, Ribonucleic acid transcriptase activity in purified wound tumor virus, *J. Virol.* **6**, 194.

Black, L. M., 1965, Physiology of virus-induced tumors in plants, *in* "Encyclopedia of Plant Physiology" (W. Ruhland and A. Lang, eds.), pp. 236–266, Springer-Verlag, New York.

Black, L. M., 1972, Plant tumors of viral origin, *Progr. Tumor Res.* **15**, 110.

Black, L. M., and Markham, R., 1963, Base pairing in the ribonucleic acid of wound tumor virus, *Neth. J. Plant Pathol.* **69**, 215.

Black, L. M., Wolcyrz, S., and Whitcomb, R. F., 1958, A vectorless strain of wound tumor virus, *Proc. 7th Int. Congr. Microbiol., Stockholm*, 255.

Black, L. M., Reddy, D. V. R., and Reichmann, M. E., 1967, Virus inactivation by moderate forces during quasi-equilibrium zonal density gradient centrifugation, *Virology* **31**, 713.

Borden, E. C., Shope, R. E., and Murphy, F. A., 1971, Physicochemical and morphological relationships of some arthropod-borne viruses to bluetongue virus—a new toxonomic group. Physicochemical and serological studies, *J. Gen. Virol.* **13**, 261.

Borsa, J., and Graham, A. F., 1968, Reovirus: RNA polymerase activity in purified virions, *Biochem. Biophys. Res. Commun.* **33**, 896.

Borsa, J., Grover, J., and Chapman, J. D., 1970, Presence of nucleoside triphosphate phosphohydrolase activity in purified virions of reovirus, *J. Virol.* **6**, 295.

Borsa, J., Sargent, M. D., Long, D. G., and Chapman, J. D., 1973a, Extraordinary effects of specific monovalent cations on activation of reovirus transcriptase by chymotrypsin *in vitro, J. Virol.* **11**, 207.

Borsa, J., Copps, T. P., Sargent, M. D., Long, D. G., and Chapman, J. D., 1973a, New intermediate subviral particles in the *in vitro* uncoating of reovirus virions by chymotrypsin, *J. Virol.* **11**, 552.

Borsa, J., Sargent, M. D., Copps, T. P., Long, D. G., and Chapman, J. D., 1973c, Specific monovalent cation effects on modification of reovirus infectivity by chymotrypsin digestion *in vitro, J. Virol.* **11**, 1017.

Bowne, J. G., and Jochim, M. M., 1967, Cytopathologic changes and development of inclusion bodies in cultured cells infected with bluetongue virus, *Am. J. Vet. Res.* **28**, 1091.

Bowne, J. G., and Jones, R. H., 1966, Observations on bluetongue virus in the salivary glands of an insect vector, *Culicoides variipennis, Virology* **30**, 127.

Bowne, J. G., and Ritchie, A. E., 1970, Some morphological features of bluetongue virus, *Virology* **40**, 903.

Brakke, M. K., 1951, Density gradient centrifugation. A new centrifugation technique, *J. Am. Chem. Soc.* **73**, 1847.

Brakke, M. K., 1953, Zonal separations by density-gradient centrifugation, *Arch. Biochem. Biophys.* **45**, 275.

Brakke, M. K., 1955, Zone electrophoresis of dyes, proteins and viruses in density gradient columns of sucrose solutions, *Arch. Biochem. Biophys.* **55**, 175.

Brcak, J., and Kralik, O., 1969, Virus and virus-like particles in gut cells of *Javesella pellucida* (F.) carrying the oat sterile virus, *Proc. 6th Conf. Czech. Plant Virol., Olomouc, 1967*, 138.

Breese, S. S., and Ozawa, Y., 1969, Intracellular inclusions resulting from infection with African horse sickness virus, *J. Virol.* **4,** 109.

Brubaker, M. M., West, B., and Ellis, R. J., 1964, Human blood group influence on reovirus hemagglutination titers, *Proc. Soc. Exp. Biol. Med.* **115,** 1118.

Burgess, R. R., 1969, Separation and characterization of the subunits of ribonucleic acid polymerase, *J. Biol. Chem.* **244,** 6168.

Casals, J., 1967, Immunological techniques for animal viruses, *in* "Methods in Virology," (K. Maramorosch and H. Koprowski, eds.), p. 113, Academic Press, New York.

Chamberlin, M., and Berg, P., 1965, Mechanism of RNA polymerase action: Characterization of the DNA-dependent synthesis of polyadenylic acid, *J. Mol. Biol.* **8,** 708.

Chang, C.-T., and Zweerink, H. J., 1971, Fate of parental reovirus in infected cells, *Virology* **46,** 544.

Chiu, R.-J., and Black, L. M., 1969, Assay of wound tumor virus by the fluorescent cell counting technique, *Virology* **37,** 667.

Chiu, R.-J., Reddy, D. V. R., and Black, L. M., 1966, Inoculation and infection of leafhopper tissue cultures with a plant virus, *Virology* **30,** 562.

Christman, J. K., Reiss, B., Kyner, D., Levin, D. H., Klett, H., and Acs, G., 1973, Characterization of a viral messenger ribonucleoprotein particle accumulated during inhibition of polypeptide chain initiation in reovirus-infected L cells, *Biochim. Biophys. Acta* **294,** 153.

Conti, M., and Lovisolo, O., 1971, Tubular structures associated with maize rough dwarf virus particles in crude extracts: electron microscopy study, *J. Gen. Virol.* **13,** 173.

Cox, D. C., and Shaw, J. E., 1970, Reovirus alteration of cellular DNA synthesis, *Ann. Okla. Acad. Sci.* **1,** 28.

Cromack, A. S., Blue, J. L., and Gratzek, J. B., 1971, A quantitative ultrastructural study of the development of bluetongue virus in Madin-Darby bovine kidney cells, *J. Gen. Virol.* **13,** 229.

Cross, R. K., and Fields, B. N., 1972, Temperature-sensitive mutants of reovirus type 3: Studies on the synthesis of viral RNA, *Virology* **50,** 799.

Dales, S., 1963, Association between the spindle apparatus and reovirus, *Proc. Natl. Acad. Sci. USA* **50,** 268.

Dales, S., Gomatos, P. J., and Hsu, K. C., 1965, The uptake and development of reovirus in strain L cells followed with labeled viral ribonucleic and ferritin-antibody conjugates, *Virology* **25,** 193.

Donoghue, T. P., and Hayashi, Y., 1972, Cytoplasmic polyhedrosis virus (CPV) of *Malacosoma disstria*: RNA polymerase activity in purified free virions, *Can. J. Microbiol.* **18,** 207.

Drouhet, V., 1960, Lesiens cellulaires provoquées par les reovirus (Virus ECHO 10). Anticorps fluorescents et étude cytochimique, *Ann. Inst. Pasteur* **98,** 618.

Dunnebacke, T. H., and Kleinschmidt, A. K., 1967, Ribonucleic acid from reovirus as seen in protein monolayers by electronmicroscopy, *Z. Naturforsch.* **22b,** 159.

Eggers, H. J., Gomatos, P. J., and Tamm, I., 1962, Agglutination of bovine erythrocytes: A general characteristic of reovirus type 3, *Proc. Soc. Exp. Biol. Med.* **110,** 879.

Els, H. J., and Lecatsas, G., 1972, Morphological studies on simian virus S.A. 11 and the "related" O agent, *J. Gen. Virol.* **17,** 129.

Els, H. J., and Verwoerd, D. W., 1969, Morphology of bluetongue virus, *Virology* 38, 213.

Emmons, R. W., Oshiro, L. S., Johnson, H. N., and Lennette, E. H., 1972, Intraerythrocytic location of Colorado tick fever virus, *J. Gen. Virol.* 17, 185.

Ensminger, W. D., and Tamm, I., 1969a, Cellular DNA and protein synthesis in reovirus-infected L cells, *Virology* 39, 357.

Ensminger, W. D., and Tamm, I., 1969b, The step in cellular DNA synthesis blocked by reovirus infection, *Virology* 39, 935.

Ensminger, W. D., and Tamm, I., 1970, Inhibition of synchronized cellular deoxyribonucleic acid synthesis during Newcastle disease virus, mengovirus, or reovirus infection, *J. Virol.* 5, 672.

Fields, B. N., 1971, Temperature-sensitive mutants of reovirus type 3. Features of genetic recombination, *Virology* 46, 142.

Fields, B. N., 1972, Genetic manipulation of reovirus—a model for modification of disease? *New Engl. J. Med.,* 287, 1026.

Fields, B. N., 1973, Genetic reassortment with reovirus mutants, *in* "Virus Research" (C. F. Fox and W. S. Robinson, eds.), pp. 461–469, Academic Press, New York.

Fields, B. N., and Joklik, W. K., 1969, Isolation and preliminary genetic and biochemical characterization of temperature-sensitive mutants of reovirus, *Virology* 37, 335.

Fields, B. N., and Raine, C. S., 1972, Altered disease in rats due to mutants or reovirus type 3, *J. Clin. Invest.* 51, 30a.

Fields, B. N., Raine, C. S., and Baum, S. G., 1971, Temperature-sensitive mutants of reovirus type 3: Defects in virus maturation as studied by immunofluorescence and electron microscopy, *Virology* 43, 569.

Fields, B. N., Laskov, R., and Scharff, M. D., 1972, Temperature-sensitive mutants of reovirus type 3: Studies on the synthesis of viral peptides, *Virology* 50, 209.

Floyd, R. W., Stone, M. P., and Joklik, W. K., 1974, Separation of single-stranded ribonucleic acids by acrylamide-agarose-urea gel electrophoresis, *Anal. Biochem.,* in press.

Foster, N. M., Jones, R. H., and McCrory, B. R., 1963, Preliminary investigations on insect transmission of bluetongue virus in sheep, *Am. J. Vet. Res.* 24, 1195.

Francki, R. I. B., and Grivell, C. J., 1972, Occurrence of similar particles in Fiji disease virus-infected sugar cane and insect vector cells, *Virology* 48, 305.

Francki, R. I. B., and Jackson, A. D., 1972, Immunochemical detection of double-stranded ribonucleic acid in leaves of sugar cane infected with Fiji disease virus, *Virology* 48, 275.

Friedman, R. M., Esteban, R. M., Metz, D. H., Tovell, D. R., and Kerr, I. M., 1972a, Translation of RNA by L cell extracts: Effect of interferon, *FEBS (Fed. Eur. Biochem. Soc.) Lett.* 24, 273.

Friedman, R. M., Metz, D. H., Esteban, R. M., Tovell, D. R., Ball, L. A., and Kerr, I. M., 1972b, Mechanism of interferon action: Inhibition of viral messenger ribonucleic acid translation in L-cell extracts, *J. Virol.* 10, 1184.

Fujii-Kawata, I., Miura, K.-I., and Fuke, M., 1970, Segments of genome of viruses containing double-stranded ribonucleic acid, *J. Mol. Biol.* 51, 247.

Fukushi, T., 1933, Transmission of virus through the eggs of an insect vector, *Proc. Imp. Acad. Jap.* 9, 457.

Fukushi, T., and Kimura, I., 1959, On Some Properties of the rice dwarf virus, *Proc. Imp. Acad. Jap.* 35, 482.

Fukushi, T., and Shikata, E., 1963a, Fine structure of rice dwarf virus, *Virology* **21,** 500.

Fukushi, T., and Shikata, E., 1963b, Localization of rice dwarf virus in its insect vector, *Virology* **21,** 503.

Furiuchi, Y., and Miura, K.-I., 1972, The 3′-termini of the genome RNA segments of silkworm polyhedrosis virus, *J. Mol. Biol.* **64,** 619.

Furiuchi, Y., and Miura, K.-I., 1973, Identity of the 3′-terminal sequence in ten genome segments of silkworm cytoplasmic polyhedrosis virus, *Virology* **55,** 418.

Furusawa, T., and Kawase, S., 1971, Synthesis of ribonucleic acid resistant to actinomycin D in silkworm midguts infected with the cytoplasmic polyhedrosis virus, *J. Invertebr. Pathol.* **18,** 156.

Gamez, R., and Black, L. M., 1967, Application of particle-counting to a leafhopper-borne virus, *Nature (Lond.)* **215,** 173.

Gamez, R., and Black, L. M., 1968, Particle counts of wound tumor virus during its peak concentration in leafhoppers, *Virology* **34,** 444.

Gamez, R., Black, L. M., and MacLeod, R., 1967, Reexamination of the serological relationship between wound tumor virus and reovirus, *Virology* **32,** 163.

Gauntt, C. J., 1972, Effect of interferon on synthesis of ss RNA in reovirus type 3-infected L cell cultures, *Biochem. Biophys. Res. Commun.* **47,** 1228.

Gauntt, C. J., and Graham, A. F., 1969, The reoviruses, *in* "The Biochemistry of Viruses" (H. B. Levy, ed.), pp. 259–291, Marcel Dekker, New York.

Gelb, L. D., and Lerner, A. M., 1965, Reovirus hemagglutination: Inhibition by N-acetyl-D-glucosamine, *Science (Wash., D.C.)* **147,** 404.

Gillies, S., Bullivant, S., and Bellamy, A. R., 1971, Viral RNA polymerases: electron microscopy of reovirus reaction cores, *Science (Wash., D.C.)* **174,** 694.

Gomatos, P. J., 1967, RNA synthesis in reovirus infected L929 mouse fibroblasts, *Proc. Natl. Acad. Sci. USA* **58,** 1798.

Gomatos, P. J., 1968, Reovirus-specific, single-stranded RNA's synthesized *in vitro* with enzyme purified from reovirus-infected cells, *J. Mol. Biol.* **37,** 423.

Gomatos, P. J., 1970, Comparison of the virion polymerase of reovirus with the enzyme purified from reovirus-infected cells, *J. Virol.* **6,** 610.

Gomatos, P. J., and Tamm, I., 1962, Reactive sites of reovirus type 3 and their interaction with receptor substances, *Virology* **17,** 455.

Gomatos, P. J., and Tamm, I., 1963a, The secondary structure of reovirus RNA, *Proc. Natl. Acad. Sci. USA* **49,** 707.

Gomatos, P. J. and Tamm, I., 1963b, Animal and plant viruses with double-helical RNA, *Proc. Natl. Acad. Sci. USA* **50,** 878.

Gomatos, P. J., and Tamm, I., 1963c, Macromolecular synthesis in reovirus-infected cells, *Biochim. Biophys. Acta* **72,** 651.

Gomatos, P. J., Tamm, I., Dales, S., and Franklin, R. M., 1962, Reovirus type 3: Physical characteristics and interactions with L cells, *Virology* **17,** 441.

Granados, R. R., Ward, L. S., and Maramorosch, K., 1968, Insect viremia caused by a plant-pathogenic virus: Electron microscopy of vector hemocytes, *Virology* **34,** 790.

Granboulan, N., and Niveleau, A., 1967, Étude au microscope electronique du RNA de reovirus, *J. Microscop.* **6,** 23.

Graziadei, W. D., and Lengyel, P., 1972, Translation of *in vitro* synthesized reovirus messenger RNAs into proteins of the size of reovirus capsid proteins in a mouse L cell extract, *Biochem. Biophys. Res. Commun.* **46,** 1816.

Green, I. J., 1970, Evidence for the double-stranded nature of the RNA of Colorado tick fever virus, an ungrouped arbovirus, *Virology* **49,** 878.

Gupta, S. L., Graziadei, W. D., III, Weideli, H., Sopori, M. L., and Lengyel, P., 1973, Selective inhibition of viral protein accumulation in interferon-treated cells; nondiscriminate inhibition of the translation of added viral and cellular messenger RNAs in their extracts, *Virology* **57,** 49.

Hand, R., and Tamm, I., 1971, Reovirus: Analysis of proteins from released and cell-associated virus, *J. Gen. Virol.* **12,** 121.

Hand, R., and Tamm, I., 1973, Reovirus: Effect of noninfectious viral components on cellular deoxyribonucleic acid synthesis, *J. Virol.* **11,** 223.

Hand, R., Ensminger, W. D., and Tamm, I., 1971, Cellular DNA replication in infections with cytocidal RNA viruses, *Virology* **44,** 527.

Harpaz, I., 1972, Maise rough dwarf, a plant-hopper disease affecting maize, rice, small grain, and grasses, Israel University Press, Jerusalem, Israel.

Hay, A. J., and Joklik, W. K., 1971, Demonstration that the same strand of reovirus genome RNA is transcribed *in vitro* and *in vivo, Virology* **44,** 450.

Hayashi, Y., and Donoghue, T. P., 1971, Cytoplasmic polyhedrosis virus. RNA synthesized *in vivo* and *in vitro* in infected midgut, *Biochem. Biophys. Res. Commun.* **42,** 214.

Hirumi, H., Granados, R. R., and Maramorosch, K., 1967, Electron microscopy of a plant pathogenic virus in the nervous system of its insect vector, *J. Virol.* **1,** 430.

Hosaka, Y., and Aizawa, K., 1964, The fine structure of the cytoplasmic-polyhedrosis virus of the silkworm, *Bombyx mori* (Linnaeus), *J. Insect Pathol.* **6,** 53.

Howell, P. G., and Verwoerd, D. W., 1971, Bluetongue Virus, Virology Monographs 9 (S. Gard, C. Hallauer, and K. F. Meyer, eds.), pp. 37–74, Springer-Verlag, Vienna.

Howell, P. G., Verwoerd, D. W., and Oellermann, R. A., 1967, Plaque formation by bluetongue virus, *Onderstepoort J. Vet. Res.* **34,** 317.

Hsu, H. T., and Black, L. M., 1973, Comparative efficiencies of assays of a plant virus by lesions on leaves and on vector cell monolayers, *Virology* **52,** 284.

Huismans, H., 1970a, Macromolecular synthesis in bluetongue virus-infected cells, I. Virus-specific ribonucleic acid synthesis, *Onderstepoort, J. Vet. Res.* **37,** 191.

Huismans, H., 1970b, Macromolecular synthesis in bluetongue virus-infected cells. II. Host cell metabolism, *Onderstepoort J. Vet. Res.* **37,** 199.

Huismans, H., 1971, Host cell protein synthesis after infection with bluetongue virus and reovirus, *Virology* **46,** 500.

Huismans, H., and Verwoerd, D. W., 1973, Control of transcription during the expression of the bluetongue virus genome, *Virology* **52,** 81.

Hukuhara, T., 1971, Variations in cytoplasmic-polyhedrosis virus, *in* "The Cytoplasmic-Polyhedrosis Virus of the Silkworm" (H. Aruga and Y. Tanada, eds.), pp. 61–78, University of Tokyo Press, Tokyo.

Iglewski, W. J., and Franklin, R. M., 1967, Purification and properties of reovirus ribonucleic acid, *J. Virol.* **1,** 302.

Ikegami, N., and Gomatos, P. J., 1968, Temperature-sensitive conditional-lethal mutants of reovirus 3. I. Isolation and characterization, *Virology* **36,** 447.

Ikegami, N., and Gomatos, P. J., 1972, Inhibition of host and viral protein synthesis during infection at the nonpermissive temperature with ts mutants of reovirus 3, *Virology* **47,** 306.

Ito, Y., and Joklik, W. K., 1972a, Temperature-sensitive mutants of reovirus. I. Patterns of gene expression by mutants of groups C, D, and E, *Virology* **50,** 189.

Ito, Y., and Joklik, W. K., 1972*b*, Temperature-sensitive mutants of reovirus. II. Anomalous electrophoretic migration behavior of certain hybrid RNA molecules composed of mutant plus strands and wild-type minus strands, *Virology* **50**, 202.

Ito, Y., and Joklik, W. K., 1972*c*, Temperature-sensitive mutants of reovirus. III. Evidence that mutants of group D ("RNA-negative") are structural polypeptide mutants, *Virology* **50**, 282.

Jensen, A. B., Rabin, E. R., Phillips, C. A., and Melnick, J. L., 1965, Reovirus encephalitis in newborn mice, *Am. J. Pathol.* **47**, 223.

Jochim, M. M., and Jones, R. H., 1966, Multiplication of bluetongue virus in *Culicoides variipennis* following artificial infection, *Am. J. Epidemiol.* **84**, 241.

Joklik, W. K., 1970, The molecular biology of reovirus, *J. Cell Physiol.* **76**, 289.

Joklik, W. K., 1972, Studies on the effect of chymotrypsin on reovirions, *Virology* **49**, 700.

Joklik, W. K., 1973*a*, The transcription and translation of reovirus RNA, *in* "Virus Research," (C. F. Fox and W. S. Robinson, eds.), pp. 105–126, Academic Press, New York.

Joklik, W. K., 1973*b*, Reovirus: A virus with a segmented double-stranded RNA genome, *in* "Viral Replication and Cancer" (J. L. Melnick, S. Ochoa, and J. Oró, eds.), pp. 123–152, Editorial Labor, S. A., Barcelona.

Joklik, W. K., and Merigan, T. C., 1966, Concerning the mechanism of action of interferon, *Proc. Natl. Acad. Sci. USA* **56**, 558.

Jordan, L. E., and Mayor, H. D., 1962, The fine structure of reovirus, a new member of the icosahedral series, *Virology* **17**, 597.

Kalmakoff, J., Lewandowski, L. J., and Black, D. R., 1969, Comparison of the ribonucleic acid subunits of reovirus, cytoplasmic polyhedrosis virus, and wound tumor virus, *J. Virol.* **4**, 851.

Kapuler, A. M., 1970, An extraordinary temperature dependence of the reovirus transcriptase, *Biochemistry* **9**, 4453.

Kapuler, A. M., 1971, Reovirus core transcriptase and ethidium bromide: A continuous fluorimetric assay for polynucleotide synthesis based on the secondary structure of mRNA, *Biochim. Biophys. Acta* **238**, 363.

Kapuler, A. M., Mendelsohn, N., Klett, H., and Acs, G., 1970, Four base-specific 5′-triphosphatases in the subviral core of reovirus, *Nature (Lond.)* **225**, 1209.

Kates, J. R., and McAuslan, B. R., 1967, Messenger RNA synthesis by a "coated" viral genome, *Proc. Natl. Acad. Sci. USA* **57**, 314.

Kawamura, H., and Tsubahara, H., 1966, Common antigenicity of avian reoviruses, *Nat. Inst. Anim. Hlth. Quart.* **6**, 187.

Kerr, I. M., 1971, Protein synthesis in cell-free systems: An effect of interferon, *J. Virol.* **7**, 448.

Kimura, I., and Black, L. M., 1971, Some factors affecting infectivity assays of wound tumor virus on cell monolayers from an insect vector, *Virology* **46**, 266.

Kimura, I., and Black, L. M., 1972*a*, The cell-infecting unit of wound tumor virus, *Virology* **45**, 549.

Kimura, I., and Black, L. M., 1972*b*, Growth of wound tumor virus in vector cell monolayers, *Virology* **48**, 852.

Kimura, I., and Shikata, E., 1968, Structural model of rice dwarf virus, *Proc. Imp. Acad. Jap.* **44**, 538. Kitajima, E. W., and Costa, A. S., 1970, Electron microscopy of pangola stunt virus infected plants and viruliferous planthopper vectors, *Proc. 7th Int. Congr. Electro. Microscopy. Grenoble* **3**, 323.

Kleinschmidt, A. K., Dunnebacke, T., H. Spendlove, R. S., Schaeffer, F. L., and Whitcomb, R. F., 1964, Electron microscopy of RNA from reovirus and wound tumor virus, *J. Mol. Biol.* **10**, 282.

Koide, F., Suzuka, I., and Sekiguchi, K., 1968, Some properties of an adenine-rich polynucleotide fragment from the avian reovirus, *Biochem. Biophys. Res. Commun.* **30**, 95.

Krug, R. M., and Gomatos, P. J., 1969, Absence of adenine-rich ribonucleic acid from purified infectious reovirus 3, *J. Virol.* **4**, 642.

Krywienczyk, J., Hayashi, Y., and Bird, F. T., 1969, Serological investigations of insect viruses. I. Comparison of three highly purified cytoplasmic polyhedrosis viruses, *J. Invertebr. Pathol.* **13**, 114.

Kudo, H., and Graham, A. F., 1965, Synthesis of reovirus ribonucleic acid in L cells, *J. Bacteriol.* **90**, 936.

Lai, K. C., and Bellamy, A. R., 1971, Factors affecting the amount of oligonucleotides in reovirus particles, *Virology* **45**, 821.

Lai, M.-H. T., and Joklik, W. K., 1973, The induction of interferon by temperature-sensitive mutants of reovirus, UV-irradiated reovirus, and subviral reovirus particles, *Virology* **51**, 191.

Lai, M.-H. T., Werènne, J. J., and Joklik, W. K., 1973, The preparatio of reovirus top component and its effect on host DNA and protein synthesis, *Virology* **54**, 237.

Langridge, R., and Gomatos, P. J., 1963, The structure of RNA. Reovirus RNA and transfer RNA have similar three-dimensional structures, which differ from DNA, *Science* (*Wash., D.C.*) **141**, 694.

Lecatsas, G., 1968, Electron microscopic study of the formation of bluetongue virus, *Onderstepoort J. Vet. Res.* **35**, 139.

Lecatsas, G., and Erasmus, B. J., 1967, Electron microscopic study of the formation of African horse sickness virus, *Arch. Ges. Virusforsch.* **22**, 442.

Lecatsas, G., and Erasmus, B. J., 1973, Core structure in a new virus, XBM/67, *Arch. Ges. Virusforschung,* in press.

Lecatsas, G., and Gorman, B. M., 1972, Visualization of the extra capsid coat in certain bluetongue-type viruses, *Onderstepoort J. Vet. Res.* **39**, 193.

Lecatsas, G., Erasmus, B. J., and Els, H. J., 1969, Electron microscopic studies on corriparta virus, *Onderstepoort J. Vet. Res.* **36**, 321.

Lecatsas, G., Erasmus, B. J., and Els, H. J., 1973, Electron microscopic studies on equine encephalosis virus, *Onderstepoort J. Vet. Res.,* in press.

Lerner, A. M., and Miranda, Q. R., 1968, Cellular interaction of several enteroviruses and a reovirus after treatment with sodium borohydride or carbohydrases, *Virology* **36**, 277.

Lerner, A. M., Cherry, J. D., and Finlay, M., 1963, Hemagglutination with reoviruses, Virology **19**, 58.

Lerner, A. M., Bailey, E. J., and Tillotson, J. R., 1966, Enterovirus hemagglutination: Inhibition by several enzymes and sugars, *J. Immunol.* **95**, 1111.

Leseman, D., 1972, Electron microscopy of maize rough dwarf virus particles, *J. Gen. Virol.* **16**, 273.

Levin, D. H., Acs, G., and Silverstein, S. C., 1970*a*, Chain initiation by reovirus RNA transcriptase *in vitro, Nature* (*Lond.*) **227**, 603.

Levin, D. H., Mendelsohn, N., Schonberg, M., Klett, H., Silverstein, S. C., Kapuler, A. M., and Acs, G., 1970*b*, Properties of RNA transcriptase in reovirus subviral particles, *Proc. Natl. Acad. Sci. USA* **66**, 890.

Levin, D. H., Kyner, D., Acs, G., and Silverstein, S. C., 1971, Messenger activity in mammalian cell-free extracts of reovirus single-stranded RNA prepared *in vitro*, *Biochem. Biophys. Res. Commun.* **42,** 454.

Levin, D. H., Kyner, D., and Acs, 1972, Formation of a mammalian initiation complex with reovirus messenger RNA, methionyl-tRNA$_F$ and ribosomal subunits, *Proc. Natl. Acad. Sci. USA* **69,** 1234.

Lewandowski, L. J., and Leppla, S. H., 1972, Comparison of the 3′-termini of discrete segments of the double-stranded ribonucleic acid genomes of cytoplasmic polyhedrosis virus, wound tumor virus, and reovirus, *J. Virol.* **10,** 965.

Lewandowski, L. J., and Millward, S., 1971, Characterization of the genome of cytoplasmic polyhedrosis virus, *J. Virol.* **7,** 434.

Lewandowski, L. J., and Traynor, B. L., 1972, Comparison of the structure and polypeptide composition of three double-stranded ribonucleic acid-containing viruses (diplornaviruses): cytoplasmic polyhedrosis virus, wound tumor virus, and reovirus, *J. Virol.* **10,** 1053.

Lewandowski, L. J., Kalmakoff, J., and Tanada, Y., 1969, Characterization of a ribonucleic acid polymerase activity associated with purified cytoplasmic polyhedrosis virus of the silkworm, *Bombyx mori, J. Virol.* **4,** 857.

Liu, H., Kimura, I., and Black, L. M., 1973, Specific infectivity of different wound tumor isolates, *Virology* **51,** 320.

Loh, P. C., and Oie, H. K. 1969, Role of lysine in the replication of reovirus. I. Synthesis of complete and empty virions, *J. Virol.* **4,** 890.

Loh, P. C., and Shatkin, A. J., 1968, Structural proteins of reovirus, *J. Virol.* **2,** 1353.

Loh, P. C., and Soergel, M., 1965, Growth charactistics of reovirus type 2: Actinomycin D and the synthesis of viral RNA, *Proc. Natl. Acad. Sci. USA* **54,** 857.

Loh, P. C., Hohl, H. R., and Soergel, M., 1965, Fine structure of reovirus type 2, *J. Bacteriol* **89,** 1140.

Long, W. F., and Burke, D. C., 1971, A comparison of interferon induction by reovirus RNA and synthetic double-stranded polynucleotides, *J. Gen. Virol.* **12,** 1.

Lovisolo, O., 1971, Maize Rough Dwarf Virus. CMI/AAB Descriptions of Plant Viruses No. 72 (A. J. Gibbs, B. D. Harrison, and A. F. Murant, eds.).

Luftig, R. B. Kilham, S., Hay, A. J., Zweerink, H. J., and Joklik, W. K., 1972, An ultrastructural study of virions and cores of reovirus type 3, *Virology* **48,** 170.

Luisoni, E., Lovisolo, O., Kitagawa, Y., and Shikata, E., 1973, Serological relationship between maize rough dwarf virus and rice black-streaked dwarf virus, *Virology* **52,** 281.

McClain, M. E., Spendlove, R. S., and Lennette, E. H., 1967, Infectivity assay of reoviruses: comparison of immunofluorescent cell output and plaque methods, *J. Immunol.* **98,** 1301.

McDowell, M. J., and Joklik, W. K., 1971, An *in vitro* protein synthesizing system from mouse L fibroblasts infected with reovirus, *Virology* **45,** 724.

McDowell, M. J., Joklik, W. K., Villa-Komaroff, L., and Lodish, H. F., 1972, Translation of reovirus messenger RNAs synthesized *in vitro* into reovirus polypeptides by several mammalian cell-free extracts, *Proc. Natl. Acad. Sci. USA* **69,** 2649.

Maramorosch, K., Shikata, E., and Granados, R. R., 1969, Multiplication and Cytopathology of a Plant Tumor Virus in Insects, National Cancer Institute Monograph No. 31, p. 493, National Cancer Institute, Bethesda, Maryland.

Martin, S. A., and Zweerink, H. J., 1972, Isolation and characterization of two types of bluetongue virus particles, *Virology* **50,** 495.

Martin, S. A., Pett, D. M., and Zweerick, H. J., 1973, Studies on the topography of reovirus and bluetongue virus capsid polypeptides, *J. Virol.* **12,** 194.

Matsuhisa, T., and Joklik, W. K., 1974, Temperature-sensitive mutants of reovirus. V. Studies on the nature of the temperature-sensitive lesion of the group C mutant *ts* 447, *Virology*, in press.

Mayor, H. D., and Jordan, L. E., 1968, Preparation and properties of the internal capsid components of reovirus, *J. Gen. Virol.* **3,** 233.

Metz, D. H., and Esteban, R. M., 1972, Interferon inhibits viral protein synthesis in L cells infected with vaccinia virus, *Nature (Lond.)* **238,** 385.

Millward, S., and Graham, A. F., 1970, Structural studies on reovirus: Discontinuities in the genome, *Proc. Natl. Acad. Sci. USA* **65,** 422.

Milne, R. G., Conti, M., and Lisa, V., 1973, Partial purification, structure and infectivity of complete maize dwarf virus particles, *Virology* **53,** 130.

Min Jou, W., Haegeman, G., Ysebaert, M., and Fiers, W., 1972, Nucleotide sequence of the gene coding for the bacteriophage MS2 coat protein, *Nature (Lond.)* **237,** 82.

Miura, K.-I., Kimura, I., and Suzuki, N., 1966, Double-stranded ribonucleic acid from rice dwarf virus, *Virology* **28,** 571.

Miura, K.-I., Fujii, I., Sakaki, T., Fuke, M., and Kawase, S., 1968, Double-stranded ribonucleic acid from cytoplasmic polyhedrosis virus of the silkworm, *J. Virol.* **2,** 1211.

Miura, K.-I., Fujii-Kawata, I., Iwata, H., and Kawase, S., 1969, Electron-microscopic observation of a cytoplasmic polyhedrosis virus from the silkworm, *J. Invertebr. Pathol.* **14,** 262.

Miyajima, S., and Kawase, S., 1969, Hemagglutination with cytoplasmic polyhedrosis virus of the silkworm, *Bombyx mori, Virology* **39,** 347.

Morgan, E. M., and Zweerink, H. J., 1974, Reovirus morphogenesis. Core-like particles in cells infected at 39°C with wild-type reovirus and temperature-sensitive mutants of groups B and G, *Virology,* **59,** 556.

Murphy, F. A., Coleman, P. H., Hansen, A. K., and Gray, G. W., 1968, Colorado tick fever virus, an electron microscope study, *Virology* **35,** 28.

Murphy, F. A., Borden, E. C., Shope, R. E., and Harrison, A., 1971, Physicochemical and morphological relationships of some arthropod-borne viruses to bluetongue virus—A new taxonomic group. Electron microscopic studies, *J. Gen. Virol.* **13,** 273.

Nichols, J. L., Bellamy, A. R., and Joklik, W. K., 1972a, Indentification of the nucleotide sequences of the oligonucleotides present in reovirions, *Virology* **49,** 562.

Nichols, J. L., Hay, A. J., and Joklik, W. K., 1972b, 5′-terminal nucleotide sequence in reovirus mRNA synthesized *in vitro, Nat. New Biol.* **235,** 105.

Nishimura, A., and Hosaka, Y., 1969, Electron microscopic study of RNA of cytoplasmic polyhedrosis virus of the silkworm, *Virology* **38,** 550.

Nonoyama, M., and Graham, A. F., 1970, Appearance of defective virions of clones of reovirus, *J. Virol.* **6,** 693.

Nonoyama, M., Watanabe, Y., and Graham, A. F., 1970, Defective virions of reovirus, *J. Virol.* **6,** 226.

Oellermann, R. A., 1970, Plaque formation by African horsesickness virus and characterization of its RNA, *Onderstepoort J. Vet. Res.* **37,** 137.

Oellermann, R. A., Els, H. J., and Erasmus, B. J., 1970, Characterization of African horsesickness virus, *Arch. Ges. Virusforsch.* **29,** 163.

Oie, H. K., and Loh, P. C., 1971, Reovirus type 2: Induction of viral resistance and interference production in fathead minnow cells, *Proc. Soc. Exp. Biol. Med.* **136**, 369.

Oie, H. K., Loh, P. C., and Soergel, M., 1966, Growth characteristics and immunocytochemical studies of reovirus type 2 in a line of human amnion cells, *Arch. Ges. Virusforsch.* **18**, 16.

Oshimo, L. S., and Emmons, R. W., 1968, Electron microscopic observations of Colorado tick fever virus in BHK 21 and KB cells, *J. Gen. Virol.* **3**, 279.

Owen, N. C., 1964, Investigation into the *p*H stability of bluetongue virus and its survival in mutton and beef, *Onderstepoort J. Vet. Res.* **31**, 109.

Pavri, K. M., 1961, Haemagglutination and haeorse-si)randed RNA in larvae of *Bombyx mori* infected with a cytoplasmic polyhedrosis virus, *Intervirology* **1**, 34.

Pett, D. M., Vanaman, T. C., and Joklik, W. K., 1973, Studies on the amino and carboxyl-terminal amino acid sequences of reovirus capsid polypeptides, *Virology* **52**, 174.

Prevec, L., and Graham, A. F., 1966, Reovirus specific polyribosomes in infected L cells, *Science (Wash., D.C.)* **154**, 522.

Prevec, L., Watanabe, Y., Gauntt, C. J., and Graham, A. F., 1968, Transcription of the genomes of type 1 and type 3 reoviruses, *J. Virol.* **2**, 289.

Reddy, D. V. R., and Black, L. M., 1966, Production of wound tumor virus and wound-tumor soluble antigens in the insect vector, *Virology* **30**, 551.

Reddy, D. V. R., and Black, L. M., 1972, Increase in wound tumor virus in leafhoppers as assayed on vector cell monolayers, *Virology* **50**, 412.

Reddy, D. V. R., and Black, L. M., 1973*a*, Estimate of the absolute specific infectivity of wound tumor virus purified with polyethylene glycol, *Virology* **54**, 150.

Reddy, D. V. R., and Black, L. M., 1973*b*, Electrophoretic separation of all components of the double-stranded RNA of wound tumor virus, *Virology* **54**, 557.

Redolfi, P., and Pennazio, S., 1972, Double-stranded ribonucleic acid from maize rough dwarf virus, *Acta Virol. (Prague)* **16**, 369.

Rhim, J. S., and Melnick, J. L., 1961, Plaque formation by reoviruses, *Virology* **15**, 80.

Rhim, J. S., Jordan, L. E., and Mayor, H. D., 1962, Cytochemical, fluorescent-antibody, and electron microscopic studies on the growwth of reovirus (ECHO 10) in tissue culture, *Virology* **17**, 342.

Rosen, L., 1968, Reoviruses, Virology Monographs 1 (S. Gard, C. Hallauer, and K. F. Meyer, eds.), pp. 73–107, Springer-Verlag, Wien.

Roy D., Graziadei, W. D., III, Lengyel, P., and Konigsberg, W., 1972, Amino-terminal sequences of several reovirus type 3 capsid proteins and identical, *Biochem. Biophys. Res. Commun.* **46**, 1066.

Sabin, A. B., 1959, Reoviruses: A new group of respiratory and enteric viruses formerly classified as Echo-type 10 is described, *Science (Wash., D.C.)* **130**, 1387.

Sakuma, S., and Watanabe, Y., 1971, Unilateral synthesis of reovirus double-stranded ribonucleic acid by a cell-free replicase system, *J. Virol.* **8**, 190.

Sakuma, S., and Watanabe, Y., 1972*a*, Reovirus replicase-directed synthesis of double-stranded ribonucleic acid, *J. Virol.* **10**, 628.

Sakuma, S., and Watanabe, Y., 1972*b*, Incorporation of *in vitro* synthesized reovirus double-stranded ribonucleic acid in virus corelike particles, *J. Virol.* **10**, 943.

Samejima, T., Hashizume, H., Imahori, K., Fujii, K., and Miura, K.-I., 1968, Optical rotatory dispersion and circular dichroism of rice dwarf virus nucleic acid, *J. Mol. Biol.* **34**, 39.

Samuel, C., and Joklik, W. K., 1974, A protein-synthesizing system from interferon-treated cells that discriminates between cellular and viral messenger RNA's, *Virology* **58**: 476.

Sato, T., Kyogoku, Y., Higuchi, S., Mitsui, Y., Itaka, Y., Tsuboi, M., and Miura, K.-I., 1966, A preliminary investigation on the molecular structure of rice dwarf virus ribonucleic acid, *J. Mol. Biol.* **16**, 180.

Schank, S. C., and Edwardson, J. R., 1968, Cytological examination of pangola grass (*Digitaria decumbens* Stent.) infected with stunt virus, *Crop Sci.* **8**, 118.

Schnagl, R. D., Holmes, I. H., and Doherty, R. L., 1969, An electron microscope study of Eubenangee, an Australian arbovirus, *Virology* **38**, 347.

Schochetman, G., and Millward, S,. 1972, Ribonucleoside diphosphate precursors for *in vitro* reovirus RNA synthesis, *Nat. New Biol.* **239**, 77.

Schonberg, M., Silverstein, S. C., Levin, D. H., and Acs, G., 1971, Asynchronous synthesis of the complementary strands of the reovirus genome, *Proc. Natl. Acad. Sci. USA* **68**, 505.

Schuerch, A. R., and Joklik, W. K., 1973, Temperature-sensitive mutants of reovirus. IV. Evidence that anamalous electrophoretic migration behavior of certain double-stranded RNA hybrid species is mutant group-specific, *Virology* **56**, 218.

Schuerch, A. R., Matsuhisa, T., and Joklik, W. K., 1974, Temperature-sensitive mutants of reovirus. VI. Mutant *ts* 447 and *ts* 556 particles that lack one or two L-genomes RNA segments, *Intervirology* (in press).

Shatkin, A. J., 1965a, Inactivity of purified reovirus RNA as a template for *E. coli* polymerases *in vitro, Proc. Natl. Acad. Sci. USA* **54**, 1721.

Shatkin, A. J., 1965b, Actinomycin and the differential synthesis of reovirus and L-cell RNA, *Biochem. Biophys. Res. Commun.* **19**, 506.

Shatkin, A. J., 1968, Viruses containing double-stranded RNA, *in* "Molecular Basis of Virology" (H. Fraenkel-Conrat, ed.), pp. 351–392, Reinhold, New York.

Shatkin, A. J., 1969, Replication of reoviruses, *Adv. Virus Res.* **14**, 63.

Shatkin, A. J., and LaFiandra, A. J., 1972, Transcriptions by infectious subviral particles of reovirus, *J. Virol.* **10**, 698.

Shatkin, A. J., and Rada, B., 1967a, Reovirus-directed ribonucleic acid synthesis in infected L cells, *J. Virol.* **1**, 24.

Shatkin, A. J., and Rada, B., 1967b, Studies on the replication of reovirus, *in* "The Molecular Biology of Viruses" (J. S. Colter and W. Paranchych, eds.), pp. 427–447, Academic Press, New York.

Shatkin, A. J., and Sipe, J. D., 1968a, RNA polymerase activity in purified reoviruses, *Proc. Natl. Acad. Sci. USA* **61**, 1462.

Shatkin, A. J., and Sipe, J. D., 1968b, Single-stranded adenine-rich RNA from purified reoviruses, *Proc. Natl. Acad. Sci. USA* **59**, 246.

Shatkin, A. J., Sipe, J. D., and Loh, P. C., 1968, Separation of ten reovirus genome segments by polyacrylamide gel electrophoresis, *J. Virol.* **2**, 986.

Shaw, J. E., and Cox, D. C., 1973, Early inhibition of cellular DNA synthesis by high multiplicities of infectious and UV-inactivated reovirus, *J. Virol.* **12**, 704.

Shikata, E., and Maramorosch, 1965, Electron microscopic evidence for the systemic invasion of an insect host by a plant pathogenic virus, *Virology* **27**, 461.

Shikata, E., and Maramorosch, K., 1966, An electron microscope study of plant neoplasia induced by wound tumor virus, *J. Nat. Cancer Inst.* **36**, 97.

Shikata, E., and Maramorosch, K., 1967a, Electron microscopy of wound tumor virus assembly sites in insect vectors and plants, *Virology* **32**, 363.

Shikata, E., and Maramorosch, K., 1967b, Electron microscopy of the formation of wound tumor virus in abdominally inoculated insect vectors, J. Virol. 1, 1052.

Shimotohno, K., and Miura, K.-I., 1973, Transcription of double-stranded RNA in cytoplasmic polyhedrosis virus in vitro, Virology 53. 283.

Silverstein, S., Bachenheimer, S. L., Frenkel, N., and Roizman, B., 1973, Relationship between post-transcriptional adenylation of herpes virus RNA and messenger RNA abundance, Proc. Natl. Acad. Sci. USA 70, 2101.

Silverstein, S. C., and Dales, S., 1968, The penetration of reovirus RNA and initiation of its genetic function in L-strain fibroblasts, J. Cell Biol. 36, 197.

Silverstein, S. C., and Shur, P. H., 1970, Immunofluorescent localization of double-stranded RNA in reovirus-infected cells, Virology 41, 564.

Silverstein, S. C., Levin, D. H., Schonberg, M., and Acs, G., 1970, The reovirus replicative cycle: Conservation of parental RNA and protein, Proc. Natl. Acad. Sci. USA 67, 275.

Silverstein, S. C., Astell, C., Levin, D. H., Schonberg, M., and Acs, G., 1972, The mechanisms of reovirus uncoating and gene activation in vivo, Virology 47, 797.

Simpson, D. H., Haddow, A. J., Woodall, J. P., Williams, M. C., and Bell, T. M., 1965, Attempts to transmit reovirus type 3 by the bite of Aedes aegypti, linnaeus, E. Afr. Med. J. 42, 708.

Skehel, J. J., and Joklik, W. K., 1969, Studies on the in vitro transcription of reovirus RNA catalyzed by reovirus cores, Virology 39, 822.

Smith, K. M., 1963, The cytoplasmic virus diseases, in "Insect Pathology," Vol. 1 (E. A. Steinhaus, ed.), p. 478, Academic Press, New York.

Smith, R. E., Zweerink, H. J., and Joklik, W. K., 1969, Polypeptide components of virions, top component and cores of reovirus type 3, Virology 39, 791.

Spendlove, R. S., Lennette, E. H., Knight, C. O., and Chin, J. H., 1963a, Development of viral antigen and infectious virus in HeLa cells infected with reovirus, J. Immunol. 90, 548.

Spendlove, R. S., Lennette, E. H., and John, A. C., 1963b, The role of mitotic apparatus in the intracellular location of reovirus antigen, J. Immunol. 90, 554.

Spendlove, R. S., Lennette, E. H., Chin, J. N., and Knight, C. O., 1964, Effect of antimitotic agents on intracellular reovirus antigen, Cancer Res. 24, 1826.

Spendlove, R. S., Lennette, E. H., Knight, C. O., and Chin, J. N., 1966, Production in FL cells of infectious and potentially infectious reovirus, J. Bacteriol. 92, 1036.

Spendlove, R. S., McClain, M. E., and Lennette, E. H., 1970, Enhancement of reovirus infectivity by extracellular removal or alteration of the virus capsid by proteolytic enzymes, J. Gen. Virol. 8, 83.

Stanley, N. F., 1961, Relationship of hepatoencephalomyelitis virus and reoviruses, Nature (Lond.) 189, 687.

Stanley, N. F., and Walters, M. N.-I., 1966, Virus induction of autoimmune disease and neoplasia, Lancet I, 962.

Stanley, N. F., Dorman, D. C., and Ponsford, J., 1953, Studies on the pathogenesis of a hitherto undescribed virus (hepato-encephalomyelitis) producing unusual symptoms in suckling mice, Aust. J. Exp. Biol. Med. Sci. 31, 147.

Stoltzfus, C. M., and Banerjee, A. K., 1972, Two oligonucleotide classes of single-stranded ribopolymers in reovirus A-rich RNA, Arch. Biochem. Biophys. 152, 733.

Stoltzfus, C. M., Shatkin, A. J., and Banerjee, A. K., 1973, Absence of polyadenylic acid from reovirus messenger RNA, J. Biol. Chem. 248, 7993.

Streissle, G., and Granados, R. R., 1968, The fine structure of wound tumor virus and reovirus, Arch. Ges. Virusforsch. 25, 369.

Suzuki, N., and Kimura, I., 1969, Purification, bioassay, properties, and seroloygy of rice viruses, in "The Virus Diseases of the Rice Plant," p. 207, Johns Hopkins Press, Baltimore, Maryland.

Svehag, S. E., 1963, Thermal inactivation of bluetongue virus, *Arch. Ges. Virusforsch.* **13**, 499.

Teakle, D. S., and Steindl, D. R. L., 1969, Virus-like particles in galls on sugar-cane plants affected by Fiji disease, *Virology* **37**, 139.

Tillotson, J. R., and Lerner, A. M., 1966, Effect of periodate oxidation on hemagglutinating and antibody-producing capacities of certain enteroviruses and reoviruses, *Proc. Natl. Acad. Sci. USA* **56**, 1143.

Toyoda, S., Kimura, I., and Suzuki, N., 1964, Rice viruses and special reference to rice dwarf virus, protein, nucleic acid, *Enzyme (Tokyo)* **9**:861.

Toyoda, S., Kimura, I., and Suzuki, N., 1965, Purification of rice dwarf virus, *Ann. Phytopathol. Soc. Jap.* **30**, 225.

Tytell, A. A., Lampson, G. P., Field, A. K., and Hilleman, M. R., 1967, Inducers of interferon and host resistance. III. Double-stranded RNA from reovirus type 3 virions (Reo 3-RNA), *Proc. Natl. Acad. Sci. USA.* **58**, 1719.

Vasquez, C., and Kleinschmidt, A. K., 1968, Electron microscopy of RNA strands released from individual reovirus particle, *J. Mol. Biol.* **34**, 137.

Vasquez, C., and Tournier, P., 1962, The morphology of reovirus, *Virology* **17**, 503.

Vasquez, C., and Tournier, P., 1964, New interpretation of the reovirus structure, *Virology* **24**, 128.

Verwoerd, D. W., 1969, Purification and characterization of bluetongue virus, *Virology* **38**, 203.

Verwoerd, D. W., 1970, Diplornaviruses: A newly recognized group of double-stranded RNA viruses, *Progr. Med. Virol.* **12**, 192.

Verwoerd, D. W., and Huismans, H., 1969, On the relationship between bluetongue, African horsesickness, and reoviruses: Hybridization studies, *Onderstepoort J. Vet. Res.* **36**, 175.

Verwoerd, D. W., and Huismans, H., 1972, Studies on the in vitro and in vivo transcription of the bluetongue virus genome, *Onderstepoort J. Vet. Res.,* **39**, 185.

Verwoerd, D. W., Louw, H., and Oellermann, R. A., 1970, Characterization of bluetongue virus ribonucleic acid, *J. Virol.* **5**, 1.

Verwoerd, D. W., Els, H. J., de Villiers, E.-M., and Huismans, H., 1972, Structure of the bluetongue virus capsid, *J. Virol.* **10**, 783.

Vidano, C., 1970, Phases of maize rough dwarf virus multiplication in the vector Laodelphax striatellus Fallén), *Virology* **41**, 218.

Wachsman, J. T., Levin, D. H., and Acs, G., 1970, Ribonucleoside triphosphate-dependent pyrophosphate exchange of reovirus cores, *J. Virol.* **6**, 563.

Wallis, C., Smith, K. O., and Melnick, J. L., 1964, Reovirus activation by heating and inactivation by cooling in $MgCl_2$ solution, *Virology* **22**, 608.

Wallis, C., Melnick, J. L., and Rapp, F., 1966, Effects of pancreatin on the growth of reovirus, *J. Bacteriol.* **92**, 155.

Walters, M. N.-I., Joske, R. A., Leak, P. J., and Stanley, N. F., 1963, Murine infection with reovirus. I. Pathology of the acute phase, *Brit. J. Exp. Pathol.* **44**, 427.

Walters, M. N.-I., Leak, P. J., Joske, R. A., Stanley, N. F., and Perret, D. H., 1965, Murine infection with reovirus. III. Pathology of infection with types 1 and 2, *Brit. J. Exp. Pathol.* **46**, 200.

Ward, R. L., and Shatkin, A. J., 1972, Association of reovirus mRNA with viral proteins: A possible mechanism for linking the genome segments, *Arch. Biochem. Biophys.* **152**, 378.

Ward, R. L., Banerjee, A. K., LaFiandra, A., and Shatkin, A. J., 1972, Reovirus-specific ribonucleic acid from polysomes of infected L cells, *J. Virol.* **9**, 61.

Warrington, R. C., Hayward, C., and Kapuler, A. M., 1973, Conformational studies of reovirus single-stranded RNAs synthesized *in vitro, Biochim. Biophys. Acta* **331**, 231.

Watanabe, H., 1967, Site of viral RNA synthesis within the midgut cells of the silkworm, *Bombyx mori*, infected with cytoplasmic-polyhedrosis virus, *J. Invertebr. Pathol.* **9**, 480.

Watanabe, Y., and Graham, A. F., 1967, Structural units of reovirus RNA and their possible functional significance, *J. Virol.* **1**, 665.

Watanabe, Y., Kudo, H., and Graham, A. F., 1967*a*, Selective inhibition of reovirus ribonucleic acid synthesis by cycloheximide, *J. Virol.* **1**, 36.

Watanabe, Y., Prevec, L., and Graham, A. F., 1967*b*, Specificity in transcription of the reovirus genome, *Proc. Natl. Acad. Sci. USA* **58**, 1040.

Watanabe, Y., Gauntt, C. J., and Graham, A. F., 1968*a*, Reovirus-induced ribonucleic acid polymerase, *J. Virol.* **2**, 869.

Watanabe, Y., Millward, S., and Graham, A. F., 1968*b*, Regulation of transcriptase of the reovirus genome, *J. Mol. Biol.* **36**, 107.

Wetter, C., Luisoni, E., Conti, M., and Lovisolo, O., 1969, Purification and serology of maize rough dwarf virus from plant and vector, *Phytopathol. Z.* **66**, 197.

Whitcomb, R. F., and Jensen, D. D., 1968, Enhancement of infectivity of a mammalian virus preparation after injection into insects, *Virology* **34**, 182.

Wiebe, M. E., and Joklik, W. K., 1973, The mechanism of interferon-induced inhibition of reovirus multiplication in L cells, *Bacteriol. Proc.* 210.

Wood, H. A., 1973, Viruses with double-stranded RNA genomes, *J. Gen. Virol.* **20**, 61.

Wood, H. A., and Streissle, G., 1970, Wound tumor virus: Purification and fractionation of the double-stranded ribonucleic acid, *Virology* **40**, 329.

Yunker, C. E., and Cory, J., 1969, Colorado tick fever virus: Growth in a mosquito cell line, *J. Virol.* **3**, 631.

Zweerink, H. J., 1974, Multiple forms of SS→DS RNA polymerase activity in reovirus infected cells, *Nature (Lond.)* **247**, 313.

Zweerink, H. J., and Joklik, W. K., 1970, Studies on the intracellular synthesis of reovirus-specified proteins, *Virology* **41**, 501.

Zweerink, H. J., McDowell, M. J., and Joklik, W. K., 1971, Essential and nonessential noncapsid reovirus proteins, *Virology* **45**, 716.

Zweerink, H. J., Ito, Y., and Matsuhisa, T., 1972, Synthesis of reovirus double-stranded RNA within virus-like particles, *Virology* **50**, 349.

Index